THIRD

P9-APQ-676

CURRICULUM DEVELOPMENT

in Nursing Education

CARROLL L. IWASIW, RN, MSCN, EdD
Professor
Co-Founding Editor, *International Journal of Nursing Education Scholarship*

DOLLY GOLDENBERG, RN, MA (ENGLISH), MSCN, PHD
Adjunct Professor
Co-Founding Editor, *International Journal of Nursing Education Scholarship*

Arthur Labatt Family School of Nursing
Faculty of Health Sciences
Western University
London, Ontario, Canada

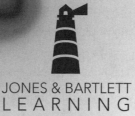

JONES & BARTLETT
LEARNING

World Headquarters
Jones & Bartlett Learning
5 Wall Street
Burlington, MA 01803
978-443-5000
info@jblearning.com
www.jblearning.com

Jones & Bartlett Learning books and products are available through most bookstores and online booksellers. To contact Jones & Bartlett Learning directly, call 800-832-0034, fax 978-443-8000, or visit our website, www.jblearning.com.

Substantial discounts on bulk quantities of Jones & Bartlett Learning publications are available to corporations, professional associations, and other qualified organizations. For details and specific discount information, contact the special sales department at Jones & Bartlett Learning via the above contact information or send an email to specialsales@jblearning.com.

Production Credits

Executive Publisher: William Brottmiller
Execuitve Editor: Amanda Martin
Associate Managing Editor: Sara Bempkins
Production Manager: Carolyn Rogers Pershouse
Production Editor: Sarah Bayle
Senior Marketing Manager: Jennifer Stiles
VP, Manufacturing and Inventory Control:
   Therese Connell

Composition: Cenveo Publisher Services
Cover Design: Kristin E. Parker
Manager of Photo Research, Rights & Permissions:
   Lauren Miller
Cover Image: © Tursunbaev Ruslan/ShutterStock, Inc.
Printing and Binding: Edwards Brothers Malloy
Cover Printing: Edwards Brothers Malloy

Library of Congress Cataloging-in-Publication Data
Iwasiw, Carroll L., author.
   Curriculum development in nursing education / Carroll Iwasiw and Dolly Goldenberg. —Third edition.
      p. ; cm.
   Includes bibliographical references and index.
   ISBN 978-1-284-02626-9
   I. Goldenberg, Dolly, author. II. Title.
   [DNLM: 1. Curriculum. 2. Education, Nursing. 3. Evidence-Based Nursing—education. WY 18]
   RT71
   610.73071′1—dc23
                                                                    2014008693

6048

Printed in the United States of America
18 17 16 15 14   10 9 8 7 6 5 4 3 2 1

Contents

Part III Preparation for Curriculum Development   77

5 Determining the Need and Gaining Faculty and Stakeholder Support for Curriculum Development   79

6 Deciding on the Curriculum Leader and Leading Curriculum Development   99

13 Creating Courses for an Evidence-Informed, Context-Relevant, Unified Curriculum   301

Part V   Implementation and Evaluation of an Evidence-Informed, Context-Relevant, Unified Curriculum   339

14 Ensuring Readiness for Curriculum Implementation   341

Part VI   Nursing Education by Distance Delivery   401

16   Curriculum Considerations in Nursing Education by Distance Delivery   403

Preface

The *Third Edition* of *Curriculum Development in Nursing Education* is once again written for everyone engaged in designing and developing curricula in baccalaureate, associate degree, and diploma nursing education. Accordingly, this includes experienced or recently appointed nursing faculty, graduate students, teaching assistants, and those who aspire to became nurse educators.

The text denotes our continuing dedication to the advancement of nursing education, and, in particular, the ongoing growth and expansion of nursing curricula. Our continuing roles as nurse educators and curriculum developers enable us to review relevancy from the second edition, as well as embrace new and contemporary information, ideas, perspectives, insights, and applications from our own experience and also from students, colleagues, and other curriculum experts and authors.

As identified in the second edition, this *Third Edition* offers information about the processes inherent in developing a curriculum for nursing education. As before, the term *curriculum* is interpreted to convey a totality, that is, the philosophical approaches, outcomes, design, courses, teaching-learning and evaluation strategies, interactions, learning climate, human and physical resources, and curricular policies. However, during the planning for this edition, it became evident that major determinants in the creation of nursing education curricula are not only the context, as previously identified, but also evidence about nursing, nursing education, and learning, and the need for curricular unity. These three premises, that is, *context-relevant, evidence-informed*, and *unified* curriculum, are pervasive throughout the text.

This edition has been significantly expanded and improved with new chapters, incorporation of updated approaches and references, and a realignment of previous parts and sections for greater clarity in the representation of the curriculum development process in nursing education. Part II is an innovative and entirely new section and addresses, in separate chapters, the fundamental or core processes of curriculum development: *faculty development, ongoing appraisal*, and *scholarship.*

While chapter configurations have remained relatively unchanged, more current nursing education ideas, perspectives, and applications have been included throughout. Several new tables and figures have been added, although those from the second edition that continue to be relevant have been retained, with some updated modifications and additions. Like the previous edition, chapters conclude with a summary, core processes and synthesis activities that comprise a hypothetical case with questions, and an additional series of questions for readers' consideration in their own setting, and chapter references. Acknowledged and reiterated once more is that nursing practice is evolving in accord with ongoing achievements and expansions in health care and general education, and with societal changes. Demographic, cultural, economic, and political forces continue to impinge upon nursing, including the number of available practicing nurses and faculty. Also unchanged are diverse values and uncertainties of life, which affect how nursing students are prepared for the roles they will assume after graduation. Therefore, restated in this *Third Edition* is that in order to present nursing as a legitimate, scholarly, evidence-informed science, nurse educators are obliged to continue to develop curricula responsive to developments in education, nursing practice, health care, and society.

Relevant definitions are included throughout the text. Of particular note are two terms. First, *professional practice* replaces the word *clinical* when referring to students' learning experiences. Whereas *clinical* conjures images of hospitals and is location specific, *professional practice* more accurately describes the learning activities in which students are engaged, and allows for the range of locations where nursing practice occurs. Secondly, *curriculum work* is used to replace the more cumbersome *curriculum development, implementation, and evaluation* where applicable.

Part I is entitled "Introduction to Curriculum Development in Nursing Education: The Evidence-Informed, Context-Relevant, Unified Curriculum." Chapter 1, *Creation of an Evidence-Informed, Context-Relevant, Unified Curriculum,* begins with definitions of curriculum generally. Then, introduced and elaborated upon is the idea that a curriculum must not only be relevant to the *context* in which it is offered (i.e., responsive to current and projected social, health and educational forces), but must also be based on *evidence* related to the circumstances that influence nursing education and practice, and be *unified,* wherein the components are logically, visibly, and consistently related to the premises of the curriculum. This conceptualization of an evidence-informed, context-relevant, unified curriculum remains pervasive throughout the text. The Model of Evidence-Informed, Context-Relevant, Unified Curriculum Development is overviewed in Chapter 1, including the core processes of faculty development, ongoing appraisal, and scholarship.

Included in "Part II: Core Processes of Curriculum Work," are the three core processes: *faculty development, ongoing appraisal,* and *scholarship.* Explication of these ideas as an integral part of curriculum work is new to the nursing education literature. These core curriculum processes are described separately in Chapters 2, 3, and 4. They are seen as continuous and necessary components of curriculum work, and therefore are incorporated into all subsequent chapters.

In Chapter 2, *Faculty Development for Curriculum Work and Change*, faculty development is described as to purpose, meaning, necessary conditions, and relationship to curriculum work Theoretical perspectives on change, their application to curriculum work, and ideas about responding to faculty resistance to change and curriculum work, are offered. Chapter 3 is *Ongoing Appraisal in Curriculum Work*. This second core process is characterized as a measurement standard and ongoing quality assurance activity fundamental to all curriculum work. The third core process is described in Chapter 4, *Scholarship in Curriculum Work*, and is portrayed as being inherent in academia and all curriculum work. Scholarliness, defined as the careful appraisal and use of relevant theory and data in curriculum work, is differentiated from scholarship—which is the purposeful, methodical creation and organization of knowledge in curriculum work, and the basis of evidence-informed nursing education practice. Included are ideas about the practical aspects of scholarship in curriculum work.

"Part III: Preparation for Curriculum Development" has been completely redesigned in Chapters 5 through 7. Chapter 5, *Determining the Need and Gaining Faculty and Stakeholder Support for Curriculum Development*, presents the rationale and need for curriculum development, situations that could precipitate curriculum development, and the extent that may be necessary. Also included are ideas about obtaining support from faculty, the school leader, students, and stakeholders. Chapter 6, *Deciding on the Curriculum Leader and Leading Curriculum Development*, expands upon Chapter 3 in the second edition. An updated and enlarged section is included on theoretical perspectives of leadership and the application to curriculum development and change. Criteria for selection of the curriculum leader and the leader's responsibilities are delineated. The chapter concludes with information about leadership in curriculum committees and development of curriculum leaders. Chapter 7, *Organizing for Curriculum Development*, is redesigned, expanded, and updated. It addresses the leader's role in organizing for curriculum development, including guiding values clarification, proposing an overall plan and faculty development activities, creating a critical path, and introducing ideas of academic freedom and scholarship within curriculum work. A section is devoted to faculty members' responsibilities in organizing for curriculum development.

In "Part IV: Development of an Evidence-Informed, Context-Relevant, Unified Curriculum," six chapters encompass pertinent previous information and incorporate current perspectives. Chapter 8, *Gathering Data for an Evidence-Informed, Context-Relevant, Unified Curriculum*, offers an overview of contextual factors: the forces, situations, and circumstances within and outside the school of nursing that influence the curriculum. Approaches for gathering contextual data are described. Chapter 9 is *Analyzing and Interpreting Contextual Data for an Evidence-informed, Context-Relevant, Unified Curriculum*. Following a clarification of terms, detailed information is included about the analysis and interpretation of contextual data. *Establishing Philosophical and Educational Approaches for an Evidence-Informed, Context-Relevant, Unified Curriculum*, Chapter 10, is a more extensive chapter in this third edition. It begins with definitions of *philosophy*, *curriculum philosophy*, and *curriculum philosophy in nursing education*. Educational philosophies, learning theories, and educational frameworks and pedagogies are summarized. An entirely new section offers information on the science of brain-based learning. Chapter 11, *Formulating Curriculum Goals or Outcomes for an Evidence-Informed, Context-Relevant, Unified Curriculum*, is greatly expanded from the second edition. Several taxonomies of learning are presented. Learning goals, objectives, outcomes, and competencies are compared, and their purposes in nursing education are described. Processes for formulating goals and outcomes are proposed. Chapter 12, *Designing an Evidence-Informed, Context-Relevant, Unified Curriculum*, is also extended and updated. Various program types, delivery, models, designs, and curriculum organizing strategies are detailed, and a larger part on interprofessional education has been included. An extensive section on designing an evidence-informed, context-relevant, and unified curriculum presents deliberations and considerations about the design process. In Chapter 13, *Creating Courses for an Evidence-Informed, Context-Relevant, Unified Curriculum*, information is provided about course details, designing courses, and planning individual classes. Creation of concept-based courses is described as well.

Part V is entitled "Implementation and Evaluation of an Evidence-Informed, Context-Relevant, Unified Curriculum." In Chapter 14, *Ensuring Readiness for Curriculum Implementation*, two concepts related to implementation are emphasized: *readiness* (the state of preparedness to introduce and enact the curriculum) and *fidelity* (the extent to which the curriculum is implemented as conceived). Involvement of faculty, students, external stakeholders, and logistical arrangements are identified as critical areas for consideration. Chapter 15, *Planning Curriculum Evaluation*, distinguishes between curriculum and program evaluation. The curriculum evaluation process is described and frameworks to assess fidelity of implementation are included.

"Part VI: Nursing Education By Distance Delivery" comprises Chapter 16, *Curriculum Considerations in Nursing Education by Distance Delivery*. Following an interpretation of *delivery of nursing education by distance*, necessary resources and ethical considerations are outlined. Curriculum considerations for course and class design are described, as well as ideas about implementing and evaluating nursing education offered by distance delivery.

Carroll L. Iwasiw and Dolly Goldenberg

Acknowledgments

We sincerely thank our families, colleagues, graduate students, and friends for their continued support and encouragement during the writing of this third edition of our text. Their patience and good humour have always been warmly appreciated.

Our appreciation is also extended to Dr. Mary Anne Andrusyszyn for the idea that scholarship is an inherent part of curriculum work and for her review of Chapter 16. We also thank Mr. Zenon Andrusyszyn for the graphics in the text.

PART I

Introduction to Curriculum Development in Nursing Education: The Evidence-Informed, Context-Relevant, Unified Curriculum

CHAPTER 1

Creation of an Evidence-Informed, Context-Relevant, Unified Curriculum

Chapter Overview

Curriculum development in nursing education is a scholarly and creative process intended to produce an evidence-informed, context-relevant, unified curriculum. It is an ongoing activity in nursing education, even in schools of nursing with established curricula. The extent of the development ranges from regular refinement of class activities and assignments to the creation of a completely original and reconceptualized curriculum. In this text, curriculum development activities are presented individually for ease of description and comprehension. However, emphasis is on the idea that the curriculum development process does not occur in ordered, sequential stages or phases. The process is iterative, with some work occurring concurrently, and with each new decision having the potential to affect previous ones.

This chapter begins with definitions of *curriculum*, and an *evidence-informed, context-relevant, unified curriculum*, followed by a description of curriculum development in nursing education. The Model of Evidence-Informed, Context-Relevant, Unified Curriculum Development is presented. It comprises a summary of the major aspects of the curriculum development process, serving as an advance organizer for this text. Additionally, attention is given to some of the interpersonal issues that can influence the curriculum development team, and hence, the completed work. The ideas about the curriculum development process introduced in this chapter are discussed more comprehensively in succeeding chapters.

Chapter Goals

- Review definitions and conceptualizations of *curriculum*.
- Ponder the meaning of curriculum as *evidence-informed, context-relevant*, and *unified*.
- Consider processes to enhance the scholarly nature of curriculum development.
- Overview the Model of Evidence-Informed, Context-Relevant, Unified Curriculum Development in Nursing Education
- Appreciate the interpersonal aspects of curriculum development.

DEFINITIONS AND CONCEPTUALIZATIONS OF CURRICULUM

Definitions of *curriculum* have been in existence since about 1820, first used in Scotland and then professionally in America a century later (Wiles & Bondi, 2007). The word comes from the Latin *currere*, to run, or to run a course (Wiles & Bondi, 2011), and originally meant the knowledge passed from one generation to the next (Wiles, 2005). A common understanding of curriculum is a program of studies with specified courses, leading to an academic certificate, diploma, or degree.

There have been so many definitions, often in response to social forces, that the scope and interpretation of *curriculum* have greatly expanded, creating some uncertainty and divergence of opinion about the meaning and intent of the word. However, definitions are important, because "they convey educators' perceptions, and in turn, these perceptions affect how a curriculum is used and indeed, even whether it is used at all" (Hensen, 2010, p. 9). Additionally, the definition specifies the scope of work to be completed by curriculum developers (Wiles & Bondi, 2011).

Oliva (2009) defines curriculum as:

> A plan or program for all the experiences that the learner encounters under the direction of the school. In practice, the curriculum consists of a number of plans, in written form and of varying scope and detail that delineate the desired learning experiences. The curriculum, therefore, may be a unit, a course, a sequence of courses, the school's entire program of studies—and may be encountered inside or outside class or school when directed by the personnel of the school. (p. 7)

Another perspective of curriculum is "a desired goal or set of values that can be activated through a development process, culminating in experiences for learners" (Wiles & Bondi, 2011, p. 5). These authors go on to state that the extent to which the experiences represent the envisioned goals is dependent on the effectiveness of the curriculum developers.

Parkay, Anctil, and Hass (2010) provide a broader description and give attention to the idea of theoretical and research bases for curricula.

> Curriculum is all of the educational experiences that learners have in an educational program, the purpose of which is to achieve broad goals and related specific objectives that have been developed within a framework of theory and research, past and present professional practice, and the changing needs of society. (p. 3)

They explain that:

- The curriculum is preplanned and based on information from many sources.
- Objectives and instructional planning should be based on theory and research about society, human development, and learning.

- Curriculum decisions should be based on criteria.
- Students play an important role in the experienced curriculum.

Many other conceptualizations exist: a written document, planned experiences, a reflection of social emphases, planned learning outcomes, hidden or visible, and living or dead (Hensen, 2010). Hensen summarizes these definitions and interpretations into three categories: *means versus ends, content versus experiences,* and *process versus plan.* Oliva (2009) also reduces the many views of curriculum to three categories. Some focus on *purpose*, what the curriculum does or is meant to achieve; the *context* in which the curriculum is implemented, possibly revealing the underlying philosophy, such as a learner-centered curriculum; and *strategy* or particular instructional or learning processes. Somewhat similarly, Wiles (2005) categorizes definitions according to the emphasis on curriculum as *subject matter,* a *plan,* an *experience,* or *outcomes.*

Lunenberg (2011) offers a category that is markedly different from those previously described: the nontechnical approach. This refers to ideas about curriculum that are more esthetic, emotional, political, and visionary, and less concerned with the how-to of curriculum development, implementation, and evaluation. For example, Diekelmann and Diekelmann (2009) propose a phenomenological, interpretative approach, termed *narrative pedagogy,* in which storytelling is the basis for interpretation and learning. The stimulation of thinking, not content, is at the heart of teacher activity. Freire (1970/2001) views education as a process of *conscientization,* the development of critical awareness of one's social reality through reflection and action, and curriculum as the creation of knowledge by learners and teachers together, within the context of their lives (Freire, 1998). Attention to political, social, gender, and/or personal perspectives is strongly evident in views such as critical pedagogy (Giroux, 2011), feminist pedagogy (Crawley, Lewis, & Mayberry, 2008; Shrewsbury, 1997), and transformative learning (Mezirow, Taylor, & Associates, 2009). The premises of the nontechnical approaches can overlap and may be combined, as exemplified in critical feminist pedagogy (Chow, Fleck, Fan, Joseph, & Lyter, 2003), often extending to include matters of race, culture, and sexuality. In descriptions of these education and learning approaches, attention is given to the underlying philosophies and to the processes of personal transformation, dialogue, reflection, inclusion, and democracy that should occur within and among students and teachers. The logistics of a formal curriculum, such as course sequencing, are not the focus of nontechnical curriculum approaches, although in professional programs, such as nursing, the nontechnical approaches can be used within the structure of a formal curriculum.

Finally, Joseph (2011) views curriculum much more broadly than any of the previous descriptions. She conceptualizes curriculum as *culture* with "complex sociopolitical,

political, and ethical layers of meaning" (p. 3), and recognizes that many cultures can exist simultaneously within an educational setting. Because curriculum is a "process for transforming educational aims and practices" (p. 3), it requires inquiry and introspection.

Despite differing definitions and conceptions, a formal curriculum is implemented with the intention that learning occurs. In professional programs, there is a written plan that usually contains philosophical statements and goals; indicates some selection, organization, and sequencing of subject matter and learning experiences; and integrates evaluation of learning. These elements, among others, are addressed as aspects of the curriculum development process in subsequent chapters.

Nursing Curriculum as Evidence-Informed, Context-Relevant, and Unified

In this text, *nursing curriculum* is defined as the totality of the philosophical approaches, curriculum goals, overall design, courses, strategies to ignite learning, delivery methods, interactions, learning climate, evaluation methods, curriculum policies, and resources. The curriculum includes all matters that affect nursing students' learning and progression and that are within the authority of the school of nursing. This conceptualization aligns with ideas of curriculum as a plan, experiences, process, means, strategy, and as being visible.

Evidence-Informed

A curriculum that is *evidence-informed* is based on systematically and purposefully gathered evidence about:

- The context in which the curriculum will be offered and graduates will practice nursing
- Students, learning, teaching, and nursing education
- Nursing practice
- Clients and their responses to health situations

The evidence that is gathered is then subject to the interpretation of curriculum developers. Plans are created, appraised according to the realities of the school of nursing, and then determined by the consensual judgment of nurse educators. As such, the curriculum is informed by evidence, but not based solely on evidence. Therefore, the term *evidence-informed* and not *evidence-based* is used.

An evidence-informed curriculum is dynamic, evolving as new evidence becomes available. Ongoing modification in response to new evidence ensures that the curriculum remains current.

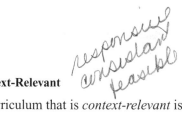

Context-Relevant

A curriculum that is *context-relevant* is:

- Responsive to students; current and projected societal, health, and community situations; and current and projected imperatives of the nursing profession
- Consistent with the mission, philosophy, and goals of the educational institution and school of nursing
- Feasible within the realities of the school and community

This type of curriculum is defined by, and grounded in, the forces and circumstances that affect society, health care, education, recipients of nursing care, the nursing profession, and the educational institution. Although there will be significant similarities in the nursing curricula of many schools, those that are most strongly contextually relevant will have unique features reflective of local and/or regional circumstances. However, a context-relevant curriculum is not simply reactive to current circumstances; it is also grounded in projections about the future. As such, a context-relevant curriculum is forward looking and prepares graduates for current nursing practice and the type of nursing practice that could or should exist now and in the future.

Unified

A curriculum that is *unified* contains curricular components that are conceptually, logically, cohesively, and visibly related, specifically:

- Philosophical approaches, professional abilities, and curriculum concepts are evident in the curriculum goals or outcomes.
- Level and course learning goals or competencies are derived from the curriculum goals or outcomes.
- Course titles reflect the philosophical approaches and curriculum concepts.
- Strategies to ignite learning and opportunities for students to demonstrate learning are consistent with the curriculum goals or outcomes, and philosophical and educational approaches.
- The language of the philosophical approaches and curriculum concepts are used in written materials and teaching-learning interactions.

The cohesion and connections between and among all aspects of the curriculum are evident. This unity is apparent in written curriculum documents and the curriculum that is enacted daily.

   In summary, a curriculum that is evidence-informed, context-relevant, and unified is grounded in evidence about nursing education, nursing practice, students, and society, and is responsive to the situation in which it is offered. The curriculum is forward looking and organized in a coherent fashion with clear relationships among the curricular elements so that its unified nature is visible.

Curriculum or Program?

Although the term *nursing curriculum* is often used interchangeably with *nursing program*, the latter is broader in scope. The nursing program is defined as the nursing curriculum; the school of nursing culture; administrative operations of the school; faculty members' complete teaching, research, and professional activities; the school's relationships with other academic units, healthcare agencies, community agencies, and professional and accrediting organizations; institution-wide support services for students and faculty; and support for the school of nursing within and beyond the parent institution. In brief, the nursing program includes activities and relationships that influence the quality and nature of the student experience but extend beyond the student experience itself.

CURRICULUM DEVELOPMENT IN NURSING EDUCATION

Curriculum development in nursing education is a scholarly and creative process intended to produce an evidence-informed, context-relevant, unified nursing curriculum. The ultimate purpose is to create learning opportunities that will build students' professional knowledge, skills, values, and identity so that graduates will practice nursing professionally and competently in changing social and healthcare environments, thereby contributing to the health and quality of life of those they serve.

Curriculum development is scholarly. It requires purposeful data gathering, logical thinking, careful analysis, presentation of cogent arguments, and precise writing. It is also creative, requiring openness to new ideas, imaginative thinking, and risk taking. The overall process is characterized by interaction, cooperation, change, and possibly conflict; comprised of overlapping, interactive, and iterative decision making; shaped by contextual realities and political timeliness; and influenced by the personal interests, styles, philosophies, judgments, and values of members of the curriculum development team.

The complex processes that lead to a substantial revision of an existing curriculum or creation of a new curriculum provide an opportunity for faculty members to expand their scholarly work, develop and implement fresh perspectives on the education of nursing students, and influence the culture of the school of nursing. Additionally, curriculum development provides an avenue to strengthen the school's impact on the community and gain support from members of the educational institution, community, and nursing profession.

The curriculum development process has neither a beginning nor end. Once developed, the nursing curriculum undergoes refinements and modifications as it is implemented, researched, and evaluated, and as new evidence becomes available about teaching, learning, students, society, health, health care, nursing education, and nursing practice. A perfect nursing curriculum cannot be achieved and remain in place without alteration. Adjustments are required over time because of changing educational, social, and health-care contexts and because nursing faculty strive to ensure that the curriculum is relevant to the context in which it is offered and in which graduates will practice nursing.

MODEL OF EVIDENCE-INFORMED, CONTEXT-RELEVANT, UNIFIED CURRICULUM DEVELOPMENT IN NURSING EDUCATION

Although written and schematic representations of curriculum development are generally linear and sequential, this is not how nursing curricula are actually developed. Curriculum development is a recursive process, with each decision influencing concurrent and subsequent choices, and possibly leading to a rethinking of previous ideas. A cohesive nursing curriculum results from ongoing communication among groups working on different aspects of curriculum development, review and critique of completed work, and confirmation of decisions. According to Scales (1985):

> In actual practice, development and implementation of the curriculum is an integrated phenomenon . . . developed in a very integrated and interrelating manner; one component . . . [does] not necessarily spring full grown and naturally from another, nor will any single component usually stand without some revision after subsequent parts are developed. (p. 3)

The iterative and recursive nature of curriculum work cannot be illustrated accurately in a two-dimensional representation. Depicting the multiple and repetitive interactions that occur between and among the individual elements of curriculum development would result in a crowded and confusing model. Therefore, like other authors before us, we present a model of the curriculum development process in nursing education that may appear linear and one-dimensional. However, chapter descriptions of each element of the model will make evident that the process is interactive.

The Model of Evidence-Informed, Context-Relevant, Unified Curriculum Development in Nursing Education depicts the overall process for nursing curriculum development and is illustrated in **Figure 1-1**. The model is multidimensional, with three core processes of curriculum work: faculty development, ongoing appraisal, and scholarship. These core processes permeate all activities leading to a sound curriculum. Included in the model are the specific activities of curriculum development, and feedback loops that

Figure 1-1   Model of Evidence-Informed, Context-Relevant, Unified Curriculum Development
© C. L. Iwasiw and D. Goldenberg. Modified from Iwasiw, C., Goldenberg, D., & Andrusyszyn, M. A. (2009). *Curriculum development in nursing education* (2nd ed.). Sudbury, MA: Jones and Bartlett.

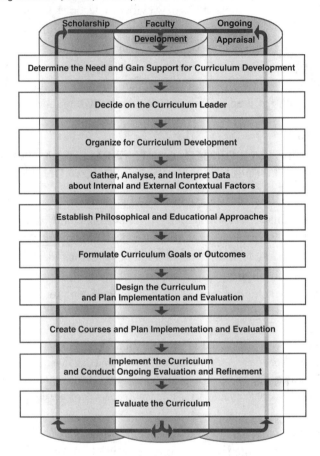

denote the dynamic nature of curriculum development, implementation, and evaluation. The model is applicable to all levels of nursing education and to all forms of curriculum delivery.

Core Processes of Curriculum Work

Faculty Development

Faculty development is necessary for all aspects of curriculum development because many nursing faculty and other stakeholders may have little or no preparation in educational theory. An evidence-informed, context-relevant, unified curriculum can result only when those developing the curriculum understand the processes involved. Therefore, deliberate and ongoing faculty development is essential to:

- Ensure that those engaged in curriculum development acquire the necessary knowledge and skills to contribute meaningfully to the processes and decisions of curriculum development
- Implement and evaluate the curriculum as intended

In addition, individuals' openness to new ideas and methods is fundamental to curriculum development, implementation, and evaluation. Their changing perspectives are indicative of personal development and the intellectual growth of all members.

Ongoing Appraisal

Ongoing appraisal of all aspects of the processes and products of curriculum development are inherent to the overall endeavor. Review and critique are necessary to ensure that:

- The processes in place are effective and satisfactory to members of the curriculum development team.
- Completed work is consistent with the basic curriculum tenets and is of an appropriate quality.

Scholarship

Scholarship is a central activity of academia, and therefore, is a core activity of curriculum development, implementation, and evaluation. This scholarship can include formal research, expository or analytical publications, and presentations. Topics could include the processes experienced, insights gained, and completed work. To engage in such activities elevates curriculum work from a local activity to knowledge development and dissemination. In this way, the science of nursing education can be advanced.

Figure 1-2 is a model of the relationship of the three core processes to curriculum work: curriculum development, implementation, and evaluation. The processes are foundational to intellectual rigor in curriculum work.

Curriculum Development Activities

Determine the Need and Gain Support for Curriculum Development

When a decision is made to open a school of nursing or to introduce a new program within an existing school, curriculum development is necessary. More typically, curriculum development begins with an acknowledgment that the existing curriculum is no longer working as effectively as desired. This recognition can arise from altered circumstances

Figure 1-2 Core Processes for Curriculum Work
© C. L. Iwasiw and D. Goldenberg

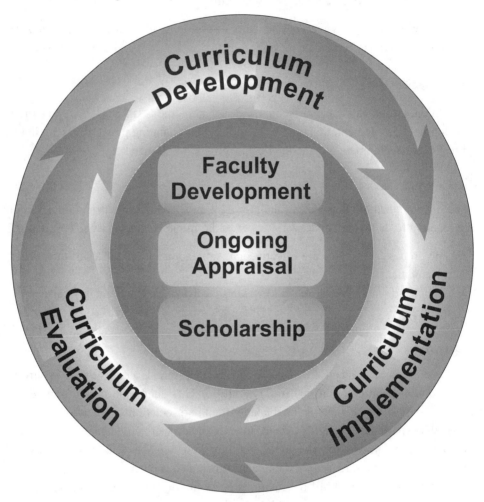

within the school (e.g., changing faculty or student profile), or outside the school (e.g., changed nursing practice or accreditation standards).

Once there is an agreement to proceed with curriculum development, support is needed from nursing faculty, educational administrators, and other stakeholders (e.g., students, graduates, nursing leaders). Gaining support for the curriculum development enterprise includes describing the logical reasons for altering the curriculum and appealing to the values held collectively by members of the school and educational institution. Faculty members' support and commitment are essential for all curriculum endeavors.

Additionally, administrative support (e.g., altered work assignments, secretarial assistance, promotion and tenure considerations) provides evidence of institutional encouragement for the initiative. Curriculum development is contingent upon adequate resources.

Decide on the Curriculum Leader

It is vital that a leader to guide the curriculum development process be determined. This individual can be appointed, elected, or given the position by consensus, according to the usual practices within a school of nursing. It is expected that the leader be knowledgeable about curriculum development, possess managerial skills to coordinate the logistics, and have the support of faculty and other stakeholders.

Organize for Curriculum Development

Attention to the logistical matters that will lead to a successful outcome is essential. Organizing for curriculum development requires consideration of, and decisions about leadership, the decision-making processes, committee structures and purposes, and approaches to getting the work done.

Gather, Analyze, and Interpret Data About Internal and External Contextual Factors

Systematic data gathering about the environment in which the curriculum will be implemented and in which graduates will practice nursing is critical to ensure that the curriculum is relevant to its context. Data are gathered about specific *contextual factors* and these are the forces, situations, and circumstances that exist both within and outside the educational institution and have the potential to influence the school and its curriculum. The contextual factors are interrelated, complex, and, at times, seamless and overlapping. Internal contextual factors exist within the school and the educational institution; external contextual factors originate outside the institution.

Typically, information is obtained about internal factors of history; philosophy, mission, and goals; culture; financial resources; programs and policies; and infrastructure. Similarly, data are gathered about the external contextual factors: demographics, culture, health care, professional standards and trends, technology, environment, and socio-politico-economics. It is necessary to determine precisely which data are required about each contextual factor, as well as the most appropriate data sources. The data are then analyzed and interpreted to deduce the core curriculum concepts and key professional abilities that graduates will need to practice nursing.

Establish Philosophical and Educational Approaches

Information about philosophical approaches used in, or suitable for nursing education, along with values and beliefs of the curriculum development team, lead to the development of statements of philosophical approaches relevant for the school and curriculum. Reaching resolution about the philosophical approaches is a critical milestone in curriculum development, because all aspects of the finalized curriculum should be congruent with espoused values and beliefs and the concepts that form the philosophical approaches. Along with the philosophical approaches is the identification of educational approaches consistent with them.

Formulate Curriculum Goal or Outcome Statements

The curriculum goal or outcome statements reflect broad abilities of graduates, each focusing on professional practice and representing an integration of cognitive, psychomotor, and affective actions. Curriculum goal or outcome statements are written to incorporate the desired abilities of graduates, philosophical approaches, and core curriculum concepts. They are a public statement of what graduates will be like.

Design the Curriculum and Plan Curriculum Implementation and Evaluation

The term *curriculum design* refers to the configuration of the course of studies. In designing the curriculum, faculty and other members of the design team determine level goals or competencies; nursing, non-nursing, and elective courses; course sequencing; relationships between and among courses; delivery methods; and associated policies. Brief course descriptions and draft course goals or competencies are prepared for nursing courses. As the curriculum is being designed, plans for its implementation are discussed concurrently to assess whether the design is likely to be feasible and how a reconceptualized curriculum can be introduced as the current curriculum is being phased out. Implementation planning also includes such matters as informing stakeholders, attending to contractual agreements and logistics, and planning ongoing faculty development.

Curriculum evaluation is an organized and thoughtful appraisal of those elements central to the course of studies undertaken by students, and of graduates' abilities. The aspects to be evaluated include the philosophical and educational approaches, curriculum goal or outcome statements, overall design, courses, strategies to ignite learning, interactions, learning climate, evaluation methods, curriculum policies, resources, and actual outcomes demonstrated by graduates. Like planning for implementation, planning curriculum evaluation should occur simultaneously with discussions about design.

Design Courses and Plan Course Implementation and Evaluation

Designing courses requires attention to the following components: purpose and description, course goals or competencies, strategies to ignite learning, concepts and content, classes, guidelines for student learning activities, opportunities for students to demonstrate learning, and evaluation of student learning. Each course must be congruent with the curriculum intent and clearly relate to intended curriculum goals or outcomes. As a mirror of the process of designing the curriculum and planning curriculum implementation and evaluation, planning for course implementation and evaluation should occur concurrently with decision making about course design.

Implement the Curriculum and Conduct Ongoing Curriculum Evaluation and Refinement

Curriculum implementation begins when the first course is introduced and continues for the life of the curriculum. Successful implementation is dependent on faculty and student adoption of the curriculum tenets and the use of congruent educational approaches and methods to evaluate learning. The curriculum evaluation plan is put into action simultaneously with curriculum implementation. Ongoing evaluation results in small refinements that smooth implementation, fill identified gaps, and/or remove redundancies.

Evaluate the Curriculum

Once completely implemented, the entire curriculum is evaluated to determine whether all elements are appropriate and congruent with one another, and to ascertain graduates' success. Internal curriculum evaluation is undertaken by members of the school of nursing, whereas external curriculum evaluation is generally conducted as a part of program evaluation by provincial, state, regional, or national approval or accrediting bodies.

Feedback Loops

The feedback loops in the model reflect the idea that at every stage of curriculum development, implementation, and evaluation, judgments are made about the appropriateness and fit of one element with previous elements, and the possibility of modification. The feedback loops signify that the curriculum is dynamic, subject to change as information about its effectiveness and appropriateness is gathered. Additionally, the feedback loops illustrate the connections among the curriculum development, implementation, and evaluation activities and the core curriculum processes, because the core processes permeate all aspects of curriculum work.

INTERPERSONAL DIMENSIONS OF CURRICULUM DEVELOPMENT

Curriculum development is not a sterile process of objective, detached decision making. Rather, it is marked by the dynamics of all interpersonal activities. Because each school of nursing has a unique set of people with their own talents, personalities, goals, knowledge, experiences, and values, the culture and dynamics vary from school to school. In general, however, learning, conflict, cooperation, resistance, eagerness, formation of group alliances, power struggles, commitment to shared goals, sadness, and satisfaction can occur during curriculum development. The human dimension is a constant factor and must be attended to even when the tasks and deadlines of curriculum development are pressing. For curriculum development to be successful, it is important that all members of the curriculum development team feel valued and appreciated for ideas they offer and work they complete.

Curriculum deliberations occur in collaboration with colleagues whose values may be divergent. Because values affect perspectives and choices, they are a powerful (although sometimes unrecognized) influence on curriculum development. Consequently, it is incumbent upon curriculum developers to reflect on their ideals and beliefs, discuss them openly with colleagues, and consider how these influence their preferences about the developing curriculum. Clarification of individual and collective values is integral to curriculum development and can be essential in times of emotional debate or apparently irresolvable conflict.

The dynamics of influence and power are also part of curriculum development and its aftermath. Faculty members with either informal or formal power in the school may influence the process in directions not supported by all, and consequently, some faculty and other stakeholders might feel devalued, resentful, or powerless. New informal leaders can emerge during curriculum development with a resulting loss of influence by others. The processes of developing and implementing a new curriculum can lead to shifts in the power dynamics within and outside the school, with associated changes in the real or perceived advantages and disadvantages experienced by individuals.

Curriculum development and implementation represent a significant change for faculty members in which they progress from known and comfortable ways of being, to a state of uncertainty, and then to new understandings and practices. Collegial support and reinforcement sustain this progress. Collectively, faculty can create and institute strategies to recognize their progress, offer encouragement to each other, and celebrate their successes. In these ways, both faculty cohesion and the curriculum are strengthened.

A full description of the interpersonal dynamics of curriculum development is beyond the scope of this text. The interpersonal dimension is a matter that requires diligent attention in all curriculum work. The success of the curriculum is dependent on the dedication of all participants, and this is most likely to develop when individuals communicate openly and supportively with one another, feel valued, and believe their ideas are contributing to quality nursing education.

CHAPTER SUMMARY

Curriculum development in nursing is a scholarly and creative endeavour that faculty members and other participants undertake with the goal of preparing graduates who will practice nursing professionally in constantly changing environments. The nursing curriculum is comprised of the totality of the philosophical approaches, curriculum goals or outcomes, overall design, courses, strategies to ignite learning, delivery methods, interactions, learning climate, evaluation methods, curriculum policies, and resources, an inclusive definition that differs from those offered by other curriculum experts. The Model of Evidence-Informed, Context-Relevant, Unified Curriculum Development in Nursing Education describes a process for developing a curriculum that is informed by evidence, relevant for the context in which the curriculum will be offered and graduates will work, and unified conceptually. Core to the model are faculty development, ongoing appraisal, and scholarship. Curriculum development begins with the recognition that a new curriculum is needed and may seem to be complete when the newly created curriculum is implemented. However, development of an evidence-informed, context-relevant, unified curriculum is really a dynamic process, because evaluation and subsequent refinement are constant features of nursing curricula, even during implementation. Successful curriculum development, implementation, and evaluation are contingent on dedicated participants whose efforts are valued and who are supported during the process.

REFERENCES

Chow, E. N. L., Fleck, C., Fan, G. H., Joseph, J., & Lyter, D. M. (2003). Exploring critical feminist pedagogy: Infusing dialogue, participation, and experience in teaching and learning. *Teaching Sociology, 31*, 259–275.

Crawley, S. L., Lewis, J. E., & Mayberry, M. (2008). Introduction—feminist pedagogies in action: Teaching beyond disciplines. *Feminist Teacher, 19*(1), 1–12.

Diekelmann, N., & Diekelmann, J. (2009). *Schooling learning teaching: Toward a narrative pedagogy.* Bloomington, IN: iUniverse Inc.

Freire, P. (1970/2001). *Pedagogy of the oppressed.* New York: Continuum International Publishing Group.

Freire, P. (1998). *Pedagogy of freedom*: *Ethics, democracy and civic courage.* Lanham, MD: Rowman & Littlefield.

Giroux, H. A. (2011). *On critical pedagogy.* London: UK. Continuum International Publishing Group.

Hensen, K. T. (2010). *Curriculum planning: Integrating multiculturism, constructivism, and education reform* (4th ed.). Long Grove, IL: Waveland Press.

Joseph, P. B. (2011). Conceptualizing curriculum. In P. B. Joseph (Ed.), *Cultures of curriculum* (2nd ed., pp. 3–22). New York: Routledge.

Lunenberg, F. C. (2011). Theorizing about curriculum. *International Journal of Scholarly Academic Intellectual Diversity, 13*(1), 1–6.

Mezirow, J., Taylor, E. W., & Associates. (2009). *Transformative learning in practice: Insights from community, workplace, and higher education.* San Francisco: Jossey-Bass.

Oliva, P. F. (2009). *Developing the curriculum* (7th ed.). Boston: Pearson Education.

Parkay, F. W., Anctil, E. J., & Hass, G. (2010). *Curriculum leadership: Readings for developing quality educational programs.* Boston: Allyn & Bacon.

Scales, F. S. (1985). *Nursing curriculum. Development, structure, function.* Norwalk, CT: Appleton-Century-Crofts.

Shrewsbury, C. M. (1997). What is feminist pedagogy? *Women's Studies Quarterly, 25,* 166–173.

Wiles, J. (2005). *Curriculum essentials: A resource for educators* (2nd ed.). Boston: Pearson Education.

Wiles, J., & Bondi, J. (2007). *Curriculum development: A guide to practice* (7th ed.). Upper Saddle River, NJ: Pearson/Merrill/Prentice Hall.

Wiles, J. W., & Bondi, J. C. (2011). *Curriculum development: A guide to practice* (8th ed.). Upper Saddle River, NJ: Pearson/Merrill/Prentice Hall.

PART II

Core Processes of Curriculum Work

CHAPTER 2

Faculty Development for Curriculum Work and Change

Chapter Overview

This chapter begins with descriptions of the purpose and meaning of *faculty development*, as well as the necessary conditions for it. The term *curriculum work* used in this chapter encompasses curriculum development, implementation, and evaluation. The relationship of faculty development, curriculum work, and change is explained to support the premise that faculty development is a core and ongoing component of all curriculum work. Faculty development for curriculum work is presented, including its purpose, goals, participants and their responsibilities, activities, and benefits. Theoretical perspectives on change are described next, with application to curriculum work. Then, strategies to support faculty during change and ideas for responding to resistance to change are offered. Synthesis activities include a case study for readers' critical analysis and questions for consideration when planning faculty development.

Chapter Goals

- Consider the purpose and meanings of *faculty development*.
- Review the conditions necessary for faculty development.
- Appreciate the necessity of faculty development as a core process of curriculum development, implementation, and evaluation.
- Gain insights into responsibilities, strategies, and benefits associated with faculty development for curriculum work.
- Relate theoretical perspectives on change to curriculum work.
- Reflect on strategies to support faculty during change.
- Ponder ideas for responding to resistance to curriculum work and faculty development.

FACULTY DEVELOPMENT

Purpose and Meaning of Faculty Development

Faculty development can be conceived of as "the theory and practice of facilitating improved faculty performance" (Halliburton, Marincovich, & Svinicki, 1988, p. 291). It is a form of continuing professional development for academics. The purpose of institution-wide faculty development generally has been improvement in teaching.

The traditional focus on the development of faculty members as teachers and evaluators of learning continues today. Currently, there is an expanded emphasis on the individual as a scholar, professional, person, and member of an organization. Therefore, development activities are aimed at all these and often include collaborative efforts and the creation of a community of learners (Brooks, 2011; Kitchen, Parker, & Gallagher, 2008; Malinsky, DuBois, & Jacquest, 2010; Taylor, 2010). However, activities related specifically to curriculum development, implementation, and evaluation consistent with curriculum tenets are not typically addressed in the literature about faculty development.

The meanings that faculty members have attributed to their own development as academics are varied and hierarchal, with each description encompassing the previous:

- Becoming more productive in their work output
- Achieving credibility and recognition
- Making ongoing improvements in their work
- Accumulating personal knowledge and skills
- Expanding the depth and sophistication of knowledge in their academic field
- Contributing to disciplinary growth or social change (Åkerlind, 2005)

From these meanings, the overall purpose of faculty development activities can be deduced as follows: to contribute to the growth and development of individuals in all their academic roles so that their capacity to advance their discipline and influence change is expanded.

Necessary Conditions for Faculty Development

Furco and Moely (2012) have listed the "conditions that are important for securing faculty buy-in and support" (p. 129) for an educational innovation. These are:

- Explicit and clearly communicated goals for the innovation, which are consistent with faculty values and concerns
- Opportunities for faculty to gain skill with the innovation and explore their questions, without excessive demands on their time
- Institutional commitment to ongoing support for the innovation
- Rewards for faculty involvement in the form of readily perceived professional development or through the faculty reward system

The development and implementation of a new or modified curriculum is a significant educational innovation, the purpose of which must be endorsed by faculty and curriculum developers after an exploration of their values. Planned faculty development activities, as a core process of curriculum work, are the ongoing embodiment of:

- The provision of opportunities for faculty and other curriculum participants to gain curriculum skills and explore questions about curriculum
- An institutional commitment to provide tangible support for curriculum work
- Professional development during curriculum work

RELATIONSHIP OF FACULTY DEVELOPMENT, CURRICULUM WORK, AND CHANGE

The processes of curriculum development, implementation, and evaluation represent a significant change in a school of nursing. There are challenges and changes to current assumptions and practices, the nature of work that is undertaken, composition of work teams, interpersonal relationships, and expectations for individuals and groups. Curriculum development and implementation of a redesigned curriculum require change from an established curriculum and familiar work patterns based on tacit assumptions, beliefs, and norms to an altered curriculum and work expectations based on expressed assumptions, beliefs, and norms that evolve and become explicit as curriculum work progresses. Thus, curriculum redesign influences and possibly changes the culture of the school of nursing.

Successful curriculum change is generally dependent upon the acquisition of new skills and perspectives by those who will implement the reconceptualized curriculum. Educational and evaluation approaches, interactions, course content, and possibly sites for professional practice teaching could be altered. Additionally, there may be shifts in interpersonal dynamics and a realignment of teaching colleagues. Similarly, curriculum evaluation can lead to some curriculum modifications, which may necessitate further change.

Because faculty members have extensive involvement in curriculum development and implementation plans, and in opportunities to introduce aspects of the redesigned curriculum into the existing one, transition to a new curriculum might be expected to occur easily and with full faculty support. Unfortunately, the change may not be smooth, because change often involves some loss and acceptance of new perspectives. Accepting and endorsing the need for change, working toward the change, and living successfully in the changed circumstances all require personal adjustment. The adjustment occurs through self-reflection, critical thinking, altered perceptions, and support and does not happen in a scheduled, linear fashion. It is determined by individual interests, motivation, and readiness.

Ongoing, systematic, and integrated professional development is necessary to ensure that the group understands a proposed change, particularly when a change in practice is a

Figure 2-1   Synchronous, intertwining, and infinite nature of curriculum development, faculty development, and change
© C. L. Iwasiw and D. Goldenberg. Modified from Iwasiw, C., Goldenberg, D., & Andrusyszyn, M. A. (2005). *Curriculum development in nursing education*. Sudbury, MA: Jones and Bartlett.

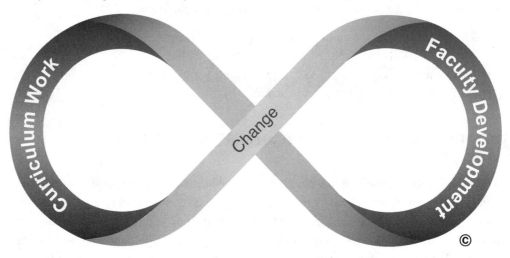

goal (Haviland, Shin, & Turley, 2010). Therefore, faculty development is a way to ensure that participants have the necessary knowledge and skills to develop, implement, and evaluate a curriculum. It is also an avenue to support participants during the changes associated with curriculum work. As such, faculty development is a core process of curriculum work. The content and nature of faculty development are defined by curriculum and change processes. In turn, learning gained during faculty development will influence the curriculum work and the change. Moreover, faculty development activities are a means to sustain change and promote continued growth within the school of nursing. **Figure 2-1** depicts the continuous, synchronous, and interrelated nature of curriculum work, faculty development, and change.

FACULTY DEVELOPMENT FOR CURRICULUM WORK

Necessity of Faculty Development for Curriculum Work

Faculty development has been described as the "essence of curriculum development" (Rush, Ouellet, & Wasson, 1991). It is essential that faculty be able to "develop coherent curriculum designs, methods for the assessment of student learning, [and] evidence-based program evaluation" (Bartels, 2007, p. 157). If faculty members are unable to do this, nursing curricula and the practice of nursing education cannot progress. Therefore, faculty development is foundational to the creation, implementation, and evaluation of a curriculum that reflects a new perspective and is true to the espoused philosophical approaches.

A core competency of the academic nurse educator is to "participate in curriculum design and evaluation of program outcomes" (National League for Nursing [NLN], 2005, p. 19). Among the components of this competency is knowledge of curriculum development: identifying program outcomes, developing competency statements, writing learning objectives, and selecting learning experiences and evaluation strategies (NLN, 2005).

However, few recent graduates of master's and doctoral programs have academic preparation in this aspect of the nurse educator role (Bartels, 2007; Benner, Sutphen, Leonard, & Day, 2010; Dearmon, Lawson, & Hall, 2011; Suplee & Gardner, 2009) because of the emphases on advanced practice roles and research in graduate nursing programs. Additionally, faculty development about the curriculum development process itself, and the creation of an evidence-informed, context-relevant, unified curriculum, is rarely planned, perhaps because of an unexamined assumption that teachers innately know how to develop curricula, or because curriculum development activities have traditionally received little (if any) credit toward promotion and tenure decisions. The result is that knowledge about nursing curriculum may be limited to personal experience, and knowledge of curriculum development processes may be absent (Goldenberg, Andrusyszyn, & Iwasiw, 2004). Thus, many nursing faculty are not equipped to undertake curriculum development or to fulfill their educator role other than in the way that they experienced it as students (Bartels, 2007).

Faculty competence in all aspects of curriculum design, implementation, and evaluation is foundational to developing an educationally sound curriculum. Because it cannot be assumed that faculty members know how to develop a curriculum, it is incumbent on school leaders to provide opportunities so that relevant knowledge and skills can be acquired. Faculty development is a core activity of curriculum work and is a catalyst for the creation and operationalization of a new vision for the curriculum. Through faculty development activities, novices can be guided to think beyond their individual areas of nursing practice expertise and their own educational experiences, to the possibilities for an entire curriculum. The interactions and synergy occurring in development sessions may also prompt seasoned faculty to consider new approaches to the nursing curriculum.

Curriculum redesign requires faculty members to look beyond their own nursing practice and teaching areas. They need to consider the future of nursing practice, the philosophical approaches and concepts that should underpin nursing practice and the curriculum, what the curriculum goals should be, and how students could achieve those goals. In addition, they must examine how all aspects of a curriculum interact and the options for curriculum design. To develop an evidence-informed, context-relevant, unified curriculum in a timely fashion, faculty and other stakeholders will likely require assistance with the curriculum development process itself, as well as with curriculum implementation and evaluation. Accordingly, it is necessary for faculty development to occur in tandem with curriculum development and to be viewed as a core component of curriculum work.

Faculty development related to all aspects of curriculum development, implementation, and evaluation is particularly timely because of the nursing faculty shortage and impending retirement of a large cohort of faculty (American Association of Colleges of Nursing, 2012; Canadian Nurses Association & Canadian Association of Schools of Nursing, 2012). Presumably, it is the older faculty members who have the most experience in curriculum work and are more likely to have formal preparation in curricular matters. Over time, therefore, there could be fewer faculty knowledgeable about curriculum work, and the mentoring or guidance they offer would not be available. Accordingly, opportunities should be created to develop or enhance the curriculum skills of novice and mid-career nurse educators.

Purpose and Goals of Faculty Development for Curriculum Work

The purpose of faculty development for curriculum work is to contribute to the growth and development of nursing faculty in all aspects of curriculum work so that their capacity to develop, implement, and evaluate an evidence-informed, context-relevant, unified curriculum is enhanced, and their ability to advance the practice of nursing education and influence future nursing practice is expanded. This purpose encompasses all aspects of curriculum work for which faculty and other curriculum participants might require additional knowledge, skills, and support.

As explicated by Bevis (2000), there are at least four goals for faculty development related to curriculum development, implementation, and evaluation. For faculty members, these include:

- Enhancing their knowledge and skills about curriculum development and curriculum evaluation
- Transforming their view of curriculum to match the perspectives of the new curriculum
- Becoming comfortable with changing roles and relationships
- Gaining skill in teaching-learning and evaluation approaches.

All are of equal importance and are achieved synergistically. Other goals can emerge in accordance with the learning needs of curriculum developers.

Enhancing Knowledge and Skills About Curriculum Development and Evaluation

Knowledge about curriculum development and curriculum evaluation processes varies among faculty members and other stakeholders. Some will know a great deal; others will be familiar with details of course planning, but not with the larger process. Some will know about course evaluation, but not about overall curriculum evaluation. To make certain that the curriculum development process is as smooth as possible, faculty development focused specifically on developing a curriculum is necessary. Knowledge of the total process will lead to an appreciation of the time required for curriculum development, work accomplished by task groups, and importance of shared understandings and consensus. Moreover, detailed information about each aspect of curriculum development and evaluation will allow task groups to develop a critical path for completion of their work and increase the likelihood that work is completed in the manner required.

Transforming the View of Curriculum

Another goal for faculty development is for faculty to transform their view of curriculum and, possibly, their view of learning, based on the philosophical approaches and learning theories chosen. It is important that faculty have opportunities to develop their understanding about the approach to curriculum that is being developed. This will be an ongoing process that will occur throughout the curriculum work and through faculty development opportunities intended to assist them in designing, implementing, and evaluating a curriculum reflecting the new view.

Becoming Comfortable with Changing Roles and Relationships

A change in faculty roles could be a consequence of curriculum redesign. A changed curriculum might mean altered relationships with students, colleagues, clients, and administrators. The role change may involve a shift in activities, power, equity, and authority, depending on the curricular philosophical approaches and goals or outcomes. If so, an exploration of these ideas and how new relationships will be enacted warrants explicit attention.

Gaining Skill in Approaches for Teaching-Learning and Evaluation of Student Learning

A necessary goal of faculty development is to become comfortable with new strategies that align with the curriculum philosophical and educational approaches, and outcomes or goals. Through development activities related to teaching and evaluation of student learning, faculty members can gain the skills necessary to:

- Implement the curriculum consistently and successfully.
- Ensure that students experience the chosen curriculum philosophical and educational approaches in all teaching-learning encounters and have opportunities to achieve curriculum goals or outcomes.
- Make certain that methods to evaluate student learning match curriculum tenets

Participants in Faculty Development Activities

Faculty members are the key players in the curriculum development, implementation, and evaluation processes, that is, in:

- Decisions to be made
- Committee work to be accomplished
- Facilitation and evaluation of student learning according to the tenets of a redesigned curriculum
- Appraisal of curriculum evaluation results

Consequently, the success of curriculum work is largely dependent upon knowledgeable and willing faculty members and development activities planned with and for them.

Importantly, others, such as students, clinicians, and administrators, who are part of the curriculum development process, should also be included in faculty development activities. Participation in these learning opportunities will expand stakeholders' knowledge and skills about curriculum processes, strengthen their commitment and connection, and deepen their understandings about the school of nursing.

Responsibility for Faculty Development

The school leader has the responsibility to invest in and support the development of faculty in order to minimize knowledge gaps in all aspects of the academic role, including curriculum work. Formal leadership confers the responsibility to act as a change agent and to operationalize professional development to "foster the future of the organization" (Kenner & Pressler, 2006, p. 2). School leaders are the primary force in initiating change, assisting faculty in their development (Smolen, 1996), creating an empowering and respectful work environment, and ensuring that stakeholders are involved in the school's activities. Identification of specific faculty development needs can be undertaken by the school leader, the curriculum leader, a faculty development committee, or individual faculty members. Typically, it is a combination of these.

Faculty members have a professional obligation to ensure they are competent in their role functions, to continue to improve as nurse educators, and to engage in activities that enhance their effectiveness (NLN, 2005) and that of others. Therefore, they have a responsibility to:

- Attend faculty development activities
- Be open to new ideas
- Participate fully in faculty development

- Commit to employing new knowledge, skills, and perspectives as they develop, implement, and evaluate the curriculum
- Contribute to the development of others

Responsibility for creating formal faculty development opportunities could rest with knowledgeable and experienced faculty members who have a solid theoretical and experiential foundation in nursing education. Their development needs may be slight, so that their participation could be to provide leadership in faculty development. They might lead formal and informal sessions, provide guidance to novices, or purposefully mentor others. These activities would spontaneously occur within a learning culture, yet may need to be formalized for faculty development for curriculum work.

Faculty Development Activities for Curriculum Work

Faculty development activities could be formal, informal, collaborative, self-managed, individual, or group based. Activities can include workshops, mentoring, group discussions, and attendance at conferences. Local sessions can be face-to-face, online, or a combination of these. Podcasts or videos of faculty development activities can be created and accessed by those unable to attend face-to-face sessions or those wanting to review information. Peer coaching can be effective for experienced faculty members (Huston & Weaver, 2008). See **Table 2-1** for examples of formal and informal strategies for faculty development. Ideas about content and processes for faculty development specific to various aspects of curriculum work are explored elsewhere in the text.

It is incumbent upon all curriculum stakeholders to reach shared understandings about curriculum work, nursing education, nursing practice and health care, the curriculum tenets, educational processes, and student–teacher–practitioner relationships. Faculty discussions of this nature serve faculty development purposes and move the curriculum development process forward.

Because faculty development is ongoing, a preliminary schedule should be agreed upon. The precise activities that are undertaken ought to be consistent with the evolving philosophy of the redesigned curriculum. It is recommended that each session's topic, format, time, location, and leader be decided early. However, schedules and topics require some flexibility so that changes can be instituted to meet participant obligations, newly identified or urgent needs, and other contingencies. The concept of just-in-time relevance is pertinent (O'Keefe, Brady, Conlan, & Wade, as cited in Myers, Mixer, Wyatt, Paulus, & Lee, 2011). If a development activity is offered at the time when members are about to engage in a particular aspect of curriculum work, they are likely to see the need for the activity and to participate willingly.

Table 2-1   Strategies for Formal and Informal Faculty Development

STRATEGIES	
Formal	**Informal**
• Audiovisual materials	• Buddy system
• Communities of interest	• Dialogue and feedback
• Conferences	• Handbooks
• Group meetings	• Learning circles
• Faculty meetings	• Luncheon meetings
• Forums	• Meetings with department heads
• Lectures by experts and/or knowledgeable colleagues	• Mentorship
• Online learning activities	• Modeling
• Peer coaching	• One-on-one discussions
• Podcasts	• Online group discussions
• Postgraduate courses	• Peer support
• Practice teaching	• Readings
• Retreats	• Shadowing
• Seminars	• Tutoring
• Tours, visits	
• Workshops	
• Videos	

In order to design a curriculum that will be acceptable to all stakeholders and relevant at the time of curriculum implementation and beyond, faculty development is necessary. When engaging in curriculum development, faculty come together, learn and grow together, accept that change is inevitable, and take ownership and pride in the future. When faculty development is enacted as a core component of curriculum work, individuals' personal investment in the curriculum and the school of nursing is increased.

Benefits of Faculty Development for Curriculum Work

Faculty development for curriculum work results in an essential benefit for the school of nursing, specifically the greatly enhanced potential for curriculum developers to:

- Create a shared vision for the curriculum (Oliver & Hyun, 2011).
- Develop an evidence-informed, context-relevant, unified curriculum.
- Implement and evaluate the curriculum in a manner consistent with the underlying tenets.

Planned and ongoing faculty development demonstrates the school's commitment to faculty and their professional growth, increases job satisfaction, and is a method to support personal and curriculum development. Curriculum developers may feel valued because of the school's investment in them. Additionally, formalized, systematic development activities can enhance faculty recruitment and retention (Heinrich & Oberleitner, 2012).

A program of faculty development can contribute to a learning culture within a school, a culture where the individual and team learning of all members (faculty, stakeholders, and students) is given attention and accorded value, and in which systems are created to support and share learning (Holyoke, Sturko, Wood, & Wu, 2012). In such an environment, members may feel secure in group learning and connected to others through shared learning, acceptance, appreciation, support, and respect.

Faculty and stakeholders who participate in development related to curriculum work have the potential, individually and collectively, to experience benefits consistent with the descriptions of development reported by Åkerlind (2005). Learning the skills of curriculum work will increase their competence and make them more efficient and effective, thereby reducing frustration and the need to redo work. Increased knowledge and skills could lead to credibility and possibly external recognition, as well as being the bases for making ongoing improvements and feeling a sense of pride in completed work. Additionally, personal skills, such as negotiation, collaboration, and consensus building, can accrue from curriculum work. There is potential to expand the depth and sophistication of knowledge about nursing education, and, if scholarship projects about curriculum work are undertaken, to influence nursing education practice beyond the school of nursing.

FACULTY DEVELOPMENT FOR CHANGE

The change associated with curriculum work can give rise to feelings and behaviors ranging from eager anticipation and full engagement, to a "wait and see" attitude with reluctant participation, to resistance involving refusal to participate and possibly sabotage. In addition to expanding participants' knowledge and skills in curriculum work, faculty development can also support faculty members' personal and professional growth during the changes associated with the curriculum work. Therefore, attention to the cognitive, psychological, and behavioral aspects of change all merit attention. Consideration should be given to how faculty might experience change, how the school's culture might influence and be affected by change, and strategies to support faculty during change. Deliberate responses intended to enhance resisters' participation in curriculum and faculty development, and their acceptance of the redesigned curriculum are also important.

Theoretical Perspectives on Change: Application to Curriculum Work

Diffusion of Innovations

This frequently cited theory gives attention to individuals and groups within a social system. According to Rogers (2003), diffusion is "a kind of social change, defined as the process by which alteration occurs in the structure and function of a social system" (p. 6). An innovation is an idea or practice that is viewed as new, and this is communicated over time among the members of the social system. Acceptance follows an S-shaped curve within a social group, with some members being slow to accept the change and others rejecting it completely. The rate of adoption is related to the following characteristics of the innovation:

- Relative advantage of the new idea over current practice
- Compatibility with existing values and past experiences of potential adopters
- Complexity of the new idea or practice
- Trialability, or the ability to test the innovation on a limited basis
- Observability of the results of the innovation to others

The interpersonal channel of communication (that is, face-to-face interaction between and among individuals of similar status) is most important in the diffusion of an innovation. Most people depend on a subjective evaluation of an innovation that is conveyed to them from individuals who have adopted the innovation.

Time is a dimension of the theory: the length of time for the innovation decision process to occur, the time for an individual to adopt the innovation, and the rate of adoption within a system. Planned dissemination can increase the rate and level of adoption more than the pace of informal dissemination (Greenhalgh, Robert, Bate, Macfarlane, & Kyriakidou, 2005). Individuals adopt the innovation at different times during a change:

- Innovators seek change and are the first to adopt the idea.
- Early adopters facilitate change.
- Early majority members prefer the status quo but provide a support system for change and accept it.
- Late majority members accept the change after most others.
- Laggards strive to maintain the status quo.
- Rejecters actively oppose and may sabotage the innovation (Rogers, 2003).

The social system is an important dimension of the theory. Communication channels, status of individuals, and decision-making processes all influence the diffusion of innovations. Greenhalgh and colleagues (2005) extend this idea: Sustainability of an innovation requires systems changes.

This theory is useful for understanding individuals' and groups' acceptance of the need for curriculum change, their commitment to it, and their readiness to engage in curriculum work and faculty development. It points to the necessity of involving respected opinion leaders in faculty development activities so they can persuade peers of the value of these endeavors, share positive evaluations of the activities, and make visible the learning they have gained. Their formal and informal diffusion of knowledge and skills relevant to curriculum work will improve the quality of the curriculum. The pace at which individuals will accept the need for curriculum redesign and faculty development may also vary. It is important to recognize that not everyone will be an innovator, early adopter, or member of the early majority. Therefore, avenues should be available to allow respectful inclusion of late majority members and laggards, and there must be a way for them to catch up through faculty development. Furthermore, it is wise to remember that curriculum change is systems change, and it is necessary that a majority will support and maintain the change.

Transtheoretical Model of Behavior Change

This model addresses behavior change of an individual as the desired outcome and incorporates changes in attitudes, intentions, and behavior. The model incorporates four theoretical concepts central to change: stages, internal processes, self-efficacy (a feeling of confidence to enact the desired behavior), and decisional balance (weighing the advantages and disadvantages of changing).

Behavioral change is conceptualized as a spiral, and this pattern represents the reality that people do not change in a straightforward, linear manner. Rather, at certain times, individuals can revert to former stages and then proceed again toward the desired change. Relapse to previous stages is considered a natural part of the change cycle. The following stages represent a continuum of motivational readiness:

- Precontemplation: Person sees no need to change.
- Contemplation: Person thinks about the benefits and losses of change and admits to desiring change, but there is no intent to act.
- Preparation: Person plans to make a specific change soon and may make small attempts at change.
- Action: Person makes an overt commitment to change and practices the new behavior over time.
- Maintenance: Person is able to avoid relapses to former stages for 6 months or more, although the temptation to relapse can persist for several years (Norcross, Krebs, & Prochaska, 2010; Prochaska & Velicer, 1997).

Participation in curriculum work and faculty development can be conceptualized as encompassing a change in faculty attitude toward the current curriculum, a decision and intention to create a new curriculum, and a change in behavior to engage in curriculum work. Curriculum implementation may require a change in attitude toward students, other faculty, and roles; behaving and interacting in new ways; and changing teaching and evaluation strategies and approach to content. Faculty development activities provide the knowledge, skills, and environment that support individual and collective change. Participation in faculty development represents action to change attitudes and behavior.

The appeal of this model of individual change is that it acknowledges that acceptance, practice, and continuation of a change are not linear processes. Rather, recycling to previous stages is seen as a natural occurrence. Reference to this theory during curriculum work provides a means to understand why some curriculum participants may question the value of new curriculum ideas that they have formerly accepted or may return to previous teaching styles during periods of stress, and then re-engage in the intent of the changed curriculum. Understanding of this model allows faculty members to be patient with each other and recognize when additional support is needed.

Organizational Change in Cultural Context (OC³ Model)

From an ethnographic analysis of change in a research-intensive university, Latta (2009) developed a model of bilateral interaction in which organizational change and culture influenced one another. According to the model, an understanding of the culture is a necessary starting point for the change process. Readiness for change can be enhanced by highlighting discrepancies between the current status and the ideal cultural commitments, and then linking a vision for change to the current and ideal cultures. Subsequently, cultural knowledge can be used to inform change initiatives and strategies. Existing norms, values, and strengths might be reinforced or built upon to move the organization toward the espoused ideals. New rituals or behaviors can be introduced, and these can contribute to a cultural shift. Tacit elements of a culture can accelerate or slow a planned change, and support or resistance to a change can be related to these, or to cultural elements that have not been taken into account. Cultural dynamics influence the outcome of the change initiative, either positively or negatively. In turn, the change process and its tangible outcomes have an effect on organizational culture.

These ideas are important to understand how culture, curriculum work, and faculty development as a change strategy can influence one another. Culture provides meaning and stability, and change jeopardizes the meaning people have about the school and the stability of their position within the culture. When a culture is at risk of change, shared learning helps a group to reduce anxiety and regain equilibrium (Schein, as cited in Owings & Kaplan, 2012).

Although a full cultural analysis is beyond the scope of those initiating or leading curriculum change, or planning and offering faculty development activities, there is merit in considering the cultural context of the school. Innovators might ask: *How might the current culture affect curriculum work and faculty development? What are the espoused and enacted norms, values, assumptions, beliefs, emotional climate, patterns of interaction, perceptions, political status, and social practices that could be built upon? What aspects of the culture might be changed or even eliminated by curriculum work and faculty development?*

Nature of Faculty Development for Change

Faculty development related to curriculum work is inherently development for change. Cognitive development and change are addressed through the acquisition of new knowledge and application of that knowledge. Practice in new behaviors, such as teaching strategies, reflects a commitment to, and support of, behavioral change. Peer support and group learning, an attitude of "we're all in this together," are indicative of attention to the psychological dimension of change.

Yet, the psychological dimension may need additional consideration. A curriculum change represents a change in the psychological contract an individual perceives to exist with the school of nursing, that is, the implicit agreements and beliefs held about the employment relationship. These include perceptions about the mutual obligations, values, expectations, and aspirations that exist outside the formal employment contract (Argyris, as cited in Owings & Kaplan, 2012). Change requires adjustments to individuals' mental maps of what should be. For some, renegotiation of the psychological contract is accepted as being a normal part of academic life; for others, there can be varying degrees of uncertainty and stress, particularly if they believe that the current curriculum and their role in it will be stable.

Therefore, faculty development activities should include attention to change processes (Fiedler, 2010) occurring in the school and acknowledgment of the feelings that change can engender. Clearly, the purpose is not to engage in psychotherapy, but rather to ensure that participants understand change, to make evident the human dimension of change, and to collaboratively plan how to offer support to one another when necessary. Additionally, by explicitly reviewing change processes, faculty and other curriculum developers acquire a means to recognize, label, and accept as normal the processes and reactions associated with change.

Activities to support faculty during curriculum work and change are suggested in **Table 2-2**. The Transtheoretical Model of Behavior change is used as the organizing framework for the table, because individuals must change and grow for real change to occur in curriculum. However, ideas are also drawn from the Diffusion of Innovations Theory (Rogers, 2003) and the OC^3 Model (Latta, 2009).

Table 2-2 Activities to Support Faculty and Curriculum Change Organized According to Stages of the Transtheoretical Model of Behavior Change	
Participants' Stage of Change	**Activities to Support Change**
Precontemplation: no intention to change	• Engage faculty in discussion about the possibility of curriculum change • Stimulate faculty discussion about frustrations and disappointments experienced within the current curriculum
Contemplation: serious consideration of a curriculum change within a specified time	• Review school and university mission and goals and discuss how strongly the current curriculum supports them • Engage faculty in consideration of the benefits of curriculum change • Share ideas about the effects of avoiding curriculum change on students, graduates, school of nursing, and educational institution • Initiate deliberations among faculty and the school leader about the possibility of removing barriers to faculty involvement in curriculum development • Encourage early adopters to share their enthusiasm
Preparation: a commitment to change the curriculum	• Engage in discussion about faculty values related to nursing education and nursing practice • Obtain group agreement to proceed with curriculum development • Identify initial faculty development needs and initiate faculty development related to curriculum development • Ensure resources to support curriculum work • Identify a curriculum leader • Organize for curriculum development • Develop a vision • Offer faculty development related to change • Provide faculty development related to the preliminary work of curriculum development

Table 2-2 Activities to Support Faculty and Curriculum Change Organized According to Stages of the Transtheoretical Model of Behavior Change (*continued*)

Participants' Stage of Change	Activities to Support Change
Action: active engagement in curriculum work and faculty development	• Provide formal and informal faculty development related to the processes of curriculum work • Plan for ongoing support and encouragement • Engage in group learning • Trial ideas from the developing curriculum in the current curriculum if possible • Provide rewards for involvement in faculty and curriculum development activities (e.g., public acknowledgment and praise, credit toward promotion and tenure) • Create rituals to acknowledge achievement of major milestones in curriculum work • Use new terminology • Disseminate information about the redesigned curriculum • Welcome late majority members and laggards
Maintenance: sustained curriculum engagement and adherence to curriculum tenets	• Publicize successes • Plan faculty development activities for aspects of curriculum implementation that are problematic • Focus on shared problem solving • Share stories about the progress achieved and new perceptions of the curriculum and the school • Identify new values and beliefs

Source: Some data from Prochaska, J. O., & Velicer, W. F. (1997). The transtheoretical model of health behavior change. *American Journal of Health Promotion*, *12*(1), 38–48; Norcross, J. C., Krebs, P. M., & Prochaska, J. O. (2010). Stages of change. *Journal of Clinical Psychology*, *67*, 143–154.

Responding to Resistance to Change

Even though members of a school of nursing collaboratively agree to proceed with curriculum development, some may be resistant to the need for curriculum redesign or faculty development. "Because change disrupts the homeostasis or balance of the group, resistance should always be expected" (Marquis & Huston, 2012, p. 169), and this may be particularly evident in academic environments where faculty members have a great deal of autonomy in their work and construct their own mini-cultures that: (1) encompass their research, teaching, and service obligations; and (2) constitute their psychological contract with the school. Curriculum change could represent a significant intrusion into these personal academic worlds.

Those who feel their academic homeostasis is being unduly disrupted may become laggards and rejecters, as described by Rogers (2003). They have the potential to undermine the momentum of the majority. This cannot be ignored. Every effort should be extended to help these resisters feel that their contributions are needed and valued, and to counteract the negativity that they might project. There is a diplomatic balance to be achieved between sensitivity to individual readiness for change and the requirement to progress with curriculum work and faculty development.

Forms of Resistance

Overt resistance is easy to identify. Some examples are:

- Openly criticizing curriculum change and faculty development activities
- Refusing to acknowledge shortcomings of the present curriculum or need for faculty development
- Predicting dire consequences of curriculum change
- Refusing to participate in curriculum and faculty development
- Actively seeking support from colleagues to stop curriculum redesign

Covert resistance can be passive, and acts of passive resistance may initially be excused. The behavior is recognized as resistance once a pattern becomes evident. Although opposed to participation in curriculum or faculty development, the passive resister does not openly state disagreement. Behavior typical of passive resistance can be:

- Lateness for or absence from meetings
- Failure to meet commitments to complete work
- Mental absence in spite of physical presence during curriculum work or faculty development
- Attempts to divert attention from the meeting purpose to trivial, peripheral, or historical matters

Covert resistance may also be passive-aggressive, and this form of resistance is sabotage. The resister may appear to support curriculum work and faculty development and is likely to be physically present but mentally uninvolved at these activities. Apparent endorsement is coupled with behind-the-scenes attempts to undermine the proposed curriculum, faculty development plans, and/or those participating in curriculum and faculty development.

Responding to Resistance

There are many possible sources of resistance to curriculum change, and although colleagues may attribute particular motivations to those opposing it, the precise reasons might never be revealed. However, it is not necessary to know the underlying rationale before confronting the unacceptable behavior. Ignoring the resistance gives license for it to continue and implicitly conveys the idea that the resister has more power than the collective will of the faculty group.

Resistance should be confronted as soon as it is recognized. The goal of supporters of curriculum redesign, the curriculum leader, or school leader is to have the resister agree to replace the unacceptable behavior with actions that are supportive of the group's efforts, or, at the absolute minimum, not undermining of the group's work and plans.

If group pressure does not lead to a modification of the resister's behavior, it will likely be necessary for the school leader to intervene. Possible strategies to respond to individual and group resistance have been proposed by a number of authors (Owings & Kaplan, 2012; Patterson, Grenny, Maxfield, McMillan, & Switzler, 2008; Patterson, Grenny, McMillan, & Switzler, 2005; Raza & Standing, 2011). All strategies should be implemented with respect, in private, and in a manner that allows the resister to feel safe and heard. The school leader might employ some or all of these measures:

- Describe the gap between the expected behavior and the observed behavior, without attributing motivation.
- Seek to understand the resister's perspectives.
- Explain the invisible consequences of the present behavior, such as diminished respect from colleagues or damage to the school's reputation.
- Be explicit and unambiguous about obligations and expectations.
- Link the desired behavior to shared values.
- Identify skills that the individual could provide during curriculum work.
- Explain the benefits of a behavior change (e.g., renewed respect, acceptance).
- Obtain a commitment to behave differently.
- Agree on an action plan and follow up to promote accountability.

The focus of the discussion is the person's behavior, not the curriculum change or the reasons for it.

Particularly troubling are reports of a faculty member's public criticism of curriculum change, faculty members, and/or faculty development. The school leader should be precise, objective, and unemotional in describing the reports and their effects on colleagues, professional practice partners, students, and the image of the school. The goal of the interaction is to obtain the resister's agreement to refrain from further public criticism. Some reasons for resistance to curriculum redesign, change, and faculty development, and possible responses, are presented in **Table 2-3**.

Table 2-3   Possible Responses to Reasons for Resistance to Change, Curriculum Redesign, and Faculty Development

Reasons for Resistance to Faculty Development and Curriculum Change	Possible Responses of Administrator, Curriculum Leader, and/or Faculty Majority
Belief in value of current curriculum and way of being	• Explore which aspects of curriculum and role are valued and why. • Suggest that involvement in curriculum and faculty development is the best way to ensure continuation of what is valued. • Make evident how aspects of current curriculum might be taken into account in curriculum redesign.
Skepticism about quality of envisioned curriculum	• Explore concerns. • Be open to possibility that resister is correct. • Acknowledge that the resistor's input has assisted in the examination of the issue, along with others' views.
Interpretation of change as personal criticism	• Validate the progressive nature of current curriculum at the time it was developed. • Emphasize that redesigning the curriculum was a collaborative group decision. • Reiterate what will be gained by a changed curriculum. • Listen actively to resister's issues (e.g., losses, fears), and if possible attempt to lessen the frequency of verbalization of concerns. • Emphasize that the resister's strengths are needed for faculty and curriculum development activities. • Validate the resister's past contributions and express confidence in ability to be successful.
Belief in own curriculum development expertise; hence no need for faculty development	• Acknowledge experience and knowledge that resister has accumulated. • Propose that resister share expertise by leading some faculty development sessions. Assign as part of workload if possible. • State consequences of nonparticipation.

Table 2-3   Possible Responses to Reasons for Resistance to Change, Curriculum Redesign, and Faculty Development (*continued*)

Reasons for Resistance to Faculty Development and Curriculum Change	Possible Responses of Administrator, Curriculum Leader, and/or Faculty Majority
Fear of reduced status or not fitting into new curriculum	• Emphasize that all faculty are uncertain about their place in the changed curriculum, particularly in the early stages when the future curriculum is undefined. • Encourage participation in curriculum and faculty development as a means of ensuring that the resister will have a valued place in the future curriculum. • Stress that faculty development activities will prepare all faculty for the envisioned curriculum.
Fear that inadequate skills and knowledge will be revealed	• Relate anecdotes from school or personal history when faculty felt they could not succeed in changed circumstances yet did achieve. • Propose the idea that many faculty may wonder if they "have what it takes" to function in the future curriculum. • Ensure that school director attends faculty development activities to underscore that everyone has learning needs and to give importance to attendance.
Lack of confidence in colleagues' ability to develop acceptable curriculum	• Agree that not all faculty are equally experienced in nursing education, generally, and in curriculum development, particularly. • Underscore that the curriculum development process is inherently a form of faculty development, and therefore colleagues will enhance skills as the project unfolds. • Emphasize that formal and informal faculty development will occur concurrently with curriculum development, thereby expanding colleagues' skills and knowledge. • Indicate that curriculum development is an opportunity for the resister to share particular expertise in nursing education, thereby becoming a model for less experienced faculty.

(*continues*)

Table 2-3   Possible Responses to Reasons for Resistance to Change, Curriculum Redesign, and Faculty Development (*continued*)

Reasons for Resistance to Faculty Development and Curriculum Change	Possible Responses of Administrator, Curriculum Leader, and/or Faculty Majority
Lack of confidence in own ability to contribute meaningfully	• Emphasize that all faculty are uncertain about undertaking curriculum development. • Remind resister that ongoing faculty development is intended to ensure that all faculty will have access to pertinent perspectives and be able to contribute to curriculum work. • Relate the strengths that resister can bring to curriculum development.
Lack of interest or disinclination to expend effort required for change, curriculum redesign, and faculty development	• Explore reasons and remove barriers if possible. • Remind resister that curriculum and faculty development are shared responsibilities for all faculty. • Discuss how resister expects to be effective in future curriculum if not involved in its creation and in faculty development. • Employ all strategies to help resister feel that contributions are needed and valued. • Consider an alternate assignment in the school of nursing as a last resort.
Concern that faculty and curriculum development will interfere with research and publication and/or progress toward tenure	• Acknowledge that faculty and curriculum development require intensive effort. • Discuss scholarship potential of curriculum work. • Describe how curriculum work can contribute to promotion and tenure. • Consider the feasibility of some faculty "opting out" of curriculum development for short periods at critical points of research activity or career progress.
Heavy workload	• Examine how workload could be altered to include participation in curriculum and faculty development activities.
Misoneism (fear of newness, innovation, or change)	• Provide as much support as possible to enhance acceptance of change.
Unrevealed personal reasons	• Accept that no one can cause another to change. • Accept that it is not possible to respond constructively to what is unknown.

An Alternate Perspective

To lessen the stress often experienced when resistance is prolonged or unrelenting, it may be helpful for faculty members to reframe the situation to make the discord or dissent seem less personal. Viewing resistance as a conflict of values, beliefs, rights, and obligations could lead to changed understandings and reactions by all involved. Presented in **Table 2-4** are possible perspectives on conflict areas about the need for faculty

Table 2-4 Possible Perspectives on Conflict Areas About Need for Curriculum Development, Faculty Development, and Change		
	Possible Perspective on Conflict Areas	
Possible Conflict Areas	**Resister**	**Faculty Majority**
Values	• Stability • Experience • Personal values	• Change • Personal growth • Shared values
Beliefs	• Quality education = current curriculum, teaching, and evaluation methods • Personal value as a teacher and nurse is expressed in current curriculum • Curriculum and faculty development and change are a repudiation of current practices • Criticism	• Quality education = new curriculum, teaching, and evaluation methods • New curriculum will enhance growth as teachers and nurses • Curriculum and faculty development will expand knowledge and skills • Critique
Interpretation of the right of academic freedom	• Individual decision making about curriculum • Maintenance of present programs	• Collegial decision making and adherence to curriculum decisions made by total faculty group • Planning and implementation of a context-relevant, evidence-informed, unified curriculum
Obligations	• Adherence to current (correct) way of doing things • Preparation of graduates for existing nursing practice	• Openness to new ideas • Preparation of graduates for future nursing practice

and curriculum development. A different view and emotional distance could make the situation more tolerable and reduce the tendency to attribute malicious motives to a resister. Explicit use of conflict resolution strategies may be in order.

Faculty members are responsible for their own reactions and behaviors. Some might choose to reject curriculum redesign and faculty development, content to remain out of step with colleagues, despite efforts to support them through change. It is wise to remember that changing another person's behavior might not be achievable. However, it is possible, and it may be necessary to change one's own reaction so as not to be consumed with anxiety, anger, and the endless creation of appeasement tactics.

Although it is antithetical to nursing's concern with individuals' wellbeing and emotional comfort, it would be wise to stop giving attention to the views of persistent resisters. It is preferable to focus on the goals and tasks of curriculum work and prepare for a reconceptualized curriculum with motivated, growth-seeking colleagues.

CHAPTER SUMMARY

Faculty development is a core process of curriculum work, that is, curriculum development, implementation, and evaluation. Identifying learning needs and planning activities to enhance knowledge and skills as participants engage in curriculum work will maximize a successful change. Change theories help to explain the processes that individuals and groups can experience during all aspects of curriculum work. A wide spectrum of faculty development activities should be considered to support faculty and stakeholders during curriculum work and change, and the most suitable should be selected. However, it is realistic to acknowledge that not all faculty members will welcome change; some might be very comfortable with maintaining the status quo. Nonetheless, a faculty development program as it relates to curriculum work and change is essential for a successful outcome and should not be delayed.

SYNTHESIS ACTIVITIES

The Aristotle College of Nursing case is an example of how members of one school of nursing responded to the provision of faculty development related to curriculum work and change. The questions following the case should help readers apply ideas from the chapter. Then, questions for consideration are provided to assist readers' considerations about faculty development for curriculum work and change in their own situations.

Aristotle College of Nursing

Aristotle College of Nursing is located in a mid-sized university that was established in 1902. The College of Nursing began as a department in the College of Medicine in 1920 and became independent in 1950. Since then, the undergraduate nursing program has had many curricula, with changes every 10 years on average. The most recent change was 11 years ago. The 28 full-time, tenured faculty members are mainly middle- and late-career individuals, and all have been at Aristotle College for 10 years or more. Seven tenure-track faculty members have been at Aristotle for 1–4 years. Additionally, there are 12 part-time faculty members who teach undergraduate theory courses and 42 part-time faculty members who teach only in professional practice courses.

Faculty members, students, and stakeholders have agreed that it is time to update the curriculum so that it has stronger emphases on patient safety, responsiveness to diversity, international perspectives, and active learning. They remain committed to the philosophical bases of the existing curriculum and envision minor changes in the curriculum goals, replacement of some existing courses with new ones, and refinement of others. The group is calling this "curriculum renewal," and they expect to have the curriculum plans finalized within 3 months. They plan to introduce the alterations 12 months after that.

The undergraduate chair, Dr. Makena Adoyo, is leading the curriculum renewal. She suggests that faculty plan a daylong retreat to review curriculum development processes and begin work on revising the curriculum goals. There is mixed reaction to this suggestion, ranging from wholehearted endorsement to comments like "we're too busy," to remarks that curriculum renewal is unnecessary. The college dean endorses the plan and approximately half of the full-time faculty commit to attending. No part-time faculty agree to be present because of teaching commitments and/or the fact that they don't consider this meeting to be paid time. Stakeholders and student leaders were not invited.

Questions and Activities for Critical Analysis of the Aristotle College of Nursing Case

1. Are the goals for the faculty retreat appropriate? Feasible? What is the rationale for saying this?
2. Was it wise to proceed with a curriculum development day for only 50% of the full-time faculty, and no part-time faculty, stakeholders, or students? Why or why not?

3. How can Dr. Adoyo link the idea of faculty development and curriculum work in a meaningful way for those who do not agree to attend the faculty development day?

4. What responses might be appropriate for those faculty members resisting change?

5. Describe the advantages and disadvantages of a 1-day retreat.

6. Decide how much faculty development, and about what topics, might be necessary for this faculty group. Explain the decisions.

7. Will faculty development about change be necessary for this group? Justify the answer with reference to theory about change.

Questions and Activities for Consideration When Planning Faculty Development in Readers' Settings

1. Who could be the best champion for the faculty development process? How can faculty development proceed if there is no strong champion?

2. What might be the anticipated and unanticipated benefits and challenges associated with initiating faculty development activities?

3. Describe the faculty development activities that faculty currently accept or reject? Hypothesize about the reasons for this.

4. How can faculty be supported to view curriculum development as an engaging, necessary, and beneficial process?

5. Analyze the congruence between faculty development for curriculum work and change and the culture of the school?

6. Consider the activities proposed in Table 2-2. Which would be most constructive in helping faculty move smoothly through the transition from the current to the envisioned curriculum? Why? Propose other suitable activities.

7. What resources (human, physical, material, fiscal) can the school access to support faculty development initiatives during curriculum development?

8. Identify the key elements of a faculty development program to support faculty and curriculum development and change.

9. Use the theoretical perspectives on change in this chapter to plan faculty development activities. Are there ideas about assisting faculty during change or about the school culture that point to the use of another change theory or framework?

10. Design a preliminary faculty development program to support curriculum work.

REFERENCES

Åkerlind, G. S. (2005). Academic growth and development—How do university academics experience it? *Higher Education, 50*, 1–32.

American Association of Colleges of Nursing. (2012). *Nursing faculty shortage.* Retrieved from http://www.aacn.nche.edu/media-relations/fact-sheets/nursing-faculty-shortage

Bartels, J. E. (2007). Preparing nursing faculty for baccalaureate-level and graduate-level nursing programs: Role preparation for the academy. *Journal of Nursing Education, 46*, 154–158.

Benner, P., Sutphen, M., Leonard, V., & Day, L. (2010). *Educating nurses: A call for radical transformation.* San Francisco: Jossey-Bass/Carnegie Foundation for the Advancement of Nursing.

Bevis, E. O. (2000). Clusters of influence for practical decision making about curriculum. In E. O. Bevis & J. Watson (Eds.), *Toward a caring curriculum: A new pedagogy for nursing* (pp. 107–152). Sudbury, MA: Jones and Bartlett.

Brooks, C. F. (2011). Toward 'hybridised' faculty development for the twenty-first century: Blending online communities of practice and face-to-face meetings in instructional and professional support programmes. *Innovations in Education and Teaching International, 47*, 261–270.

Canadian Nurses Association & Canadian Association of Schools of Nursing. (2012). *Registered nurses education in Canada statistics 2009–10.* Retrieved from http://www.cna-aiic.ca/~/media/cna/page%20content/pdf%20en/2013/07/26/10/41/education_statistics_report_2009_2010_e.pdf

Dearmon, V., Lawson, R., & Hall, H. R. (2011). Concept mapping a baccalaureate nursing program: A method for success. *Journal of Nursing Education, 50*, 656–659.

Fiedler, S. (2010). Managing resistance in an organizational transformation: A case study from a mobile operator company. *International Journal of Project Management, 28*, 370–383.

Furco, A., & Moely, B. E. (2012). Using learning communities to build faculty support for pedagogical innovation: A multi-campus study. *Journal of Higher Education, 83*, 128–153.

Goldenberg, D., Andrusyszyn, M. A., & Iwasiw, C. (2004). A facilitative approach to learning about curriculum development. *Journal of Nursing Education, 43,* 31–35.

Greenhalgh, T., Robert, G., Bate, P., Macfarlane, R., & Kyriakidou, O. (2005). *Diffusion of innovations in health service organizations: A systematic literature review.* Oxford: BMJ Books/Blackwell.

Halliburton, D., Marincovich, M., & Svinicki, M. (1988). Strengthening professional development. *Journal of Higher Education, 59,* 291–304.

Haviland, D., Shin, S-H., & Turley, S. (2010). Now I'm ready: The impact of a professional development initiative on faculty concerns with program assessment. *Innovations in Higher Education, 35*, 261–275.

Heinrich, K. T., & Oberleitner, M. G. (2012). How a faculty group's peer mentoring of each other's scholarship can enhance retention and recruitment. *Journal of Professional Nursing, 28*, 5–12.

Holyoke, L. B., Sturko, P. A., Wood, N. B., & Wu, L. J. (2012). Are academic departments perceived as learning organizations? *Journal of Case Studies in Education, 2*, 1–20.

Huston, T., & Weaver, C. L. (2008). Peer coaching: Professional development for experienced faculty. *Innovations in Higher Education, 33*, 5–20.

Kenner, C., & Pressler, J. I. (2006). Successfully climbing the academic leadership ladder. *Nurse Educator, 31*(1), 1–3.

Kitchen, J., Parker, D. C., & Gallagher, T. (2008). Authentic conversation as faculty development: Establishing a self-study group in a faculty of education. *Studying Teaching Education, 4*, 157–171.

Latta, G. F. (2009). A process model of organizational change in cultural context (OC³ Model). *Journal of Leadership & Organizational Studies, 16*(1), 19–37.

Malinsky, L., DuBois, R., & Jacquest, D. (2010). Building scholarship capacity and transforming nurse educators' practice through institutional ethnography. *International Journal of Nursing Education Scholarship, 7*, Article 33.

Marquis, B. L., & Huston, C. J. (2012). *Leadership roles and management functions in nursing: Theory and application* (7th ed.). Philadelphia: Wolters Kluwer/Lippincott Williams & Wilkins.

Myers, C. R., Mixer, S. J., Wyatt, T. H., Paulus, T. M., & Lee, D. S. (2011). Making the move to blended learning: Reflections on a faculty development program. *International Journal of Nursing Education Scholarship, 8,* Article 20.

National League for Nursing. (2005). *The scope of practice of academic nurse educators.* New York: Author.

Norcross, J. C., Krebs, P. M., & Prochaska, J. O. (2010). Stages of change. *Journal of Clinical Psychology, 67,* 143–154.

Oliver, S. L., & Hyun, E. (2011). Comprehensive curriculum reform in higher education: Collaborative engagement of faculty and administrators. *Journal of Case Studies in Education, 2,* 1–20.

Owings, W. A., & Kaplan, L. S. (2012). *Leadership and organizational behavior in education: Theory into practice.* Boston: Pearson Education.

Patterson, K., Grenny, J., Maxfield, D., McMillan, R., & Switzler, A. (2008). *Influencer: The power to change anything.* New York: McGraw-Hill.

Patterson, K., Grenny, J., McMillan, R., & Switzler, A. (2005). *Crucial confrontations: Tools for resolving broken promises, violated expectations, and bad behavior.* New York: McGraw-Hill.

Prochaska, J. O., & Velicer, W. F. (1997). The transtheoretical model of health behavior change. *American Journal of Health Promotion, 12*(1), 38–48.

Raza, S. A., & Standing, C. (2011). A systemic model for managing and evaluating conflicts in organizational change. *Systems Practical Action Research, 24,* 187–210.

Rogers, E. M. (2003). *Diffusion of innovations* (5th ed.). New York: Free Press.

Rush, K., Ouellet, L., & Wasson, D. (1991). Faculty development: The essence of curriculum development. *Nurse Education Today, 11,* 121–126.

Smolen, D. (1996). Constraints that nursing program administrators encounter in promoting faculty change and development. *Journal of Professional Nursing, 12,* 91–98.

Suplee, P. D., & Gardner, M. (2009). Fostering a smooth transition to the faculty role. *Journal of Continuing Education in Nursing, 40,* 514–520.

Taylor, K. L. (2010). Understanding the disciplines within the context of educational development. *New Directions for Teaching and Learning, 122,* 59–67.

CHAPTER 3

Ongoing Appraisal in Curriculum Work

Chapter Overview

Ongoing appraisal is an inherent part of all curriculum work, from initiation of the idea of curriculum change, to evaluation of a fully implemented curriculum. This core process of curriculum work is a means of quality assurance. In this chapter, a definition of ongoing appraisal is presented, followed by descriptions of its purposes and processes, including the inherent cognitive processes. Criteria are offered for ongoing appraisal of curriculum work. Finally, attention is briefly given to the interpersonal aspects of ongoing appraisal. The chapter concludes with a summary, a case for analysis, and questions for readers to consider in their own settings.

Chapter Goals

- Understand *ongoing appraisal* as a core process in curriculum development, implementation, and evaluation.
- Appreciate the purposes of ongoing appraisal.
- Recognize the cognitive processes inherent in ongoing appraisal in curriculum work.
- Value the role of professional judgment in ongoing appraisal.
- Consider interpersonal aspects of ongoing appraisal.

DEFINITION OF ONGOING APPRAISAL

Ongoing appraisal is the deliberative, continuous, repeated, and careful critique of curriculum ideas, products, and processes during and after their creation, implementation, and evaluation. It involves constant analytical comparison between what is new and what has already been decided to identify areas of coherence and inconsistency.

This appraisal is dependent on:

- A commitment to the development, implementation, and evaluation of an evidence-informed, context-relevant, unified curriculum
- Knowledge of:
  - Curriculum development, implementation, and evaluation processes
  - The context in which the curriculum will be offered
  - The philosophical and educational approaches of the curriculum
  - The conceptual bases of the curriculum
  - Students for whom the curriculum is being developed
  - Decisions already made about the curriculum
- Professional judgment

Ongoing appraisal is a core process of curriculum work, although it is generally unlabelled and its purpose not explicated. It is part of a scholarly approach to all curriculum work, both while the work is in progress and after it is completed. It is important that this core process be an expected, explicit, and visible part of curriculum work.

PURPOSES OF ONGOING APPRAISAL

Ongoing appraisal is a quality assurance process in curriculum development, implementation, and evaluation and is the basis of the recursive nature of curriculum work. The purposes of ongoing appraisal are to ensure that:

- An evidence-informed, context-relevant, unified curriculum is developed.
- The curriculum is implemented and evaluated in a manner true to the curriculum intent.
- Decisions and processes inconsistent with the curriculum intent are identified early, and the necessary revisions are made.
- The curriculum work is of a suitable quality.

ONGOING APPRAISAL PROCESSES IN CURRICULUM WORK

As the term *ongoing* implies, the appraisal process is continuous during all curriculum work. It begins with an understanding of the context in which the curriculum will be offered and the curriculum decisions that have been made. Then, as curriculum development teams work together, individual members judge ideas that are proposed. The team discusses the ideas, examining and informally appraising them. The ongoing appraisal results in revisions and improvements during the creation of ideas. Once the team feels its task is completed, members review and appraise the completed work to ensure that it is consistent with prior curriculum decisions, the curriculum context, and so forth. This constant consideration and reconsideration of the work at hand is essential to achieve quality, but appraisal only by those who created the ideas may not be sufficient to achieve a feasible and unified curriculum.

Also needed is more formal review of completed work to ensure that it meets the desired criteria and standards. Although one curriculum development team may view its own work as appropriate, the work must be appraised in light of all other developing work to ensure that the concurrent work is consistent. Therefore, it is recommended that a mechanism for formal appraisal of the developing curriculum be in place. This appraisal could be conducted by members representing several development teams, or by a critique committee. Formal appraisal is essential to ensure that all aspects of the curriculum, singly and together, are unified and consistent with the curriculum intent. A depiction of the ongoing appraisal process is provided in **Figure 3-1**.

Figure 3-1   Ongoing appraisal
© C. L. Iwasiw

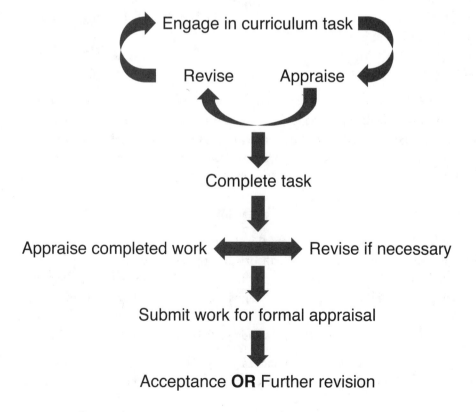

Similarly, ongoing appraisal is necessary during curriculum implementation. Ongoing appraisal is essential to ensure that the curriculum intent is reflected in the strategies to ignite learning and methods to evaluate student achievement. Also, student learning is continuously appraised. During curriculum evaluation, it is necessary to continually appraise whether the evaluation procedures are consistent with the curriculum philosophical approaches, and whether the procedures are providing necessary and important information upon which to judge the entire curriculum.

The process of ongoing appraisal might result in a rethinking or reaffirmation of past decisions, and possibly adjustments to past or newly completed work, whichever is not fully congruent with the curriculum intent. Importantly, intentional ongoing appraisal should lead to the development, implementation, and evaluation of an evidence-informed, context-relevant curriculum whose elements are conspicuously unified.

COGNITIVE PROCESSES INHERENT IN ONGOING APPRAISAL

Experienced nurse educators will recognize that the intellectual work of ongoing appraisal includes cognitive processes common in nursing education, research, and practice. A few of these interwoven and overlapping processes are briefly described, along with their application to curriculum work.

Critical Thinking

The consensus definition of the American Philosophical Association is that critical thinking is "purposeful, reflective judgment which manifests itself in reasoned consideration of evidence, context, methods, standards, and conceptualizations in deciding what to believe or what to do" (Facione, 2013). It is composed of a constellation of core cognitive skills: interpretation, analysis, inference, explanation, evaluation, and self-regulation (Facione, 2013).

Curriculum developers must constantly do the following:

- Interpret evidence, theories, and philosophical approaches.
- Consider and explain the evidence and theory underlying proposed ideas.
- Take into account the context in which the curriculum will be implemented, the philosophical bases of the curriculum, and the goals or outcomes they want students to achieve.
- Establish and review their methods and standards for the curriculum work itself.

In so doing, they interpret information and ideas, analyze the congruence with other curriculum decisions, predict the outcomes of their ideas, explain how new ideas fit into the developing curriculum and are consistent with its tenets, and evaluate the quality and merit of individual ideas and constellations of ideas. This all requires being alert to one's biases and assumptions, and being open to the ideas and reasoning of others.

Constant Comparison

Constant comparison is a process used in the analysis phase of grounded theory research. The procedure includes the constant comparison of new data to previously developed categories to assess whether the data fit or whether new data codes are necessary (Polit & Tatano Beck, 2012). In curriculum work, new ideas, decisions, products (i.e., written documents), and processes are constantly compared to previous decisions and completed work to ensure there is logical, conceptual, and philosophical unity.

Evaluation

Evaluation is a process of judging the quality or worth of something. It entails three steps. First, a standard is established. Then, data about the phenomenon of interest are assembled or observed and compared to the established standard. Finally, a judgment is made about whether the observed data represent an acceptable level.

Throughout curriculum work, ongoing appraisal is a form of evaluation. Curriculum developers repeatedly ask whether their ideas meet the explicated and unexplicated criteria and standards that they hold as individuals and as a group. When implementing the curriculum, faculty members, students, and external stakeholders constantly make judgments about the quality of teaching and learning. Similarly, as formal evaluation of the curriculum is planned and undertaken, the evaluation planners continually judge their efforts against a standard: *Will the evaluation procedures tell us what we need to know about the curriculum?* Finally, when the evaluation data are available, the total curriculum is judged.

Reflection

Reflection-in-action is a "reflective conversation with the situation" (Schön, 1983, p. 76), a process in which every action becomes a local experiment and the responses to the action become the impetus for further development, reframing of the situation, or deeper analysis. Reflection-in-action includes elements of intuitive knowing and artistry. Reflection-on-action, in contrast, is a retrospective examination of a situation (Schön, 1983). Mezirow (1991) furthered these ideas by identifying that it is possible to reflect on *content* (perceptions, thoughts, feelings, or actions), *process* (how we perceive, think, act, or feel), and *premises* (why we perceive, think, act, or feel as we do).

Curriculum development requires constant individual and collective reflection-in-action and reflection-on-action. As curriculum developers propose and accept ideas, they constantly appraise and revise them in response to group discussion and assessment of the ideas' congruence with the curriculum intent and their own standards. Similarly, during curriculum implementation, faculty monitor responses to the teaching-learning situation and modify their teaching as necessary on the spot. Their subsequent reflection on action results in course refinements. During curriculum evaluation, the procedures are monitored to ensure that pertinent information is being obtained. Throughout the curriculum development, implementation, and evaluation processes, decisions and actions are reviewed concurrently and retrospectively with a view to improving the ideas and processes. In this ongoing appraisal, the questions asked and the comments offered are representative of reflection on content, process, and premises.

Professional Judgment

Professional judgment is "the ability to make considered decisions or come to sensible conclusions" (Stevenson, 2010). According to Murphy (2006), people have different perspectives on the information available when making a judgment, some attending mainly to the *range* (time orientation from historical to future), some to the *scope* (breadth), and others to the *depth* of information. The point of view influences the conclusions that are reached.

In curriculum work, the quality of the judgments reached is improved by curriculum development teams whose members have different perspectival emphases. For example, those with an historical perspective will know what has worked in the past. Members with a future orientation will see the possible consequences of ideas and what nursing practice and education could and should be. Those with a broad scope might integrate knowledge of curriculum development, students' characteristics, and nursing practice. Participants who focus on depth of knowledge can add important information unknown to the others. Therefore, when completed work is being judged, interactive critical reflection and team consensus are likely to be more useful than the professional judgment of any one individual. In addition, a curriculum team's professional judgment, based on a variety of perspectives, is more likely to be acceptable to a larger group than the views of one person alone.

Although much information is gathered in advance of creating and implementing a curriculum, there is no absolute formula for interpreting and prioritizing the data, and then transforming it into a nursing curriculum. The data and ideas that arise are concurrently:

- Interpreted
- Considered within contextual realities of the school, educational institution, and community
- Combined with curriculum development teams' imagination and artistry

- Viewed in relation to curriculum tenets
- Examined in light of team members' experience and expertise

Ultimately, each curriculum represents the best consensual professional judgment of those who developed it. Their sensible conclusions become the nursing curriculum.

CRITERIA FOR ONGOING APPRAISAL IN CURRICULUM WORK

Curriculum developers, implementers, and evaluators determine the criteria and standards for the curriculum work, and this can include acceptance of externally imposed standards. They create processes and products, and monitor the quality of the work. The processes, products, and quality all require discussion when the group is organizing for curriculum development.

In all curriculum work, five major criteria to ensure a quality curriculum and against which curriculum work is appraised are:

- Relevance for the context in which it will be implemented
- Consistency with current evidence about nursing practice, nursing education, and learning
- Congruence with the curriculum intent
- Logical progression
- Unity

The sections that follow provide some questions that reflect ongoing appraisal during curriculum work.

Curriculum Development

While engaging in deliberative ongoing appraisal during curriculum development, faculty and stakeholders repeatedly ask themselves such questions as:

- Is this work consistent with the philosophical approaches?
- Do these ideas fit the context?
- Is our language reflective of the curriculum's philosophical approaches and major concepts?
- What is the evidence, rationale, or theoretical base for deciding this?
- How well does this work align with previous decisions and completed work?
- Will these plans give opportunity for students to achieve the stated goals or outcomes?
- How can ideas or processes be improved to be more consistent with the curriculum intent?

- Is this curriculum work of the quality that we expect of ourselves?
- Is this curriculum work of the quality that will likely be acceptable to external reviewers?

Curriculum Implementation

During curriculum implementation, some questions faculty, students, and professional practice partners might ask are:

- What are the premises that underlie decisions about teaching-learning events?
- Are the strategies to ignite learning consistent with the agreed-upon philosophical and educational approaches?
- Are strategies to evaluate student learning consistent with the philosophical and educational approaches?
- Are the methods suitable for the context?
- Is the language reflective of the curriculum's philosophical approaches and major concepts?
- How well do students understand the main ideas of the curriculum?
- How well do course processes provide opportunities for students to achieve the stated goals or competencies?
- Are the expectations of students reasonable?
- How can ideas or processes be improved to be more consistent with the curriculum intent?

Curriculum Evaluation

During curriculum evaluation, appraisal questions about the evaluation process might include:

- Are the curriculum evaluation strategies consistent with the philosophical approaches?
- Are the evaluation strategies providing information that will be useful in making a judgment about the curriculum?
- Are all relevant stakeholders involved?
- How can the curriculum evaluation strategies be improved?

INTERPERSONAL ASPECTS OF ONGOING APPRAISAL

Ongoing appraisal is a deliberative, continuous, repeated, and careful critiquing of ideas throughout curriculum development, implementation, and evaluation, and this constant critique is part of a scholarly approach to curriculum development. The ongoing creation, critique, and refinement of ideas during curriculum work can be intellectually stimulating for team members. Indeed, the work relationships themselves "can be a generative source of enrichment, vitality, and learning that helps individuals, groups, and organizations grow, thrive, and flourish" (Ragins & Dutton, 2006, p. 3).

However, not all curriculum teams are sources of mutual support and enrichment, and even in such groups, ideas that are proposed must be handled with care. Curriculum ideas do not present themselves in the middle of a table, fully formed, and unconnected to individuals. They originate with people who may have a large emotional investment in the ideas they offer. Therefore, appraisal, no matter how strongly it is grounded in the curriculum tenets, may not be perceived as objective or constructive. It may be viewed as personal criticism or an attack of a highly-valued viewpoint.

Verbal appraisal of ideas requires attention to the sensitivities of the originator and to careful use of language. Important is a collective attitude of, *How can we make it align more closely with the curriculum tenets?* or, *How can we make it better?* As in all other academic work, there will be divergence of views, and groups must manage these to reach a consensus that will lead to the best curriculum possible, while preserving and possibly enhancing relationships within the groups.

When a team has submitted its work for formal appraisal, team members' self-esteem is at stake. The formal appraisal can be perceived as a *pass or fail situation*. If the curriculum team is asked to revise its work substantially, members may believe they have failed in the eyes of their colleagues. If the work is deemed acceptable with minor changes or no changes, they may believe the team has passed. In all circumstances of informal and formal ongoing appraisal, it is vital that members treat each person and their suggestions with care and respect, so that everyone feels valued for their ideas and efforts, and remains committed to the curriculum work.

CHAPTER SUMMARY

Ongoing appraisal is the deliberative, repeated, and careful critique of curriculum ideas, products, and processes during and after their creation and implementation. It is a core process of all curriculum work, contributes to the scholarliness of the endeavor, and is a form of quality assurance. Ongoing appraisal incorporates processes such as critical thinking, constant comparison, evaluation, reflection, and professional judgment. The appraisal requires careful attention to curriculum team members' self-esteem. In curriculum work, ongoing appraisal occurs continuously within curriculum teams and more formally when each portion of curriculum work is completed. A formal appraisal contributes to the unity of the curriculum. Ultimately, the conclusions reached by the curriculum development teams become the curriculum.

SYNTHESIS ACTIVITIES

The Shakespeare University College of Nursing case is presented to illustrate the main ideas about ongoing appraisal in curriculum work. It is followed by questions to guide a critical analysis of the case. Then, questions are offered that might assist readers when considering how to incorporate ongoing appraisal into curriculum work.

Shakespeare University College of Nursing

Shakespeare University has a 40-year history of providing nursing education. Initially, it offered certificate programs in public health and nursing administration. Current programs include a baccalaureate program for registered nurses, an upper-division baccalaureate program, an 18-month accelerated program for students with prior degrees, and a nurse practitioner program.

Following considerable discussion, the faculty members have agreed that they should offer a 4-year integrated baccalaureate program to replace the upper-division baccalaureate program. Although it took considerable lobbying within the university, the College of Nursing did receive permission to introduce a 4-year program.

Faculty members, students, and stakeholders of the Shakespeare University College of Nursing have been working on curriculum development. They are excited about the prospect of this approach to nurse preparation and most recognize the potential for students' stronger acculturation into professional nursing. Following agreement about the philosophical and educational approaches, curriculum outcomes, and overall design, course development teams were formed.

There are two nursing courses in the first semester of the program, *Nursing and Society* and *Communication Skills for Nursing Practice*. In the second semester, there are three nursing courses. *Introduction to Nursing Practice* will give students opportunities to learn about assessment throughout the lifespan. In the course, *Nursing of Developing Families: Theoretical Perspectives*, students will learn about family theory and nursing care of young families. The third course is *Nursing Interventions with Developing Families*. In this course, students will visit young families to complete growth and development assessments, practice communication skills, and identify the health-promoting activities of young families.

Dr. Sophia Alexiou, Dr. Abraham Danziger, and Dr. Jill Summers are either leaders or members of the course development teams as described in **Table 3-1**. All are experienced nurse educators who have participated in curriculum development

		PROFESSORS	
COURSES	**Dr. Alexiou**	**Dr. Danziger**	**Dr. Summers**
Nursing and Society	Leader		Member
Communication Skills for Nursing Practice		Member	Leader
Introduction to Nursing Practice	Leader		Member
Nursing of Developing Families: Theoretical Perspectives	Member	Leader	
Nursing Interventions with Developing Families		Leader	Member

Table 3-1 Involvement in Course Development

in the past. Other faculty, students, and clinicians are also part of the development teams. Each team has three to five members. Only Drs. Alexiou, Danziger, and Summers are working on more than one course in the first year of the program. They each believe they have a firm understanding of the curriculum intent, prior decisions, context, and standards. Accordingly, they interpret these to other team members who have not been actively involved in the planning. Concurrently, course development for second-year courses is beginning with different development teams.

James Blackenstock, a faculty member on the course development team for *Nursing and Society*, suggests that there be regular meetings among the course leaders and one additional member of each course team (making a group of eight). The purpose of the meetings would be to review the work completed by each team to ensure that ideas about the courses are complementary and consistent with the curriculum intent. He believes this is important while the courses are being developed and that a final review is necessary once the course development is completed. Moreover, he suggests it would be prudent to meet with those developing the second-year courses so there is continuity in the curriculum.

Dr. Alexiou allows that this idea might be good *in theory* but asserts that this is unnecessary because she and the other course leaders are experienced curriculum developers, talk frequently, and know what should be in the courses. She also says that additional meetings are out of the question because everyone is too busy.

Questions and Activities for Critical Analysis of the Shakespeare University College of Nursing Case

1. What could be the value of James Blackenstock's suggestion for the curriculum and for the course developers?
2. Determine how the development team might be influenced by Dr. Alexiou's statement that the course leaders know what should be in the courses.
3. How might the course development teams be affected by the fact that some members have not been involved in previous decision making about the curriculum?
4. Describe how ongoing appraisal may be built into the course development procedures even if there are no formal meetings to review the work of all teams.
5. What insights can be gained from Dr. Alexiou's and James Blackenstock's views of formal, ongoing evaluation?

Questions and Activities for Consideration When Planning Ongoing Appraisal in Readers' Settings

1. How can ongoing appraisal be explained as a core process of curriculum work?
2. What rationale can be offered about the value of ongoing appraisal?
3. In what ways can deliberative ongoing appraisal be built into curriculum work?
4. Propose processes to ensure that all members feel free to contribute to interactive, ongoing appraisal.
5. Suggest a feasible process to develop explicit standards against which to judge the curriculum work.
6. Who could or should be involved in ongoing appraisal of curriculum work?
7. At what points of the curriculum development processes should formal ongoing appraisal occur?
8. How can the curriculum leader ensure that ongoing appraisal is a core process of curriculum work and that it contributes to quality assurance of the nursing curriculum?

REFERENCES

Facione, P. A. (2013). *Critical thinking: What it is and why it counts*. Retrieved from http://www
.insightassessment.com/pdf_files/what%20and%20why%202007.pdf
Mezirow, J. (1991). *Transformative dimensions of adult learning*. San Francisco: Jossey-Bass.

Murphy, T. P. (2006). Judgment: The foundation of professional success. *Consulting Psychology Journal: Practice and Research, 58,* 185–194.

Polit, D. F., & Tatano Beck, C. (2012). *Nursing research: Generating and assessing evidence for nursing practice* (9th ed.). Philadelphia: Wolters Kluwer/Lippincott Williams & Wilkins.

Ragins, B. R., & Dutton, J. E. (2006). Positive relationships at work: An introduction and invitation. In J. E. Dutton & B. R. Ragins (Eds.), *Exploring positive relationships at work: Building a theoretical and research foundation* (pp. 3–25). New York: Lawrence Erlbaum Associates, Taylor & Francis Group.

Schön, D. A. (1983). *The reflective practitioner: How professionals think in action.* New York: Basic Books.

Stevenson, A. (Ed.). (2010). Professional judgement. *Oxford Dictionary of English* (3rd ed.). Retrieved from http://www.oxfordreference.com/view/10.1093/acref/9780199571123.001.0001/m_en_gb0433600?rskey=rdf9E7&result=2&q=

CHAPTER 4

Scholarship in Curriculum Work

Chapter Overview

Scholarly work is an expectation in schools of nursing and the essential foundation of an evidence-informed, context-relevant, unified curriculum. In curriculum work, *scholarliness* is the careful appraisal and use of relevant theory and data. This is the basis of scholarship, the advancement of knowledge. Scholarship is a central activity of academia and curriculum work, which is a central activity of schools of nursing. Therefore, scholarship and curriculum work are logically and inextricably linked, and scholarship must be a core process of all curriculum work. Scholarship related to curriculum work is foundational to expanding the evidence base for nursing education practice.

This chapter begins with descriptions of *scholarliness* and *scholarship* in curriculum work. Examples of curriculum scholarship projects, based on Boyer's (1990, 1995) conceptualizations of five types of scholarship are offered. Then, ideas relevant to moving from curriculum work to scholarship, including thinking and acting like a scholar, practical matters, and authorship, are presented. Synthesis activities conclude the chapter.

Chapter Goals

- Differentiate between *scholarliness* and *scholarship* in curriculum development, implementation, and evaluation.
- Understand scholarship as a core curriculum process.
- Identify practical issues in scholarship related to curriculum work.
- Consider authorship of scholarship projects based on collaborative curriculum work.

SCHOLARLINESS IN CURRICULUM WORK

All aspects of curriculum work (i.e., development, implementation, and evaluation) require a scholarly approach. *Scholarliness* is the careful appraisal and use of relevant theory and data in curriculum work. It requires faculty to be immersed in the literature and be knowledgeable about current trends, priorities, and evidence in the following:

* Curriculum development, implementation, and evaluation
* Higher education, generally
* Nursing education, specifically
* Nursing practice
* Health and health care
* Societal and political trends

The quality of the curriculum will depend on the depth and breadth of curriculum developers' knowledge and understanding about these matters. Thoughtful appraisal and professional judgment are applied as curriculum developers use their knowledge in a deliberative fashion to create, implement, and evaluate a curriculum. In other words, scholarliness in curriculum work is careful intellectual work. It involves assessing and applying the evidence base for nursing curriculum, contextualizing the evidence for a school of nursing and its environment, and ensuring that the curriculum is conceptually unified. The result is an evidence-informed, context-relevant, unified curriculum.

SCHOLARSHIP IN CURRICULUM WORK

Scholarship in Academia

Scholarship is the purposeful and methodical creation of knowledge, organization of the knowledge in a way that is meaningful to others, and distribution of the knowledge for peer review and critique (Iwasiw, 2013). Glassick, Taylor Huber, and Maeroff (1997) have identified six standards of quality in scholarship: clear goals, adequate preparation, appropriate methods, significant results, effective presentation, and reflective critique.

Scholarship is a central activity of academia and has traditionally been understood as research. However, Ernest L. Boyer (1990, 1995) proposed an expanded view of scholarship as being composed of five interrelated components: the scholarships of discovery, integration, application, teaching, and engagement. The *scholarship of teaching* was later described as the *scholarship of teaching and learning* (Hutchings & Shulman, cited in Hutchings, Taylor Huber, & Ciccone, 2011). The five types of scholarship are:

- Scholarship of discovery: generation of new knowledge
- Scholarship of integration: "making connections across the discipline, . . . illuminating data in a revealing way" (Boyer, 1990, p. 18); "interpretation, fitting . . . research into larger patterns" (p. 19)
- Scholarship of application: use of new or specialized knowledge to solve problems (Boyer, 1990)
- Scholarship of teaching and learning: creation of "bridges between the teacher's understanding and the student's learning" (Boyer, 1990, p. 23); "transforming and extending" (p. 24) knowledge of the discipline and "ideas about teaching the field" (Hutchings & Shulman, cited in Hutchings et al., 2011, p. 2)
- Scholarship of engagement: creation of connections between the university and significant social, civic, and ethical problems; this requires continuous communication between academic and civic communities to enrich the quality of life of all (Boyer, 1995)

The goal of scholarship is to advance knowledge through rigorous and systematic inquiry, replication of previous work, and/or creation of new ideas. Scholars study a topic or problem, and/or create new conceptualizations, explanations, theories, models, or processes. Then, the work is disseminated and its quality examined by knowledgeable peers who critique the scholarship products. For peer review and critique to occur, dissemination must be in a public forum, typically conference presentations and published articles. In essence, then, scholarship in academia is the creation of knowledge, organization of the knowledge, and distribution of the knowledge for others to review. It is dissemination and peer critique that elevate local scholarly activities to public academic scholarship.

Scholarship in Curriculum Work

Scholarship in curriculum work is the planned development and dissemination of knowledge about curriculum development, implementation, and evaluation. It is dependent on, but extends beyond, scholarliness. Because curriculum development, implementation, and evaluation are essential and pervasive activities in academic nursing, it is logical to view scholarship as a core process of all curriculum endeavors.

Scholarship is the basis of evidence-based nursing education practice, which Emerson and Records (2008) identify to be "today's challenge and tomorrow's excellence" (p. 359). Scholarship is the means through which a knowledge base will be developed "that could guide nurse educators to develop high quality, relevant, and cost-effective models of education that produce graduates who can make a difference in the health system" (Broome, 2009). It is the foundation that will shape the direction for change (Chinn, 2011) in nursing education.

Further to these ideas, we posit that evidence-informed nursing education practice is built on scholarship and knowledgeable judgment about all aspects of curriculum development, implementation, and evaluation. This includes processes, participants, products, contexts, and outcomes. This scholarship is foundational to developing and extending the evidence base for nursing education practice (Iwasiw, Goldenberg, & Andrusyszyn, 2005).

Research about pedagogical practices and learning is a form of curriculum scholarship that may be seen as the only research necessary to achieve evidence-based nursing education. However, beyond pedagogy, Emerson and Records (2008) view teaching as including "curricular development, student advisement, creation of learning environments, and administrative activities that influence teaching and learning" (p. 361), and these require study. Tanner (2010) proposes a need for research into the effectiveness of the multiple pathways to nursing licensure and the curricular structures suitable for students in accelerated programs. Additionally, Tanner, Bellack, and Harker (2009) have identified a number of areas requiring attention through scholarship: faculty retention and development, evaluation of educational innovations and reform, effective approaches for today's students, and education that aligns with healthcare reforms and social justice. These examples are illustrations of research that encompasses all phases of curricular development, implementation, and evaluation, as well as the categories of Boyer's (1990, 1995) typology of scholarship.

To achieve excellence in nursing education practice, nursing faculty must give attention to the scholarships of discovery, integration, application, teaching and learning, and engagement as part of all curriculum work. The overlapping nature of Boyer's five types of scholarship means that one project might fulfill the description of more than one type of scholarship. For example, a study of students' experiences in curriculum development is easily identified as the scholarship of teaching and learning. It might also represent the scholarship of discovery.

"Multiparadigmatic, multimethod, multipedagogical research is necessary for building the science of nursing education" (Young, 2008, p. 94), and this is possible within the full spectrum of curriculum work. Each school should identify the paradigms and methods most aligned with the philosophical approaches of its curriculum, and its members can then plan scholarship projects accordingly. Further, the National League for Nursing (n.d.) has called for multi-site studies, a missing feature of most nursing education research, but something that is feasible among schools using similar curriculum models, philosophical approaches, educational approaches, and evaluation methods.

A listing of the five types of scholarship elucidated by Boyer (1990, 1995) is presented in **Table 4-1**, along with ideas about their application to curriculum work. The examples in

Table 4-1   Scholarship Definitions and Their Application to Curriculum Work

Scholarship Definitions	Application to Curriculum Work	Examples of Scholarship Projects
Scholarship of discovery: generation of new knowledge (Boyer, 1990)	Inquiry into curriculum, development, implementation, and evaluation processes	Faculty and stakeholders' responses to curriculum development processes
Scholarship of integration: "making connections across the discipline; . . . illuminating data in a revealing way" (Boyer, 1990, p. 18); "interpretation, fitting . . . research into larger patterns" (p. 19)	Development of interprofessional courses with members of other health science disciplines	Outcomes and meaning of interprofessional practice placements for students in nursing, medicine, and physical therapy
Scholarship of application: use of new or specialized knowledge to solve problems (Boyer, 1990)	Adoption and integration of theories or concepts into the curriculum to address particular issues related to student learning or issues within nursing practice	Analysis of factors facilitating students' learning in particular professional placements and the relationship of the factors to learning and organizational theories
Scholarship of teaching and learning: creation of "bridges between the teacher's understanding and the student's learning" (Boyer, 1990, p. 23); "transforming and extending" (p. 24) knowledge	Development, implementation, and testing of teaching strategies consistent with the philosophical approaches and goals of the curriculum	Faculty members' knowledge of, and self-efficacy for, teaching practices consistent with the curriculum
Scholarship of engagement: creation of connections between the university and significant social, civic, and ethical problems; this requires continuous communication between academic and civic communities to enrich the quality of life of all (Boyer, 1995)	Active participation of professional and community partners, students, and consumers to create an evidence-informed, context-relevant curriculum that addresses the professional and health needs of society	Critical analysis of facilitators of stakeholders' involvement in nursing curriculum development, implementation, and/or evaluation

Source: Some data from Boyer, E. L. (1990). *Scholarship reconsidered: Priorities of the professoriate*. Princeton, NJ: The Carnegie Foundation for the Advancement of Teaching; Boyer, E. L. (1995). The scholarship of engagement. *Bulletin of the American Academy of Arts and Sciences*, *49*(7), 18–33.

the table represent different paradigms and methods. Some examples might fit the description of more than one type of scholarship because the categories are not mutually exclusive. One example only is given for each scholarship category.

Faculty members' responsibilities associated with curriculum extend beyond its development, implementation, and evaluation. There is a responsibility to advance and disseminate knowledge about curriculum processes, participants, products, contexts, and outcomes. "Being a nurse academic and scholar is a privileged position which brings with it special obligations to ensure the responsible development, dissemination and application of new knowledge in the field of nursing" (Johnstone, 2012, p. 113), and this obligation extends to all aspects of curriculum work in schools of nursing.

FROM CURRICULUM WORK TO SCHOLARSHIP

Thinking and Acting Like a Scholar

To move beyond the scholarly work of curriculum development, implementation, and evaluation to scholarship requires nursing faculty individually and collectively to, first and foremost, think like scholars. A nursing scholar is someone who:

- Is dedicated to knowledge development and dissemination
- Views self as having a personal and ongoing obligation to advance knowledge
- Is steeped in the literature
- Questions constantly
- "Maintain(s) an interactive connection between theory and practice" (Robert & Pape, 2011, p. 41)
- Thinks strategically about scholarship when undertaking curriculum development, implementation, and evaluation.

Thinking like a scholar requires extensive and critical reading of the literature, careful observation and analysis of nursing education practice, and constant questioning about what is known and not known. The questions that arise from this approach spark ideas for scholarship projects and are relevant to all aspects of curriculum work.

What do we know? What don't we know that we should know? What are our assumptions, and what is the evidence for those assumptions? How could we do things differently or better to elicit the desired results? Answering these questions requires knowledge of nursing education practice and literature, as well as higher education literature. Identification of what is established knowledge and what requires further development, explication, or examination is essential so that efforts are directed at advancing knowledge.

What aspects of our curriculum development work could be relevant for a wider audience? Who is that audience? Answers to these questions will influence the scholarship projects that are undertaken and the venues for dissemination.

What is (are) the relevant theory(ies) or model(s)? Theory- or concept-based scholarship is essential to advance knowledge in nursing education. Because scholarship could be about faculty members and stakeholders, learning by students and/or faculty, processes employed, outcomes, partnerships, as well as many other topics, familiarity with theories, models, and concepts from a broad range of disciplines is important for the curriculum development team. A theoretical base is necessary for the scholarliness of the project, and its absence may preclude the credibility or utility of the project outside the school of nursing. Further, publication of work that lacks a theoretical foundation may not be possible.

In addition to thinking like a scholar, Glassick and colleagues (1997) assert that the actions of scholars must reflect the qualities of integrity, perseverance, and courage. Simply put, scholars must be honest in reporting their work and its results, be truthful in presenting dissenting views, persist in scholarly work in spite of competing pressures, and "risk disapproval in the name of candor" (p. 65). In curriculum work, scholars must be honest in reporting, for example, literature that does not support personal or theoretical preferences, learning outcomes that do support hypotheses, or aspects of the educational context that are not ideal. It is vital that they persist with their scholarship plans and efforts, even though the results are not what they desired or are not popular with some colleagues.

Attending to Initial Practical Aspects of Scholarship

The importance of scholarship projects arising from curriculum development, implementation, and evaluation processes ought to be discussed and agreed to in advance by all participants. Some projects can be determined at the outset of curriculum development; others will arise as curriculum work progresses. It is recommended that dialogue about scholarship occur early and repeatedly, because many scholarship projects, conference presentations, and manuscripts can be generated as part of curriculum development. Scholarship should be seen as an integral part of curriculum work that will strengthen the curriculum and the school, expand team members' skills and professional profile, and contribute to career success.

Another consideration is the timing of each project. Some projects should be undertaken concurrently with the curriculum development activities; some can be completed retrospectively. Although many projects could be proposed, it is necessary to think about the number that are reasonable while time and attention are being given to curriculum development itself. Similarly, many projects could be completed retrospectively, such as an analysis of the overall process, but thoughtful consideration is required about how to sustain momentum for this work.

Some scholarship projects could require the approval of an institutional ethics board, and informed consent by participants for formal data collection. If projects of this nature are being contemplated, the length of time required for formal approval and the timing of data collection have to be taken into account.

Because scholarship is rarely a solo event in nursing, decisions about scholarship projects and the people to be involved are important strategic decisions. Collaborative projects allow for skills and knowledge to be pooled and scholarship developed, in spite of competing demands and resource limitations (Thompson, Galbraith, & Pedro, 2010). The quality of relationships, individuals' skills and commitment, and the nature and amount of intellectual synergy will determine the success of the projects.

As project ideas and teams are created, there will be myriad matters of design, logistics, writing, motivation, dissemination, and authorship to be addressed early. Curriculum development teams are urged to recognize, acknowledge, and confront these matters. If they are openly discussed, frustrations can be reduced and the rewards of scholarship experienced.

As the school is organizing for curriculum development, it is beneficial to have a discussion about scholarship in curriculum work to ensure that all members of the curriculum development team:

- Are aware that scholarship is an expected part of the process
- Understand definitions and descriptions of scholarship
- Identify possible scholarship projects
- Know which types of projects will require approval from an ethics board
- Consider their interest in participating in particular projects
- Accept the responsibilities and expectations of scholarship project participants
- Value the ethics of authorship, and therefore,
    - Appreciate when individuals are entitled to authorship designation, acknowledgment as a contributor, or no recognition at all
    - Recognize that honorary authorship (Kovacs, 2012) and authorship order based on status (American Psychological Association [APA], 2010) are antithetical to academic integrity
- Comprehend the career implications of scholarship activities and authorship designation
- Feel free to raise questions about scholarship and authorship as curriculum development unfolds.

Deciding on Authorship

Many faculty members and stakeholders contribute to curriculum development, implementation, and evaluation as part of the teaching mission of the school and not specifically as part of the scholarship mission. In curriculum work, there typically is not a small team comprised of a principal investigator and co-investigators who conceptualize the overall design of the curriculum, apply for funding, and execute the implementation in a manner analogous to research development and conduct. Rather, groups work collaboratively, building on each others' ideas to design, implement, and evaluate a curriculum. What does this mean for authorship when the scholarship projects are being written up, reported, and disseminated?

Widely accepted for research publications are the conditions specified for authorship by the International Committee of Medical Journal Editors (ICMJE, n.d.): "Authorship should be based on: 1) substantial contributions to conception and design, acquisition of data, or analysis and interpretation of data for the work; and 2) drafting the article or revising it critically for important intellectual content; and 3) final approval of the version to be published; and 4) agreement to be accountable for all aspects of the work" (¶2).

Each scholarship team should discuss authorship as soon as practicable and how the order of authorship is linked to the contributions made to the project (APA, 2010, pp. 18–19). When more than one publication or conference presentation can result from the project, discussions about the order of authorship may arise repeatedly, and it is helpful to have a process for reaching decisions. Questions about authorship that could be discussed are: *What types of contribution warrant first authorship and coauthorship? How many coauthors are reasonable? What level of contribution warrants an acknowledgment, but not authorship? What is the link between authorship of a conference presentation and subsequent manuscript preparation of the same, but expanded topic?* Ideas about these and other questions may evolve as the curriculum work progresses and scholarship projects emerge.

It is reasonable that each scholarship project team determines its leader, the order of authorship, authorship responsibilities, deadlines, and accountabilities (Erlen, Siminoff, Sereika, & Sutton, 1997). Nonetheless, it is important to give thought to how extensively the work of the entire curriculum development team formed the basis for individual projects, whether others' efforts should be recognized, and, if so, how this can be accomplished.

When scholarship, such as a manuscript describing the finalized curriculum, is based on the collaborative efforts of many faculty and stakeholders, two fundamental questions may arise: *Who owns the curriculum that has resulted from the thought and collaborative efforts of many?* And, therefore, who is entitled to prepare a manuscript and publish the completed work? The curriculum products of faculty and stakeholders are not the same as data provided by study participants. Rather, the curriculum is the intellectual product of many. Accordingly, discussion about authorship of presentations and manuscripts related to work that was completed by individuals beyond the scholarship project team or by the total group should occur with as many members as possible. Ideas to consider are:

- People to be involved in the preparation of presentations and manuscripts
- Authorship and authorship order
- Recognition of those who contributed to the curriculum work, but not specifically to the scholarship project, either in an acknowledgment note or within the text of a publication
- The possibility of group authorship (e.g., The X School of Nursing Curriculum Development Team).

If there is to be group authorship, the ICMJE (n.d.) requires that the corresponding author for the manuscript list the group name and all individual authors. Group authorship could conceivably include everyone who participated in curriculum development, and this might be 20 or more people. Ultimately, decisions about authorship of the completed curriculum should rest with those who created it.

CHAPTER SUMMARY

Scholarship is a core process of curriculum work. It is the purposeful and methodical creation of knowledge, organization of the knowledge in a way that is meaningful to others, and distribution of the knowledge for peer review and critique (Iwasiw, 2013). Based on a scholarly approach to all curriculum work, the goal of scholarship is to advance knowledge. Boyer's (1990, 1995) five categories of scholarship are possible throughout curriculum work, and all contribute to the science of nursing education. Curriculum developers must think like scholars, both individually and collectively, to identify and complete scholarship projects. Identification of scholarship projects, logistics, and authorship should be addressed openly and early.

SYNTHESIS ACTIVITIES

The White Cliffs University School of Nursing case is an example of how faculty members at one school of nursing responded to the idea of including scholarship as a core component of curriculum work. Questions for critical analysis of the case may provide ideas relevant to readers' situations. Following the case questions are further ideas that might assist readers when consideration is given to the core curriculum process of scholarship.

White Cliffs University School of Nursing

White Cliffs is an established university whose School of Nursing has had an upper-level, nursing major bachelor of science in nursing program for 10 years. Since its inception, enrollment in the program has grown to 600 students. There are 25 full-time faculty, of whom 12 are doctorally prepared, 5 are enrolled in doctoral programs (2 in nursing education programs), and the remaining 8 are master's-prepared and not intending to further their education. Twenty master's-level nurse clinicians have part-time contracts and contribute to teaching in the classroom and/or in professional practice courses. Approximately 50 baccalaureate-prepared nurses have part-time, short-term contracts to facilitate learning in professional practice courses in the upper-level courses. The School has a solid track record in funding and publications about care of individuals with acute illnesses and families of children with acute and chronic illnesses.

Two of the PhD faculty, Dr. Joseph Green and Dr. Ercilia Garcia, have degrees in higher education and have been mentors to the two faculty members enrolled in Nursing Education PhD programs, Angela McLeod and Soraya Tavana. Together, these four are an informal nursing education group who have published expository and research articles about educational practices, such as the learning outcomes of simulated practice experiences. Their funding has been limited in comparison to the researchers who study nursing care, and they believe that their scholarship has not been accorded the same respect as is given to projects supported by large grants. They have hope that this attitude will change as an emphasis on scholarship related to evidence-informed nursing education gains prominence.

Most full-time members of the School have agreed that it is time for curriculum renewal. They are satisfied with the underlying premises of the curriculum but believe that updating of content and a stronger emphasis on evidence-informed practice is necessary. In addition, the nursing education group would like the unity among the philosophical approaches, course goals, and course descriptions to be strengthened. Dr. Garcia has been asked to lead the curriculum renewal process, and she would like curriculum scholarship to be part of the renewal process.

Eighteen full-time and seven part-time faculty are meeting to hear Dr. Garcia's ideas about curriculum renewal processes. Dr. Green, Angela, and Soraya are present. Dr. Garcia asks for ideas about how to proceed with curriculum renewal and discussion follows. This discussion concludes with one member's statement, "Ercilia, we want to update the curriculum. You develop a plan and let us know what we have to do. Let's get it done as quickly and painlessly as possible."

Dr. Garcia says she will develop a plan if that is what the group wants, and that plan will include attention to scholarship associated with curriculum work. The response from one full-time faculty member is, "The nursing education group can take care of that. I'm already too busy with my own research."

Questions and Activities for Critical Analysis of the White Cliffs University School of Nursing Case

1. How can Dr. Garcia link the idea of scholarliness, scholarship, and curriculum work in a meaningful way to gain support for curriculum scholarship?
2. Propose ways Dr. Garcia can capitalize on the research history in the School to advance the idea that scholarship become part of curriculum renewal for faculty not identified as part of the nursing education group.
3. What other reactions might arise to Dr. Garcia's suggestion that scholarliness and scholarship become part of curriculum renewal, in addition to the response that it is the responsibility of the nursing education group?
4. How might the nursing education group respond to objections about incorporating scholarship into curriculum renewal?
5. Describe how Dr. Garcia can present scholarship related to curriculum as a credible undertaking when funds for nursing education research are limited.

Questions and Activities for Consideration When Planning Curriculum Scholarship Activities in Readers' Settings

1. In what ways is scholarliness in curriculum work valuable to faculty members and stakeholders?
2. How can scholarship be explained as a core process in curriculum development in a way that will be meaningful to colleagues?
3. Consider the best approach for identifying possible scholarship projects.
4. Propose suggestions to generate interest in scholarship projects among colleagues and stakeholders.

5. Suggest how a discussion of authorship issues and ethics be initiated and facilitated among curriculum participants.
6. Who should lead scholarship projects related to curriculum? How should this decision be achieved?
7. What might the school of nursing gain by engaging in scholarship projects during curriculum development, implementation, and evaluation? Evaluate whether there might be disadvantages to engaging in scholarship related to curriculum work.
8. Develop a feasible plan to incorporate scholarship into curriculum development, implementation, and evaluation.

REFERENCES

American Psychological Association. (2010). *Publication manual of the American Psychological Association* (6th ed.). Washington, DC: Author.

Boyer, E. L. (1990). *Scholarship reconsidered: Priorities of the professoriate.* Princeton, NJ: The Carnegie Foundation for the Advancement of Teaching.

Boyer, E. L. (1995). The scholarship of engagement. *Bulletin of the American Academy of Arts and Sciences, 49*(7), 18–33.

Broome, M. E. (2009). Building the science for nursing education: Vision or improbable dream. *Nursing Outlook, 57*, 177–179.

Chinn, P. (2011). Editorial: The role of scholarship in shaping the future of nursing. *Advances in Nursing Science, 34*, 91.

Emerson, R. J., & Records, K. (2008). Today's challenge, tomorrow's excellence: The practice of evidence-based education. *Journal of Nursing Education, 47*, 359–370.

Erlen, J. A., Siminoff, L. A., Sereika, S. M., & Sutton, L. B. (1997). Multiple authorship: Issues and recommendations. *Journal of Professional Nursing, 13*, 262–270.

Glassick, C. E., Taylor Huber, M., & Maeroff, G. I. (1997). *Scholarship assessed: Evaluation of the professoriate.* San Francisco: Jossey-Bass.

Hutchings, P., Taylor Huber, M., & Ciccone, A. (2011). *The scholarship of teaching and learning reconsidered: Institutional integration and impact.* San Francisco: Jossey-Bass.

International Committee of Medical Journal Editors. (n.d.). *Defining the role of authors and contributors.* Retrieved from http://www.icmje.org/recommendations/browse/roles-and-responsibilities/defining-the-role-of-authors-and-contributors.html

Iwasiw, C. L. (2013). *How to turn the academic project, clinical project, or term paper into a publishable paper.* Workshop presented at the Labatt Family School of Nursing, London, Ontario.

Iwasiw, C. L., Goldenberg, D., & Andrusyszyn, M. A. (2005). Extending the evidence base for nursing education (Editorial). *International Journal of Nursing Education Scholarship, 2*, 1–3.

Johnstone, M.-J. (2012). Academic freedom and the obligation to ensure morally responsible scholarship in nursing. *Nursing Inquiry, 19*, 107–115.

Kovacs, J. (2012). Honorary authorship epidemic in scholarly publications? How the current use of citation-based evaluative metrics make (pseudo)honorary authors from honest contributors of every multi-author article. *Journal of Medical Ethics, 39*(8), 509–512.

National League for Nursing. (n.d.). *NLN Research Priorities in Nursing Education 2012–2015.* Retrieved from http://www.nln.org/researchgrants/researchpriorities.pdf

Robert, R. R., & Pape, T. M. (2011). Scholarship in nursing: Not an isolated concept. *MEDSURG Nursing, 20,* 41–44.

Tanner, C. A. (2010). The future of nursing: Leading change, advancing health. *Nursing Education Perspectives, 31,* 347–353.

Tanner, C. A., Bellack, J. P., & Harker, J. (2009). The new wave of nursing education scholarship. *Journal of Nursing Education, 48,* 1–3.

Thompson, C. J., Galbraith, M. E., & Pedro, L. W. (2010). Building collaborative scholarship in an academic community. *International Journal of Nursing Education Scholarship, 7,* Article 37.

Young, P. K. (2008). Toward an inclusive science of nursing education: An examination of five approaches to nursing education research. *Nursing Education Perspectives, 29,* 94–99.

PART III

Preparation for Curriculum Development

Determining the Need and Gaining Faculty and Stakeholder Support for Curriculum Development

Chapter Overview

This chapter provides insight into considerations that precede a decision to undertake curriculum redesign and that can lead to faculty and stakeholder support for curriculum development. Although creation of a completely reconceptualized curriculum or revision of an existing one may seem the obvious answer to rectify identified curriculum shortcomings or to incorporate changes into nursing education practice, it is advisable to give thoughtful consideration to the support that can be obtained from those who would be involved. Because faculty members have the main responsibility for curriculum development, their support is essential.

The rationale for curriculum redesign, extent of the curriculum development to be undertaken, the timeframe for completion, and strategies to gain support, are addressed. The core processes of curriculum work, as related to the chapter topics, are described, followed by a chapter summary. Synthesis activities include a case exemplifying reasons for curriculum development and ideas for analysis of the case. The chapter concludes with questions designed to help readers decide if circumstances are suitable to begin the formal process of curriculum development in individual settings.

Chapter Goals

- Consider factors and influences that precipitate curriculum development or revision.
- Reflect on the extent of curriculum development necessary.
- Identify stakeholders in curriculum development.
- Propose strategies to gain faculty and stakeholder support for curriculum development.
- Assess faculty and stakeholder readiness and support for curriculum development or revision.
- Consider the core processes of curriculum work in relation to the need and support for curriculum development.

DETERMINING THE NEED FOR CURRICULUM DEVELOPMENT

The idea of engaging in curriculum development generally arises among a small group of faculty members and possibly other stakeholders (e.g., practitioners, administrators, educational and community partners, students, graduates) who have a vested interest in the school of nursing, its curriculum, and graduates. This group believes that the current curriculum is no longer adequate to prepare students to practice competently in the healthcare and societal contexts they will encounter when they graduate. Identifying reasons why curriculum development is necessary, the extent of the curriculum development that might be required, participants, and possible timelines are important ideas to present to colleagues when seeking their support for curriculum development.

Reasons for Curriculum Development

The purpose of nursing programs is to graduate nurses who will practice competently in a changing healthcare environment and thereby contribute to the health and quality of life of the individuals, families, groups, and/or communities they serve. Situations that impede the ability of the school of nursing to achieve this purpose might, as a consequence, threaten its stability, success, or reputation, and precipitate thoughts of modifying the curriculum or creating a new one.

Ongoing changes within the school of nursing context can influence faculty to consider the possibility of curriculum development. Some changes might include alterations in:

- Availability of resources
- Faculty numbers or expertise
- Student profiles
- Introduction of new ideas by stakeholders
- General discontent with the status quo
- Results of internal curriculum evaluation
- Results of external program or school reviews

Changing circumstances within the context of the parent educational institution might also lead to a belief that curriculum development is timely. Some probable examples might be changes in:

- Academic policy directions or priorities
- Institutional budget
- Educational technologies
- Library resources and services
- Faculty and staff contracts

Similarly, altered situations outside the educational institution can be important signals to faculty and other stakeholders that curriculum development is required to ensure that the curriculum is context-relevant. Changes might occur in:

- Nursing and educational paradigms
- Organization of nursing education throughout a state or province
- Graduates' success rates on licensure or registration exams
- Competition from other schools
- Enrollment demand
- New graduates' ability to meet employer expectations
- Accreditation or approval standards
- Profile of the nursing workforce
- The healthcare environment and provision of health care
- Health profile of the population
- Professional and/or governmental standards, regulations, and priorities
- Priorities of health agencies

A compelling single situation, or a combination of circumstances, can result in the view that the existing curriculum is no longer working as effectively as desired, is outmoded in some way, or is not as responsive to the context as it should be. The consideration of curriculum development or revision can arise gradually when the following occur:

- New ideas and educational methods emerge.
- It becomes apparent that a series of alterations in the curriculum has resulted in a loss of curriculum unity.

Alternatively, curriculum development can be unavoidable and even urgent because of profound contextual changes within the school of nursing, parent institution, or the environment outside the educational agency.

Continual changes in health and healthcare systems, technologies, population profiles, expectations, demands, and predictions about the future of health care have led to the realization that the education of nurses, and, therefore, nursing curricula, must be subjected to evaluation, revision, and maybe even dramatic change (Benner, Sutphen, Leonard, & Day, 2010; Institute of Medicine, 2010). Nursing faculty are challenged and required to develop relevant, evidence-informed curricula to prepare nurses for new and future roles and responsibilities consistent with population health, global perspectives, and dynamic healthcare systems. Because the pace of societal and healthcare change is rapid, the challenge and obligation are continuous. The desire to create and maintain an evidence-informed, context-relevant, unified curriculum arises from faculty members' professional imperative to ensure that graduates will be able to practice nursing competently and contribute meaningfully to the health and wellbeing of clients and society in local and global contexts.

Extent of Curriculum Development

Those initiating the idea of curriculum development should give thought to the extent of development they believe necessary to achieve an evidence-informed, context-relevant, unified curriculum that will build students' professional knowledge, skills, attitudes, and judgment. The scope of curriculum development can encompass:

- Creation of a completely new and reconceptualized curriculum that is not based upon an existing curriculum
- Significant revision of an existing curriculum, so that many curriculum elements are substantially modified and curriculum unity is preserved or achieved
- Limited revision to correct identified gaps or overlaps in the existing curriculum

A revision extends well beyond the ongoing curriculum refinement (i.e., fine-tuning activities such as the annual updating of course content and readings) in which faculty members routinely engage. Rather, curriculum development entails dedicated effort by the total faculty group and committed stakeholders. Therefore, it is wise to give careful thought to which aspects of the current curriculum are working well, which are outmoded, and/or which are redundant. This analysis is important when trying to gain support for curriculum development.

Should the existing curriculum be revised, or should a new curriculum be created? There is no formulaic answer to this question. The response results from a comprehensive and holistic assessment of many factors and the application of faculty and stakeholder judgment about the appraisal. These factors include, but are not limited to:

- The time period since the curriculum was originally created or significantly revised
- The nature and extent of altered circumstances in the school and beyond
- Faculty members' and stakeholders' emotional and intellectual investment in the existing curriculum
- Energy for change
- Results of ongoing curriculum evaluation
- Areas of the existing curriculum that have led to satisfaction or discontent among faculty, students, graduates, or stakeholders

In general, a desire for extensive change in a major element of the curriculum, such as its philosophical approaches (and the resultant curriculum goal or outcome statements, educational approaches, and evaluation methods), leads to the creation of a new curriculum. Similarly, significant changes in the nature and availability of professional practice placements could bring forth ideas of starting anew with curriculum development.

In contrast, a conviction that, for example, altered course sequencing could yield better results for students, would likely result in curriculum revision. In the same vein, the recognition that students are not achieving a particular curriculum goal or outcome would probably lead to revision within the existing curriculum, but not necessarily to the development of a new curriculum. However, an important aspect of this revision is that the final product must be appraised within the context of the total curriculum to ensure that it is logical, conceptually unified, and consistent with the basic curriculum tenets. See **Table 5-1** for examples of the extent of curriculum development and the purposes of each.

Timeframe for Curriculum Development

The timeframe for completion of the work is another consideration when proposing curriculum revision or the development of an entirely new curriculum. How quickly is the redesigned curriculum needed? When might the new or revised curriculum be implemented? These and other factors require examination when thinking about the start and completion dates for the curriculum development project. Each must be assessed within the context of all the other ideas presented in this chapter.

Table 5-1 Extent and Purposes of Curriculum Development	
Extent of Curriculum Development	**Purposes**
Curriculum Revision	
• *Within one course*: significant changes to one or more major course elements (e.g., goals or outcomes, concepts, content, evaluation of student achievement)	• To correct gaps or redundancies
• *Within two or more courses*: significant changes to one or more major course elements	• To align or sequence learning experiences more logically
Major Curriculum Revision	• To incorporate current and anticipated contextual realities
Changes to one or more curriculum foundation(s) (concepts, goals or outcomes, philosophical approaches, educational approaches) with resultant modifications to all courses	• To include current perspectives
	• To "modernize" a successful curriculum
	• To achieve curriculum integrity and unity
Creation of a New Curriculum	To build an evidence-informed, unified curriculum relevant for current and future contexts

First is the urgency of the curriculum redesign. This is influenced by the factors that prompted consideration of curriculum development initially. If, for example, two successive groups of graduates have had a high failure rate on licensing examinations, then there is pressure to improve the curriculum quickly. Similarly, a change in services in local healthcare agencies may necessitate an immediate refocusing of professional practice courses. Conversely, the immediacy of altering an undergraduate curriculum to reflect a slowly changing trend in local demographics may not be as great.

Faculty and stakeholder understanding of the nature of an evidence-informed, context-relevant, unified curriculum and their knowledge of curriculum development processes also have an effect on a probable timeframe. If extensive faculty development will be necessary, time must be allotted for this.

The annual work cycle of the school of nursing and the number of full-time faculty members will influence the schedule for beginning and completing the curriculum development process. Is there a semester when full-time faculty members are less busy with teaching and able to devote concentrated time to curriculum development? If so, consideration should be given to the amount of work that could be achieved in those time periods. If not, the amount of curriculum development time that can be integrated into the ongoing work of the school requires assessment.

A critical factor to review when contemplating a timeframe is the culture of the school and parent institution. Because "readiness for change is culturally embedded" (Latta, 2009, p. 25), it is worthwhile to contemplate whether innovation is a feature of the institution, or whether change occurs at a measured pace. The shared meaning that faculty members give to change and the current curriculum, and the shared meaning within the institution about the value and meaning of change, innovation, and stability (Latta, 2009) will affect views about curriculum change, and thus, the time to develop and implement a redesigned curriculum.

The nature and rapidity of institutional decision-making processes give an indication of the time to completion. Do curriculum decisions need to be approved by several committees within and beyond the school of nursing, or are decisions made relatively quickly and locally, with the expectation that implementation will soon follow? The usual time period from initial decisions to enactment of the decisions will affect the interval allotted for curriculum development and implementation.

Finally, when thought is given to a timeframe for curriculum development, a mindful review should be conducted of the people who might be involved in order to identify those likely to be supporters and resisters. How much time can the supporters realistically be expected to give to curriculum development? How much time will be taken up with overcoming resistance and winning support? The motivation and time commitments of those who will be involved will affect the expected completion. Preparation of a tentative schedule for curriculum development will give participants some idea of the amount of time and work being asked of them, and this can affect their support.

GAINING FACULTY AND STAKEHOLDER SUPPORT FOR CURRICULUM DEVELOPMENT

Although a small group of faculty and stakeholders may initiate the idea of curriculum development, it is ultimately the decision of the total group of faculty, administrators, and possibly other stakeholders about whether to undertake curriculum development, and, if so, the extent of development and the timelines for completion. The decision about whether to proceed with curriculum development is influenced mainly by the depth of discontent with the existing curriculum and by beliefs about how a redesigned curriculum could influence the success of the school and individual members. Other factors that influence the decision are faculty members' level of knowledge about curriculum development and nursing education, practice, and research, and the resources available for curriculum development. Attention to these ideas forms the basis for gaining support for curriculum development.

Curriculum development cannot proceed on the conviction of only a few faculty members. In general, all those who will be affected by a change should be involved in the planning (Marquis & Huston, 2012). Because curriculum development, and the subsequent implementation, represents a significant change in the work activities and interactions of faculty and stakeholders, it cannot proceed without their support. The commitment and effort of all faculty and many other stakeholders are essential for success.

First and foremost is support from faculty colleagues, particularly full-time faculty, because they will assume the largest responsibility for curriculum development and implementation. Next, the school leader's support is prerequisite to formally starting the intensive work of curriculum development.

Moreover, advocates can seek support from students, professional colleagues, educational partners, healthcare clients, and administrators. The endorsement of representatives from each group strengthens the case for proceeding with curriculum development, because all are participants in the school of nursing and its curriculum. There is no set sequence for gaining stakeholder support after preliminary agreement from faculty colleagues and the school leader. However, stakeholder involvement in early and subsequent stages of curriculum development strengthens bonds between schools of nursing and those involved (Cambers, 2010) and can result in a curriculum with wide support.

Gaining Support from Faculty Colleagues

Gaining faculty colleagues' support for curriculum development involves an appeal to logic and values. Neither alone is sufficient. The precise approach will, of course, be dependent on the organization and the people involved.

First, those proposing curriculum development must be able to articulate clearly why they believe curriculum development is necessary. It is important to present factual data about how deficiencies (Wilkin & Dyer, cited in Latta, 2009) in the current curriculum are evident, the consequences of those deficiencies, and the thinking that led to the conclusion that curriculum modification is necessary. Presenting general ideas about possible alternate curricula can extend colleagues' thinking and increase their acceptance of the idea of redesigning the curriculum.

Second, the perceived need for curriculum development can be linked to values held by faculty, students, and graduates of the school of nursing, and/or the educational institution itself. For example, if the institution takes pride in being innovative, responsive to diversity, and a leader in education, then curriculum development can be presented as a means to support those values. In **Table 5-2**, ideas are offered that could be helpful in convincing colleagues that curriculum development is needed. Innovations (or the possibility of an

Table 5-2 Examples to Convince Colleagues of Need for Curriculum Development	
Appeal to Logic	**Appeal to Values**
Need for curriculum change or development, such as:	Opportunity to shape the curriculum
• Deficiencies in current curriculum	Desire for:
• Unsatisfactory external and/or internal evaluations	• Professional and personal growth of students and curriculum developers
• Trends requiring new approaches	• Competent graduates
• Evidence from literature to support change	• Enhancement of School's prestige
Requirement to provide a curriculum responsive to healthcare and societal needs	• Status as innovators, leaders
Suggestions about possible alternative curricula	Opportunity for:
Possible positive consequences of curriculum development:	• Personal prestige
	• Innovation and transformation
1. Strengthened congruence with:	• Organizational preeminence
• Organizational mission and values	• Enhanced reputation of individuals and school
• Personal and professional values	Possible negative consequences of avoiding curriculum development:
2. Favorable external and internal evaluations	
3. Student satisfaction, leading to enhanced work environment for faculty	• Decreased appeal and marketability of the school to applicants, students, and faculty
4. Increased employability of graduates	• Decreased marketability of graduates to employers
Enhanced appeal of the school to potential faculty members and applicants	• Unrealized funding opportunities
Possibility of obtaining funding for curriculum development	• Unfavorable internal and/or external reviews
	• Diminished prestige

innovation) are most likely to be accepted if the new idea is consistent with the values and culture of the organization and its members, and with the ideal cultural commitments (Greenhalgh, Robert, Bate, Macfarlane, & Kyriadidou, 2005; Latta, 2009).

It is important to consider the best way to seek support. Should colleagues be approached individually or collectively? Clearly, there are advantages and drawbacks to both. (See **Table 5-3** for an analysis of approaching colleagues individually or collectively.) A combination may be appropriate, first talking with colleagues individually to gain the acceptance of informal leaders, and then presenting ideas to a larger group. Involvement of informal leaders is a means to share the leadership for introducing the idea

Table 5-3 Advantages and Disadvantages of Approaching Colleagues Individually or Collectively to Gain Support for Curriculum Development

Approach	Advantages	Disadvantages
Individual	Freer expression and exploration of ideas	One viewpoint; no collective ideas
	Less threatening	Lack of support for persons proposing change
	Quick response or possible decision	
	Greater willingness to share experiences	Time required to collect and compile ideas from individuals
	In-depth, thoughtful response possible	Discomfort resulting from disagreement
	Personal consultation valued	Pressure to conform
Collective	Group response more broad	Delayed response or decision (many ideas before consensus)
	Sharing of many ideas	
	Opportunity to use democratic or consensual process, which strengthens a decision to proceed	Time required to share all experiences relative to decision
	Increased awareness of others' strengths	Potential group veto of curriculum change
	Opportunity to learn from others' feedback	Undue influence by strong group members
	Improved faculty bonding by uniting to reach common goal	Group think
	Shared thinking for responses, resulting in a stronger position	
	Less time-consuming	
	Opportunity for group to make more informed assessments of need for curriculum development	

of curriculum development, a strategy consistent with producing "leadership through interactions" (Denis, Langley, & Sergi, 2012, p. 214). The decision about how to introduce the idea of curriculum development to colleagues will be influenced by knowledge of individual faculty members, interpersonal dynamics in the school, and the credibility of those seeking support for curriculum change.

The importance of listening to colleagues when seeking support cannot be overemphasized. Their perspectives are important and worthy of attention, because they are being asked to take on a large endeavor. Colleagues need to feel that their concerns have been accurately heard and taken into account in subsequent decision making. Careful listening is a means to gain information from colleagues whose support is needed, and the act of listening, in itself, positively affects the influence of the listener (Ames, Maissen, & Brockner, 2012). Therefore, it is wise for those desirous of curriculum development to give opportunity for the views of others to be expressed, and to give careful attention to those views when discussing the possibility of curriculum development with individuals or groups.

Gaining Support from the School Leader

The support of the school leader is necessary before curriculum work can proceed, no matter how much endorsement exists among the faculty and other stakeholders. Matters to address with the school leader are listed in **Table 5-4**. Precise information about each

---

Table 5-4   Matters to Discuss with the School Leader

1. Need for curriculum development
2. Extent of faculty support
3. Leadership of curriculum development
4. Estimated time for development and implementation of redesigned curriculum
5. Effect on other work:
   - Teaching (classroom, professional practice, laboratory)
   - Student advisement
   - Scholarship
6. Faculty, student, and stakeholder involvement
7. Resources needed:
   - Faculty release time
   - Support personnel
   - Materials
   - Technological equipment
   - Physical space
   - Funding
8. Positive consequences of curriculum development for the school

point will not be available at an initial meeting. Yet, thoughtful identification of the academic and administrative aspects of curriculum development will increase the credibility of those proposing this possibility to the school leader. The initial goal is to gain support for the idea of initiating curriculum development and a commitment to examine ways to provide resources for the undertaking. Endorsement from the school leader is essential for curriculum work to begin.

However, verbal endorsement will not be sufficient for the processes of curriculum development, implementation, and evaluation. Institutional resources are essential for curriculum change (Oliver & Hyun, 2011). Indeed, without resources, the curriculum work cannot proceed.

Gaining Support from Community and Healthcare Stakeholders

When schools of nursing are contemplating curriculum development, they are usually experiencing challenges that are known to community and healthcare partners, and shared by the partners, such as overcrowded student placements. Simultaneously, those partners are experiencing their own challenges and anticipating new ones as political and funding landscapes change.

It can be productive to arrange individual appointments with the nursing leaders of the school's largest partners to solicit preliminary support for curriculum development. At this stage, it is important to emphasize the following:

- Curriculum development is being considered.
- The purpose of the meeting is to determine whether there is initial support by the school's partners for a changed nursing curriculum.

Topics that might be addressed during the meeting include:

- Shared challenges
- The school's recognition of limitations and challenges within the current curriculum, particularly those most relevant to the nursing leader's organization
- Factors that will affect a decision to proceed with curriculum development, including stakeholder support
- The nursing leader's general ideas about the knowledge, skills, and abilities required for nursing practice in the future
- The desired involvement of members of partner organizations if curriculum development is undertaken

The meeting can end with a request for the nursing leader's endorsement for curriculum development. Furthermore, this is an opportunity to alert the leader that more detailed information gathering about the knowledge, skills, and abilities required of nurses in the future will be sought if a decision to undertake curriculum development is reached.

Gaining Support from Students

Students have many ideas about how the curriculum they are experiencing can be improved, and often they expect changes to be made as soon as they voice those ideas. Therefore, their support for curriculum development is usually readily given, with the implicit expectation that their concerns about gaps or overlaps are corrected and their ideas about new areas to include are realized.

Student support for curriculum development can be sought through the nursing student council or in brief meetings during class time. It is important to emphasize that if curriculum development proceeds, time will be necessary to gather data (including data from them) and for the development work, and that changes will not be instantaneous. Therefore, they are being asked to support the idea of curriculum redesign for future students.

Some may argue that requesting student support early is unnecessary and raises expectations of immediate change. Our view is that students are the ones most affected by curriculum. They are the recipients of educational decisions and are required to function within the boundaries of those decisions. Therefore, just as clients are entitled to participate in decisions about all aspects of their care (including the possibility of changes in care), so too are students entitled to be informed and involved in educational planning and decision making.

RESPONDING TO INITIAL OBJECTIONS

Although some faculty members may be enthusiastic about the idea of curriculum development, others may have a different view. It can be expected that some will feel hesitant and others may resist the possibility of curriculum development, and thus, change. Overcoming initial objections is foundational to winning faculty and stakeholders' support. To ignore opposition will likely result in a failure to proceed and/or in slow and resentful involvement. Therefore, it is wise to anticipate, recognize, and respond to objections promptly.

First, challenges about the accuracy of information that illustrates the need for curriculum development, or the conclusions drawn, can be anticipated. This may reflect an honest, intellectual disagreement, a deeply held belief in the value of the current curriculum, a general response to change, or opposition to those proposing curriculum development.

When reasons for curriculum development are questioned, it is tempting to invite challengers to explain their position. This is a strategy to be used with caution, because a protracted dispute about who is right or which facts are correct is not productive. Such disagreements can annoy or even alienate others, who might then view curriculum development as a potentially endless series of conflicts. In the face of criticism about the reasons for curriculum development, it is more constructive to respond that the reasons to proceed are compelling and to acknowledge that not all might share that view.

Further, it may be necessary to enumerate the potential risks of avoiding curriculum development. These can include the possibility of unfavorable external reviews by approval or accrediting bodies, decreased ability to attract students and faculty, difficulty retaining faculty, and unrealized funding opportunities.

Some faculty may feel so overstretched with their current workloads that even the *idea* of curriculum development and the work it will entail is overwhelming. The time required for this endeavor can seem daunting and could be a real barrier. It is important, therefore, to recognize and acknowledge that curriculum development is a large undertaking, and that the reality of workloads and available time needs to be explored thoroughly with the school leader and faculty members. It may be that competing demands make curriculum development impossible. If so, would the school leader be open to having some members delay or give up some responsibilities, at least for a short period, to allow the process to unfold?

To win the support of particular individuals, it is wise to identify the criticisms they have voiced about the current curriculum and acknowledge the aspects they value. Through individual or small-group meetings, participants can be reminded that curriculum development is an opportunity to alter or eliminate the weaker aspects of the current curriculum. Additionally, it is essential to emphasize that their active involvement in the curriculum development process could also lead to maintaining or updating cherished parts of the existing curriculum. Affirming that strengths of the present curriculum may be retained, if this is deemed appropriate by the curriculum development team, might induce cooperation.

Financial constraints will be a concern for the school leader and may also be raised by other faculty members. Curriculum development takes time, and faculty and staff time is costly. Therefore, an acknowledgment that resources are needed for curriculum development and an assurance that this matter will be discussed with the school leader, and subsequently with faculty and stakeholders, will go a long way in gaining support. It is also helpful to identify possible funding sources for curriculum development, such as internal university funds or foundations known to support innovations in nursing education. Certainly, adequate system resources are needed for change to occur and be sustained (Greenhalgh et al., 2005; Oliver & Hyun, 2011).

Another reason some may object to the idea of curriculum development is that those proposing it do not have the respect of colleagues. It is essential that those advocating curriculum development have good relationships with colleagues and are seen as having credible views about curriculum. If not, the proposal for curriculum change may be rejected. Identifying whether personalities are the reason for opposition is a painful process. Those recommending curriculum development might consider if their ideas are usually sought and supported by colleagues, and if others generally choose to work with them. In the event that personality seems to be a reason for objections, it would be wise to leave the initiation of the idea to others who are respected within the faculty and stakeholder group. If this is not possible, some interpersonal work must be done before support will be gained. Objections that may be raised to the idea of curriculum development and possible responses are summarized in **Table 5-5**.

Table 5-5 Responses to Initial Objections to the Idea of Curriculum Change	
Nature of Objections	**Responses**
Challenge to evidence for curriculum development	Respond that reasons are compelling.
Satisfaction with current curriculum	Emphasize the: • Importance of offering a curriculum that will maximize student learning and graduates' success • Opportunity to be on the cutting edge of change and transformation in nursing education • Personal and professional growth potential inherent in curriculum development
Fear that treasured part of the curriculum will be lost	Affirm that as curriculum work proceeds, aspects of the current curriculum may be retained. Comment that active involvement is the only means to ensure a satisfactory curriculum.
Time commitment required for curriculum development	Present possible funding opportunities for curriculum development. Comment that there will be discussion with the school leader about possible altered work assignments. State that individuals' involvement will influence the curriculum development process, and thus the time required.
Fear that curriculum development will negatively affect scholarship	Comment that there will be discussion with the school leader about possible altered work assignments. State that curriculum development is a responsibility of the academic role. Underscore that scholarship is an inherent part of development, implementation, and evaluation.
Apparent lack of resources to support curriculum development	Respond that resources will be discussed with the school leader and faculty members.
Lack of support for faculty proposing change	Allow credible faculty to initiate the idea of curriculum development.

DECIDING TO PROCEED WITH CURRICULUM DEVELOPMENT

It is unlikely that all objections to curriculum development will be overcome or that all faculty members will enthusiastically endorse proceeding with curriculum development. Nonetheless, once potential curriculum team members have individually and collectively considered the reasons for and against curriculum development, a majority concurs that curriculum development is necessary, and the school leader supports the idea, the curriculum development process should be ready to proceed. Because faculty members will assume the greatest responsibility for the work of curriculum development, their support is the foundation upon which the quality of the curriculum development process will rest. Therefore, faculty members' endorsement of the decision to proceed is essential. The decision may be reached by consensus, or it may be formalized by a motion that specifies a timeline for implementation of a redesigned curriculum, depending on the typical decision-making procedures in the school of nursing.

Once a decision about moving forward has been reached, it is usual to advise students and stakeholders, some of whom may subsequently become involved in the curriculum development process. Informing others beyond the school of nursing makes public the intention to proceed with curriculum development and creates an expectation of change.

CORE PROCESSES OF CURRICULUM WORK

Faculty Development

Faculty development during individual and group discussion about the need for curriculum development is most likely to be informal. Some members will want to know what the process of curriculum development entails. Similarly, stakeholders outside the school of nursing may require information about what curriculum redesign might mean for them. Provision of this information will expand their understanding of what they are being asked to endorse.

Ongoing Appraisal

During the phase of determining the need and gaining support for curriculum development, the initiators constantly appraise others' reactions to their ideas and approaches, both simultaneously and retrospectively. They then revise their approach as necessary until a decision is reached about whether or not to proceed with curriculum development.

Scholarship

It is unlikely that a scholarship project will be planned about gaining support for curriculum development. However, a retrospective report and analysis of the processes that led to the proposal for curriculum redesign, and subsequent endorsement, could be prepared for submission to a journal. An article such as this could be helpful to faculty members elsewhere who wish to initiate the idea of curriculum redesign. In addition, a retrospective qualitative study could be undertaken to determine how the process was experienced by those whose support was being sought and whether there were particular features that were salient in their decision to support curriculum redesign.

CHAPTER SUMMARY

Faculty and stakeholder support for curriculum development is essential for the process to begin and for the achievement of a successful outcome. Endorsement of curriculum development is accomplished through open and thoughtful consideration of the reasons for curriculum development and the factors that might be limiting. Attention to the values of individual and collective faculty and stakeholders, the scope of curriculum development that might be necessary, and the timeframe envisioned for the undertaking will influence whether approval is gained. The impetus and decision to proceed must be thoughtfully reviewed, because curriculum development is intensive and requires ongoing faculty and stakeholder dedication and involvement. Throughout the processes of determining the need and gaining support for curriculum development, the initiators engage in informal faculty development and ongoing appraisal. Scholarship related to this phase of curriculum development can be undertaken, likely retrospectively.

SYNTHESIS ACTIVITIES

The Castlefield University School of Nursing case illustrates some ideas about the need for curriculum development and support for undertaking curriculum work. The questions following the case can guide a critical analysis of the situation. Questions are then provided that might assist readers as they consider the need and support for curriculum development in their settings.

Castlefield University School of Nursing

Castlefield University School of Nursing offers a 4-year, integrated baccalaureate nursing program, with professional practice beginning in the second semester of the first year. The current curriculum was introduced 12 years previously and modifications have occurred periodically throughout the years.

Several faculty members of Castlefield University School of Nursing are considering the need for changes to the undergraduate nursing curriculum. In particular, two relatively new faculty members, William and Martha, who obtained their nursing doctorates 2 years ago and then began teaching on a full-time basis in the second year of the program, are especially vocal about the relevance of the curriculum. They are also concerned about reports from healthcare agency staff that Castlefield nursing students and graduates seem unable to meet practice expectations.

Their concerns were brought forth at the monthly meeting of the Undergraduate Curriculum Committee, which comprised faculty from all 4 years of the program. One committee member, who has taught at Castlefield for 4 years, appeared sympathetic. However, those with 12 or more years of experience in the nursing program felt there is no need for change because they believe that the present nursing curriculum is up to date. This latter group has enjoyed excellent relationships with the school leader, Dr. Virginia Higgins, who has facilitated their attendance at workshops and conferences on newer curriculum approaches involving feminist, caring, and student-centered approaches. Following these workshops, some minor curriculum revisions were made.

William and Martha continue to present their case for curriculum revision. They staunchly propose that the current nursing program seems no longer relevant for the times and requires changes. They argued that, from their perspective and that of other faculty and stakeholders with whom they have consulted, there is very little stated or included in the curriculum about evidence-based nursing practice and patient safety. Martha also added that there is insufficient content in the curriculum about the clients who are served and the community as a whole. William continued that, while he had been eager to become a member of the school of nursing 2 years previously, he has yet to identify the relationship of the nursing program to the university's broad goals. Both William and Martha questioned if, indeed, the nursing program really represents an evidence-informed, context-relevant, unified curriculum.

Two other committee members added their concern about unsatisfactory reports from healthcare agencies about some students and graduates. All faculty had been shocked to learn that this year, nearly 20% of the graduates were unsuccessful on the National Council Licensure Examination (NCLEX). That particular group of graduates had also been quite vocal about their displeasure with the Castlefield nursing program and with some of the nursing faculty. They had previously met with William and Martha, and with several nursing staff with whom they had worked as students, to discuss what they could do to improve their chances for success on the next NCLEX examination. However, in spite of the NCLEX failure rate and apparent agency disappointment about some Castlefield students and graduates, there is increasing pressure from the university's senior administrators to increase enrollment, as well as research funding and publication rates.

In view of administrators' pressure, the concerns of some nursing faculty and several healthcare employers, and the scheduled approval and accreditation reviews within 3 years, Dr. Higgins is convinced that the time is right for a significant curriculum revision or the development of a new curriculum. After speaking further with William and Martha, some more experienced nursing faculty members, and interested stakeholders, Dr. Higgins calls a special meeting to discuss whether curriculum revision or development is needed.

Questions and Activities for Critical Analysis of the Castlefield University Case

1. Analyze the factors or influences that would propel Castlefield nursing faculty toward a review of the present curriculum and consideration of change. Propose other methods Martha and William might have used to raise their concerns and analyze the possible effectiveness of the methods.

2. Describe the rationale that William, Martha, and other committed faculty members can provide to convince others of the need to develop an evidence-informed, context-relevant, and unified curriculum. How could their ideas be proposed?

3. Suggest how support for this rationale could be obtained. What could be the sources of support for curriculum development? Sources of resistance?

4. How can Dr. Higgins and the committed nursing faculty members obtain strong enough support for curriculum development? Which stakeholders can be recruited to participate?

5. Hypothesize about how experienced nursing faculty might respond to William and Martha's criticisms of the curriculum. What are some possible responses?

6. Recommend a means to diplomatically caution nursing faculty to consider whether allegiance to their nursing practice specialties might overshadow the broader perspectives of nursing required in contemporary undergraduate nursing education.

7. How might Dr. Higgins's initiation of the idea of curriculum development influence faculty members' decision about whether or not to proceed? How can she assess faculty members' acceptance of the need and readiness to support the process for development of an evidence-informed, context-relevant, and unified curriculum?

8. What would be a suitable timeframe for revising the curriculum in light of the rationale for change and the upcoming approval and accreditation reviews?

Questions and Activities for Consideration of the Need and Support for Curriculum Development in Readers' Settings

1. Explain why curriculum development is necessary now. What is the evidence for proposing that curriculum work proceed? How compelling are the ideas?
2. From whom is support needed for the idea of curriculum development? Who are the stakeholders, and how can their support be gained?
3. Propose ideas to gain faculty support. Determine the advantages and disadvantages of approaching colleagues individually or collectively.
4. How can evidence be presented about the necessity for curriculum development so it is convincing to faculty colleagues?
5. Consider how extensive curriculum development should be. Might the development be a revision of the current curriculum or a completely new curriculum? Develop rationale for the proposal about the extent of curriculum development.
6. What could be the impact of participation in curriculum development on faculty members' other commitments?
7. Hypothesize about possible objections to curriculum development and develop responses to the objections. List the potential risks associated with not proceeding with curriculum development at this time.
8. In addition to the need for curriculum development, what else should be discussed with the school leader in a preliminary way?
9. Describe the resources required to be successful with curriculum development. What funding sources are available outside the school of nursing?
10. Are there sufficient resources (people, time, physical, material) to proceed with curriculum development now?
11. Is informal agreement to proceed sufficient, or would a formal motion be preferable? Why?
12. If agreement to proceed is obtained, which stakeholders should be informed of the decision? Should they be invited to become members of the curriculum development team?
13. What other considerations require thoughtful attention?
14. Propose scholarship activities that might be considered.

REFERENCES

Ames, D. B., Maissen, L. B., & Brockner, J. (2012). The role of listening in interpersonal influence. *Journal of Research in Personality, 46*, 345–349.

Benner, P., Sutphen, M., Leonard, V., & Day, L. (2010). *Educating nurses: A call for radical transformation.* San Francisco: Jossey-Bass.

Cambers, W. (2010). Collaboration and curriculum design—a stakeholder symposium. *Mental Health Nursing, 30*(2), 14–15.

Denis, J. L., Langley, A., & Sergi, V. (2012). Leadership in the plural. *The Academy of Management Annals, 6*, 211–283.

Greenhalgh, T., Robert, G., Bate, P., Macfarlane, R., & Kyriakidou, O. (2005). *Diffusion of innovations in health service organizations: A systematic literature review.* Oxford: BMJ Books/Blackwell Publishing.

Institute of Medicine. (2010). *The future of nursing: Leading change, advancing health.* Washington, DC: National Academies Press.

Latta, G. F. (2009). A process model of organizational change in cultural context (OC^3 Model): The impact of organizational culture on leading change. *Journal of Leadership and Organizational Studies, 16*(1), 19–37.

Marquis, B. L., & Huston, C. J. (2012). *Leadership roles and management functions in nursing: Theory and application* (7th ed.). Philadelphia: Wolters Kluwer/Lippincott Williams & Wilkins.

Oliver, S. L., & Hyun, E. (2011). Comprehensive curriculum reform in higher education: Collaborative engagement of faculty and administrators. *Journal of Case Studies in Education, 2*, 1–20.

CHAPTER 6

Deciding on the Curriculum Leader and Leading Curriculum Development

Chapter Overview

Theoretical perspectives on leadership and their application to curriculum work and change are presented in this chapter. Criteria for selection of a curriculum leader and the possibility of internal or external appointees are presented as a basis for deciding on this leader. Presented next is information about the responsibilities of the curriculum leader and leadership within curriculum teams. Development of curriculum leaders and ideas about the core processes of curriculum work in relation to curriculum leadership conclude the chapter. Following the chapter summary, the synthesis activities include a case study and questions to illustrate the foremost points of the chapter. Finally, questions are posed to assist readers with determination of curriculum leadership in individual settings.

Chapter Goals

- Review theoretical perspectives on leadership and their application to curriculum work and change.
- Consider criteria and processes for selection of a curriculum leader.
- Address the curriculum leader's responsibilities.
- Examine leadership activities within curriculum teams.
- Contemplate the development of curriculum leaders.
- Reflect on the core processes of curriculum work related to curriculum leadership.

THEORETICAL PERSPECTIVES ON LEADERSHIP: APPLICATION TO CURRICULUM WORK AND CHANGE

Leadership is a socially constructed process that arises, is enacted, and is responded to through interpersonal inactions (Uhl-Bien, 2006). All parties influence the interaction, and thus, the leadership process. The interactions and relationships can arise from a formal arrangement in which the leader has an identified and sanctioned role within an organization. Alternately, there can be a relationship of informal leadership, in which the leader has no official role, yet influences others in a significant fashion. In both situations, the goal is to influence people to accomplish explicit or implicit goals.

Whether leadership is formal or informal, components of effective leadership in a culture of change include having a vision and moral purpose, being flexible, building relationships, creating and sharing knowledge, understanding change, and expanding others' capacity for change (Patterson, McAuley, & Fleet, 2013; Stefancyk, Hancock, & Meadows, 2013). Moreover, for sustainable change to occur, the leader must be able to influence the group to give ongoing attention and commitment to the collective purpose, the achievement of the curriculum work, group relationships, and the maintenance of a changed culture.

Following a systematic review of leadership styles of formal leaders and the outcome patterns for the nursing workforce and work environments, Cummings and colleagues (2010) concluded that transformational (vision-based with emphasis on capacity-building) and relational (people-focused, with all members developing and benefiting) leadership yielded better results than transactional leadership (task-focused, power-based). Among the results associated with transformational and relational leadership were nurses' increased levels of job satisfaction, organizational commitment, health, productivity, effectiveness, and improved collegial relationships. Despite differences between staff nurses and nursing faculty, and between healthcare and academic environments, it seems reasonable to conclude that transformational and relational leadership would lead to similar positive results during curriculum work in schools of nursing.

Transformational Leadership

Transformational leaders motivate others to perform to their full potential over time, by influencing a change in perceptions, providing a challenging vision and sense of direction, and involving group members in participatory decision making about how to achieve the vision (Robbins & Davidhizar, 2007). Bass & Bass (as cited in Owings & Kaplan, 2012) have identified four factors associated with transformational leadership:

- Idealized influence (charisma)
- Inspirational motivation (ability to communicate a motivating vision)

- Intellectual stimulation (encouragement of creative problem solving)
- Individualized consideration (coaching and mentoring)

Transformational leaders use mentoring and intellectual satisfaction in the group, and engage with others so that they and the group members raise each other to higher levels of motivation and ethical decision making. They are visible and accessible to those they lead (Clavelle & Drenkard, 2012). Leaders focus on collective purpose and mutual growth and development, articulate a vision, behave as change agents, and empower others to expend extra effort beyond performance expectations. Team members have improved job satisfaction, productivity, enthusiasm, team spirit, organizational commitment, and efficacy (Avolio, Walumbwa, & Weber, 2009; Clavelle & Drenkard, 2012).

Working with faculty and stakeholders, transformational leaders develop a vision of the curriculum, create a strategy to achieve the vision, and identify specific actions to progress to the vision. They model the behaviors that are consistent with the curriculum tenets. In addition, they provide assistance to groups as necessary, identify faculty development needs, and plan for faculty to expand their capacity for curriculum work. Importantly, transformational leaders keep the vision in the forefront, are optimistic about people's ability to achieve the vision, and ensure that vision is realized through small, planned successes.

Transformational leaders are responsive to members. This means that they recognize when individuals and groups are ready to move ahead with change, feel overburdened by the curriculum work, or are resistant to particular ideas. They adapt their strategies to ensure that motivation is maintained or reignited to facilitate the success of the curriculum work. For example, if the curriculum group becomes discouraged, the transformational leader offers ideas to help the group reframe or reinterpret the situation and encourage group participation in determining processes for moving forward (Boga & Ensari, 2009).

Authentic Leadership

Authentic leadership theory is based in positive psychology and emphasizes positive and developmental interactions between leaders and followers. The ultimate outcome is genuineness in relationships through greater self-awareness and self-regulated behavior, both of which foster positive self-development. Authentic leaders put the concerns of others ahead of their self-interest. The four components of authentic leadership behavior are:

- Balanced processing: objectively analyzing relevant data before making a decision
- Internalized moral perspective: being guided by moral standards that regulate behavior

- Relational transparency: presenting one's true self by sharing information and revealing feelings as appropriate
- Self-awareness: understanding own strengths, weaknesses, and meaning making (Avolio et al., 2009)

These leader behaviors contribute to a positive organizational climate of trust and integrity, and to followers' psychological capital—that is, a positive state of development based on self-efficacy, optimism, hope, and resilience. In an extensive review of authentic leadership research, Gardner, Cogliser, Davis, and Dickens (2011) identified the outcomes of authentic leadership. The outcomes include those reported for transformational leadership, positive leader modeling, followers' trust in the leader, psychological wellbeing, reduced burnout, increased psychological capital, and personal identification with the leader. Further, creativity (Rego, Sousa, Marques, & Pina e Cunha, 2012) and work engagement (Giallonardo, Wong, & Iwasiw, 2010) have been reported as outcomes of authentic leadership. In curriculum work, authentic leaders are genuinely interested in the development of their colleagues. They model productive, open relationships and behaviors consistent with the curriculum tenets. Because they are confident and self-aware, they are consistent in their approach to individuals and groups, able to recognize and share their curriculum knowledge, acknowledge their limitations, and give recognition to others' curriculum and relational strengths. Moreover, the leader analyzes curricular and interpersonal matters in an objective manner, using relevant data and knowledge about curriculum, change, and interpersonal relationships. Therefore, the authentic curriculum leader is able to view situations of disagreement in a dispassionate way, making a decision when necessary, or guiding the group to a balanced decision. Similarly, this leader is able to assess colleagues' progress in the change process and respond appropriately.

DECIDING ON THE CURRICULUM LEADER

Development, implementation, and evaluation of a curriculum are large undertakings that require leadership and organization for successful completion. Because of the importance of the work for a school's success, a curriculum leader is usually given responsibility for guiding the process. This leader creates a situation in which faculty and stakeholders feel connected to the curriculum (Buchanan, 2008) through a combination of curriculum expertise, relational and organizational/managerial skills, and knowledge of change processes.

Criteria for Selection of the Curriculum Leader

Curriculum Expertise

A key criterion when deciding on the curriculum leader is curriculum expertise. Importantly, the curriculum leader must be knowledgeable about nursing education and curriculum development, implementation, and evaluation. This leader should also be thoroughly immersed in the literature, practice, and governance of nursing education in order to bring essential ideas to the group and have credibility with members.

The curriculum leader also requires knowledge about the type of program for which the curriculum is being developed, such as associate, baccalaureate, or graduate degree. An understanding of the nature of such programs, the expectations of graduates, and approval and accreditation requirements will allow the curriculum leader to guide novices in curriculum work to suitable resources, processes, and decisions.

Relational Skills

Curriculum work is interpersonal work. Therefore, the human dimension is a constant and requires ongoing attention, even when the tasks and deadlines of curriculum development are pressing. The quality of the curriculum leader's relationships with everyone involved in curriculum work is foundational to the quality of the curriculum produced. Therefore, this leader must possess excellent interpersonal skills. These will garner respect from the curriculum team and be the foundation upon which the emotional tone of the curriculum work will proceed.

Organizational/Managerial Skills

An intent to develop a curriculum is insufficient to bring it to fruition. The processes that lead a curriculum from conception to implementation and to evaluation require planning and organizational structure. The curriculum leader requires organizational and managerial skills to ensure that a suitable plan for the work is in place and that the work proceeds in a timely manner.

Knowledge of Change Processes

Leading curriculum work means leading a change process. Accordingly, it is incumbent on the curriculum leader to have knowledge of change processes; how to support individual, group, and culture change; and how to recognize individual and group reactions to change. Because change is not always a smooth, steady process, the leader needs to have accurate "*emotional aperture*, that is, the ability to perceive various shared emotions that exist within a collective" (Sanchez-Burks & Huy, 2009, p. 22), and then to implement strategies that will assist members to respond effectively to change and achieve the final goal.

Institutional Knowledge

Knowledge of the educational institution, its academic policies, and approval processes is also important. However, if the potential leader does not possess this information, familiarity with institutional operations can be readily acquired through documents, websites, and academic leaders.

Appointment from Within the School of Nursing

Typically, the curriculum leader comes from within the school of nursing. In general, selection of the curriculum leader occurs in a manner congruent with usual practices in the school of nursing. Most frequently, the school leader consults with faculty members; uses his or her judgment about individuals' curriculum knowledge, interpersonal relationships, and capacity for leadership; and then comes to a decision about an appropriate choice. Alternately, the curriculum leader can be either informally chosen through consensus in recognition of an individual's knowledge and credibility, or formally elected. If curriculum development leadership is already a part of the role description of the undergraduate chair or curriculum committee chair, there may be no decision to be made.

Whatever the means of choosing a curriculum leader, formal appointment ultimately rests with the school leader. Because of the time required to fulfill the responsibilities of the position, there are implications for work assignments within the school and only the school leader can manage these.

Appointment from Outside the School of Nursing

It is possible to advertise for and appoint a curriculum leader who has not been part of the school of nursing. In this case, the appointment is typically for 2 or 3 years to allow time for the curriculum to be developed, for implementation to begin, and for evaluation to be planned. An external appointment can be a suitable approach when there is no one within the school able to take on the position. However, it is an approach to be considered carefully.

A new appointee will not know the school's history, culture, values, and internal politics. This can be advantageous or problematic, depending on the situation within the school and the reasons there was no internal appointment. The new curriculum leader will require time to develop relationships inside and beyond the school and to become acquainted with the institutional policies and culture. It can be expected that this leader will need to establish credibility with the group before unity can be established and mutual goals endorsed.

An alternative is to seek direction from a curriculum consultant, who might be appointed for a short term. Consultants should be chosen carefully according to their area of curriculum expertise and to the needs of faculty. Typically, external consultants are short-term adjuncts to curriculum development, rather than an integral part of the daily activities.

Announcement of the Appointment of a Curriculum Leader

The school leader should make a formal announcement of the appointment of a curriculum leader to members of the school, to appropriate members of the academy, and to healthcare and community partners. This announcement gives legitimacy to the position and to the curriculum leader's activities. It is essential for all who will be involved in curriculum work to understand the curriculum leader's responsibilities, authority (if any), and accountabilities.

CURRICULUM LEADERSHIP

The curriculum leader has three categories of responsibility and accountability: relational, curricular, and organizational/managerial. These operate synergistically and must be fulfilled simultaneously. The quality of the leader's relationships with curriculum team members and stakeholders, in combination with his or her curriculum skills, is essential to the accomplishment of curriculum work. However, the curriculum work can proceed only when the leader has developed sound logistical and organizational scaffolding to support it. Interpersonal, conceptual, and behavioral complexity underpin successful curriculum leadership.

Relational and Change Leadership

The curriculum leader must work effectively with individual faculty members, curriculum teams, and external stakeholders. As the figurehead and champion of curriculum development, the leader represents both the school and the developing curriculum. Therefore, leadership based on excellent relationships is mandatory. Specific relational leadership activities consistent with transformational and authentic leadership theories and with change theories would be to:

- Project a sense of agency, self-confidence, and optimism
- Model exemplary interpersonal skills
- Demonstrate confidence in colleagues' ability and respect for their ideas
- Facilitate discussion to shape a vision of the curriculum
- Initiate and lead respectful discussions about curriculum and underlying assumptions and values
- Liaise with the school leader, curriculum advisory committee, nursing community, and other academics
- Engage stakeholders in curriculum work
- Foster creativity and support task completion
- Build capacity through formal and informal teaching, and through mentoring
- Offer a positive outlook on progress
- Take all relevant data into account before reaching decisions and while facilitating participative decision making
- Maintain focus on agreed-upon vision and goals

- Provide opportunities for group reflection about change
- Be alert and responsive to interpersonal dynamics and to individual and group emotions
- Recognize individual and group stage of change and offer support when appropriate
- Lead discussion about changes in the school culture
- Be visible and accessible in the curriculum process
- Acknowledge own knowledge gaps and act to correct them
- Mediate conflict in a manner that leads to a balanced resolution
- Plan for recognition of milestone achievements
- Behave in a consistent, reliable, authentic manner

Curricular Leadership

The curriculum leader's expertise in curriculum processes is essential to the success of curriculum work. However, the leader must tread a careful line between conveying information that will move the work forward and directing the outcome. The outcome of the work is not the leader's decision. Although the leader is knowledgeable about the curriculum development process and the substance and relevance of the work to be done, the authority for curriculum decisions rests with the faculty and school leader.

Curricular leadership takes several forms that range from listening to ideas, to offering possible ideas, to providing clear information about curriculum matters and processes. At all times, the enactment of relational leadership skills is essential. Specific examples of curricular leadership are to:

- Listen to ideas about curriculum and pose questions to stimulate further thinking about values, assumptions, or consequences
- Consult with curriculum groups and offer ideas for their consideration
- Critique the completed work of curriculum groups and provide feedback
- Provide formal and informal faculty development sessions related to curriculum development, implementation, and evaluation
- Identify matters requiring discussion, such as the need to review academic policies to ensure they remain relevant for a changed curriculum
- Alert curriculum developers to potential problems, for example, plans that might conflict with institutional policies
- Provide technical information or resources related to specific aspects of curriculum development, for instance, formulating curriculum goals or outcomes
- Model behavior consistent with the curriculum philosophical approaches
- Arrange for faculty development activities as needed
- Participate in planning for curriculum implementation and evaluation

Organizational and Managerial Responsibilities

Curriculum work requires organizational and managerial oversight; therefore, there are attendant responsibilities associated with curriculum leadership. The curriculum leader organizes and manages the *processes* of curriculum work and not the curriculum team members. Typically, there is no supervisory role in curriculum leadership. The curriculum leader is responsible to:

- Serve as an ex officio member of the curriculum committee (if not already a member)
- Initiate organization of the curriculum development work
- Propose committees to be formed
- Develop a communication strategy
- Ensure that curriculum development activities proceed in a timely fashion to meet agreed-upon deadlines
- Negotiate with the school leader for adequate resources for curriculum development
- Initiate discussion (and perhaps negotiate) with other departments about non-nursing courses
- Prepare reports and finalize documents for institutional approval of the curriculum
- Participate in planning for strategies to inform stakeholders of curriculum redesign
- Assist in publicizing the redesigned curriculum

LEADERSHIP WITHIN CURRICULUM TEAMS

Although there is a curriculum leader for the overall curriculum work, that individual is not the designated leader of the many committees, task groups, and/or curriculum development teams that are formed during curriculum development. Usually, an individual from within each group assumes a leadership role. Additionally, informal leadership can develop as the curriculum work progresses. Consequently, leadership for curriculum work is distributed among faculty members and stakeholders.

Within curriculum teams it is usual to have an identified leader (or chair) or co-leaders. These individuals are accountable for completion of their task and should use relational, curriculum, and organizational/managerial skills to do so. Their responsibilities mirror those of the curriculum leader, although on a smaller scale. Typically, they seek guidance and information from the curriculum leader.

Curriculum team membership is optimal for the development and exercise of informal leadership. Because leadership arises through relationships, interactions, and communication (Uhl-Bien, 2006), the collaborative relationships in small groups allow individuals to feel comfortable about offering ideas that influence the task. As group members work together productively, leadership may be shared, with different individuals emerging as leaders for different aspects of the work (Denis, Langley, & Sergi, 2012), even though there is a nominal leader. The informal leadership within groups may not be recognized or acknowledged, but it contributes significantly to curriculum work.

The value of informal leadership in task completion and change should not be underestimated. Informal social networks among faculty members and stakeholders, whether or not they are working on the same curriculum task, affect attitudes toward the curriculum endeavor. The influence of informal leaders on perspectives that develop outside of formal meetings has a profound effect on the success of curriculum work.

Curriculum development, implementation, and evaluation require an investment of time, effort, and leadership by many individuals. Some will demonstrate leadership for a short period of time or in relation to a specific task. Others will demonstrate leadership in a continuous fashion and may have potential to be designated as curriculum leaders in the future.

DEVELOPMENT OF CURRICULUM LEADERS

Most leaders do not spring forth, fully confident, and effective. Rather, they undergo a process of growth and maturation in the leader role, usually with the guidance of a mentor. Unfortunately, a process of planned growth and maturation is not typically true of nursing curriculum leaders, for whom there is no defined developmental or career path. Being mentored to become a curriculum leader and gradually assuming more experience and wisdom are not common.

Young, Pearsall, Stiles, Nelson, and Horton-Deutch (2011) reported that nursing faculty leaders gained their formal leadership positions (including curriculum leadership) by being "thrust" into the position because they possessed particular expertise needed in the school, or because of longevity and having earned the respect of colleagues. Others became leaders because of a history of risk-taking in educational practices or speaking forthrightly about needed change in the school or educational institution. In each situation, the leaders felt unprepared for their new roles, yet were perceived as leaders by colleagues.

Importantly, deliberative preparation for curriculum leadership is essential as educational and healthcare systems become more complex, with concomitant expanded expectations of nursing graduates. The future of nursing education, and thus, the practice of nursing, should be in the hands of those with preparation in nursing education processes, leadership, and research. To advance curriculum leadership, it is necessary that:

- All nursing faculty have (at minimum) preparation in nursing education theory and practice, including learning theories and philosophies, teaching and evaluation methods, and course design.
- This preparation is a condition of hiring or contract renewal.

- Specific attention is given to all aspects of curriculum development, implementation, and evaluation in graduate programs in nursing education.
- *Curriculum leadership*, including change leadership, is a specific course in doctoral programs in nursing education.
- Knowledgeable nursing curricularists are named as curriculum mentors and coaches in schools of nursing.
- Opportunities for discussion and reflection about curriculum processes and leadership are created in schools of nursing.
- Aspects of curriculum leadership (e.g., course redesign) are recognized as part of nursing faculty members' career development.
- Schools of nursing support faculty members to attend conferences and workshops related to nursing curriculum and curriculum leadership.
- Planning for curriculum leadership development and curriculum leadership succession is instituted in schools of nursing.

The minimum level of education could be accomplished through graduate certificate programs. If all faculty members had at least this level of preparation, there would be immediate improvements in curriculum implementation and informed participation in curriculum work. Mentorship about all aspects of curriculum work is essential to expand faculty members' knowledge and skill in curriculum. It is important, however, that curriculum experts do not merely clone themselves. Innovation and change will be limited if the protégé does not have freedom to introduce and test new ideas and methods (Burke, 2008). The importance of scholarly attention to, and scholarship about, curriculum development, implementation, and evaluation in graduate programs is self-evident.

Of paramount importance is attention to curriculum leadership (including theory, purposeful observation, guided practice with feedback, and research) in doctoral programs in nursing education. Once a faculty position is secured, the required education in nursing curriculum leadership could be followed by the assumption of progressively more demanding curriculum responsibilities, preferably with ongoing mentoring by a curriculum leader. This will help to build an individual's self-concept as a curriculum leader and will contribute to the goal of having curriculum leaders who are prepared educationally, experientially, and personally for their roles, not merely thrust into the position.

Opportunities for curriculum work should be available, valued, and rewarded in schools of nursing, in the same way as research opportunities. It is not proposed that the development of curriculum leaders within schools of nursing supplant the development of researchers, but rather that more evident importance and visibility be accorded to the ongoing preparation of those who will lead the education of future nurses and who will conduct the research about nursing education and its outcomes.

CORE PROCESSES OF CURRICULUM WORK

Faculty Development

Preparing leaders for the curriculum development process is essential to the success of this undertaking and for the future of nursing education. If only a few among the faculty have sufficient preparation to be leaders in curriculum development or curriculum leadership, faculty development preparation would be appropriate for the faculty group.

Faculty development activities could initially focus on what leadership is, leadership development and approaches, acceptance of leadership responsibilities, and, importantly, specific information about what would be involved in leading aspects of curriculum development. Attention could be given to the responsibilities associated with chairing curriculum groups. Practicing curriculum leadership behaviors through role-playing might facilitate learning in these sessions.

If members with leadership and curriculum development experience are available, these persons could be called upon to offer faculty development opportunities and mentor those without experience. Mature leaders (both formal and informal) feel obligated to embrace the role of mentor and pass on their wisdom (Bennis, 2004) about curriculum work to novice colleagues. By doing so, experienced faculty members fulfill their responsibility to nurture the next generation of curriculum leaders.

Ongoing Appraisal

Ongoing appraisal of curriculum leadership is multi-pronged. The curriculum leader engages in self-appraisal. In addition, everyone involved in curriculum work appraises the curriculum leader and their own leadership activities within groups. Some questions that curriculum leaders might ask themselves are:

- Am I consistently acting in a way that is true to my values?
- Am I providing the emotional and technical support that facilitates the curriculum work? What is my evidence?
- Is the organization of the curriculum work sufficient or is more needed?
- How are faculty and stakeholders responding to me and to my leadership?
- What else could or should I be doing?
- Are we accomplishing quality curriculum work?

Wise curriculum leaders will periodically ask faculty and stakeholders how well they are doing and what they could be doing differently or additionally.

In their appraisal of the curriculum leader, curriculum team members will consider:

- How respectful of my ideas is the leader? How respectful of others' ideas is the leader?
- How satisfied am I with the way the leader functions?

- How well does the leader know how to make the curriculum work happen?
- Does it seem that the leader is helping us to get our work accomplished?
- How credible is the leader? How extensive is the leader's curriculum knowledge?
- How well is the leader attending to the group's need for information and development?

Curriculum team members who consider their own leadership activities within groups might consider:

- Am I expressing ideas in a way that captures the group's attention and stimulates further thinking?
- Do I demonstrate informal leadership frequently enough to believe that I am contributing meaningfully to the group's productivity and collegial relationships?
- Am I ready to take on a more formal role in the curriculum development process?

Periodic appraisal of the curriculum leader by curriculum groups and the school leader can be important to ensure the ongoing success of curriculum work. The curriculum leader needs to know how the curriculum groups are responding to the leadership strategies so that necessary adjustments can be made. The school leader should assess the success of the appointment and offer feedback and guidance as necessary.

Scholarship

Many scholarship projects related to curriculum leadership are possible. Some examples are:

- A study of the lived experiences of formal curriculum leaders (Ylimaki, 2011)
- An enquiry into the meaning of curriculum leadership by leaders and curriculum participants (Ylimaki, 2011)
- An examination of effective and ineffective curriculum leadership strategies from the perspectives of curriculum leaders and participants
- An analysis of the processes, challenges, and results experienced by curriculum leaders
- A study of the career paths of designated curriculum leaders

CHAPTER SUMMARY

Effective leadership is of paramount importance in curriculum work. Determining who the curriculum leader will be and the responsibilities inherent in the position is foremost in providing the groundwork for success. Leadership in curriculum work requires expert knowledge of the curriculum process, organizational and managerial skills, and the ability to work productively with others.

In this chapter, theoretical perspectives on leadership, that is, transformational and authentic leadership, are presented as applied to curriculum work and change, followed by criteria for selecting the curriculum leader and appointment of this leader. Curriculum development leadership and leadership within curriculum groups are overviewed. Development of curriculum leaders and attention to the core processes of curriculum work as they relate to curriculum leadership conclude the chapter.

SYNTHESIS ACTIVITIES

The Northern Lights University School of Nursing case contains some ideas about curriculum leadership, and the questions that follow provide a basis for consideration of the situation. Then, questions are offered that might assist readers when contemplating formal and informal curriculum leadership in their own settings.

Northern Lights University School of Nursing

Northern Lights University School of Nursing is about to embark on a significant revision of its 4-year undergraduate nursing degree program. Dr. Isabel Purset, the school leader, with the agreement of undergraduate nursing faculty and senior administrators, has decided on a formal appointment to the position of curriculum leader from within the school of nursing.

Dr. Sylvia Kraus, who has been in the School for 22 years, is the current curriculum chair. Eight years previously she led the development and implementation of the current accredited curriculum. Through that process and her subsequent work as curriculum chair, Dr. Kraus has developed sound relationships with university administrators and professional practice partners.

Dr. Purset considers Dr. Kraus to be an obvious choice for the position of curriculum leader, and she makes a formal announcement to the nursing faculty, stakeholders, university administrators, and to healthcare and community partners that Dr. Kraus will lead the curriculum work. She comments that she is confident that Dr. Kraus's curriculum knowledge and experience, as well as her excellent interpersonal relationships within and beyond the School of Nursing, will ensure a timely and successful completion of the curriculum revision.

Dr. Kraus willingly accepts the appointment, in view of the support of the school leader and faculty colleagues. Additionally, she believes her familiarity with the institution's academic policies and approval processes will be an asset to the curriculum endeavour. In her acceptance remarks to the nursing faculty and stakeholders, Dr. Kraus clearly articulates the responsibilities she has in the role and asks for continued support and a commitment from the faculty and stakeholder members to participate in the curriculum work.

Dr. Kraus's appointment is warmly endorsed by most faculty members. However, a few privately voice reservations about the appointment of someone so strongly associated with the current curriculum.

Questions and Activities for Critical Analysis of the Northern Lights University School of Nursing Case

1. What factors or influences led the school leader, Dr. Purcet, to appoint the current curriculum chair, Dr. Kraus, to undertake the additional responsibilities of leading curriculum development?
2. Analyze the merits of Dr. Purcet's decision and the merits of the reservations about Dr. Kraus's appointment. What conclusion can be drawn about the wisdom of Dr. Purcet's decision?
3. How could Dr. Purcet announce the appointment of Dr. Kraus as leader of curriculum redevelopment to institutional administrators, nursing faculty, and community leaders?
4. How can Dr. Purcet and committed faculty and stakeholders obtain support from nonsupportive members for Dr. Kraus's appointment? How can Dr. Kraus herself overcome the reservations of some colleagues?
5. Propose strategies for Dr. Kraus to demonstrate her ability and commitment to leading curriculum redevelopment.
6. Suggest how Dr. Kraus can contribute to the development of her colleagues' curriculum leadership skills while leading curriculum revision.

Questions and Activities for Consideration of Curriculum Leadership in Readers' Settings

1. Are there important criteria for selection of a curriculum leader in addition to those described in the chapter? If so, what are they?
2. Which aspects of the curriculum leader's responsibilities are most relevant? Why? Who might best fulfill the expectations and responsibilities?
3. Could the role of curriculum leader be shared if there is not a candidate able to fulfill all of them? Explain your response.

4. How have curriculum leaders been selected in the past? Suggest the best approach for deciding on a curriculum leader now.

5. Describe the discussion and negotiation a candidate for curriculum leadership might want to undertake with the school leader.

6. Assess the effects of support or nonsupport for the curriculum leader on the task of curriculum development.

7. If objections are raised about a possible curriculum leader, what can be done and by whom to overcome the resistance?

8. Suggest contingencies that might affect the selection and/or choice of a curriculum leader.

9. Who could contribute to faculty development for curriculum leadership? Describe the needed faculty development.

10. Create a plan to appraise the leadership effectiveness of a formal curriculum leader, committee chairs, and team members.

11. Outline scholarship projects that could be undertaken in relation to curriculum leadership.

REFERENCES

Avolio, B. J., Walumbwa, F. O., & Weber, T. J. (2009). Leadership: Current theories, research, and future directions. *Annual Review of Psychology, 60,* 421–449.

Bennis, W. G. (2004). The seven ages of the leader. *Harvard Business Review, 82*(1), 46–53.

Boga, I., & Ensari, N. (2009). The role of transformational leadership and organizational change on perceived organizational success. *The Psychologist-Manager Journal, 12,* 235–251.

Buchanan, M. T. (2008). Curriculum management: Connecting the whole person. *Issues, 82,* 41–44.

Burke, W. W. (2008). *Organizational change: Theory and practice.* London: Sage.

Clavelle, J. T., & Drenkard, K. (2012). Transformational leadership practices of chief nursing officers in Magnet® organizations. *Journal of Nursing Administration, 4,* 195–201.

Cummings, G. G., MacGregor, T., Davey, M., Lee, H., Wong, C. A., Lo, E., . . . Stafford, E. (2010). Leadership styles and outcome patterns for the nursing workforce and work environment: A systematic review. *International Journal of Nursing Studies, 47,* 363–385.

Denis, J. L., Langley, A., & Sergi, V. (2012). Leadership in the plural. *The Academy of Management Annals, 6,* 211–283.

Gardner, W. L., Cogliser, C. C., Davis, K. M., & Dickens, M. P. (2011). Authentic leadership: A review of the literature and research agenda. *Leadership Quarterly, 22,* 1120–1145.

Giallonardo, L. M., Wong, C. A., & Iwasiw, C. L. (2010). Authentic leadership of preceptors: Predictor of new graduate nurses' work engagement and job satisfaction. *Journal of Nursing Management, 18,* 993–1003.

Owings, W. A., & Kaplan, L. S. (2012). *Leadership and organizational behavior in education.* Boston: Pearson Education.

Patterson, C., McAuley, E., & Fleet, A. (2013). Leading change from the inside: A braided portrait. *Reflective Practice, 14*(1), 58–74.

Rego, A., Sousa, F., Marques, C., & Pina e Cunha, M. (2012). Authentic leadership promoting employees' psychological capital and creativity. *Journal of Business Research, 65,* 429–437.

Robbins, B., & Davidhizar, R. (2007). Transformational leadership in health care today. *Health Care Manager, 26,* 234–239.

Sanchez-Burks, J., & Huy, Q. N. (2009). Emotional aperture and strategic change: The accurate recognition of collective emotions. *Organization Science, 20*(1), 22–34.

Stefancyk, A., Hancock, B., & Meadows, M. T. (2013). The nurse manager: Change agent, change coach? *Nursing Administration Quarterly, 37*(1), 13–17.

Uhl-Bien, M. (2006). Relational leadership theory: Exploring the social processes of leadership and organizing. *Leadership Quarterly, 17,* 654–676.

Ylimaki, R. M. (2011). *Critical curriculum leadership.* New York: Routledge.

Young, P. K., Pearsall, C., Stiles, K. A., Nelson, K. A., & Horton-Deutch, S. (2011). Becoming a nursing faculty leader. *Nursing Education Perspectives, 32,* 222–228.

CHAPTER 7

Organizing for Curriculum Development

Chapter Overview

This chapter provides practical guidelines about organizing for curriculum development. Once a decision has been made to proceed with curriculum development, both the curriculum leader and faculty members have specific responsibilities in preparing for this undertaking. The leader is responsible for guiding faculty to consensus about values and beliefs, proposing an overall plan for curriculum and faculty development, clarifying the relationship of curriculum development and implementation to academic freedom, introducing the possibility of scholarship projects, and negotiating for resources. Faculty members have responsibility for participating on committees to complete curriculum development tasks, welcoming stakeholders, seeking input, and considering scholarship projects. A discussion of activities associated with organizing for curriculum development is followed by ideas about faculty development, ongoing appraisal, and scholarship related to the initial organization. The synthesis activities that conclude the chapter comprise a case study, questions to guide case analysis, and activities to organize for curriculum development in readers' settings.

Chapter Goals

- Consider the curriculum leader's and faculty members' responsibilities in organizing for curriculum development.
- Identify matters to be discussed when organizing for curriculum development.
- Review activities to organize for curriculum development.
- Contemplate the core processes of curriculum work related to organizing for curriculum development.

CURRICULUM LEADER'S RESPONSIBILITIES IN ORGANIZING FOR CURRICULUM WORK

The curriculum leader has the responsibility for leading the faculty group in the decision making that is necessary to prepare for the intensive work of curriculum development. The leader's curriculum, relational, and organizational skills are foremost as the faculty group is guided to prepare for curriculum development.

Guiding Values Clarification

Individual and collective values are an important influence on curriculum development. The perceived need for curriculum development is linked to values held by faculty members. As faculty begin to prepare for curriculum development, it is important that a shared base of values and beliefs is established. Therefore, the wise curriculum leader will guide faculty and participating stakeholders to consider and reach consensus about:

- The purpose and processes of nursing education
- What nursing practice could and should be
- What constitutes excellence in nursing curricula
- The role of the nursing curriculum in supporting the institutional mission and priorities

Consensus about these matters will provide a solid foundation to move forward with curriculum development. The discussion about values provides the groundwork for future decisions about curriculum goals and educational and philosophical approaches. A discussion about excellence is the basis for determining what acceptable quality is, as the developing curriculum is appraised. A dialogue about values and beliefs forms the basis of a vision of the curriculum. Moreover, agreement to link the curriculum to the institutional mission explicitly could strengthen future requests for budgetary support. Finally, agreements about values and beliefs become a touchstone during future curriculum discussion when divergent views might sometimes seem irreconcilable.

Proposing an Overall Plan

It is incumbent on the curriculum leader to present an overall plan for the accomplishment of the curriculum work. The plan should take into account the proposed date for curriculum implementation, the realities of faculty workloads, and the time that faculty members can regularly give to curriculum work. Importantly, the plan ought to incorporate the activities necessary to create or revise a curriculum. Bringing some order to curriculum development activities expedites the subsequent work and helps to make the process seem possible to novices. The presentation of a tentative plan with timelines makes real the work that is ahead and to which faculty are committed.

Leading Discussion About the Plan and Other Pertinent Matters

The curriculum leader has the responsibility of ensuring that matters pertinent to the undertaking are raised, discussed, and agreed upon. Depending on the culture of the school, the leader might provide information, propose ideas, and ask for endorsement of decisions, or lead discussion about all or some of them. Typically, the matters are discussed in a relatively seamless fashion as the overall plan is presented.

Selection of a Change Theory

Selection of a change theory to guide the overall processes of curriculum development and implementation, and the attendant culture change, will allow curriculum developers to have a framework for the progress of their work and for the reactions that individuals might experience. Group attention to choosing a change theory will give a common frame of reference for the curriculum work and the processes that faculty experience individually and collectively.

Participants in Curriculum Development

The National League for Nursing (2003) has stated, "faculty, students, consumers and nursing service personnel must work in partnership to design innovative educational systems that meet the needs of the healthcare delivery system now and in the future" (p. 1). Therefore, participants in curriculum development comprise more than faculty members.

Faculty involvement, and the nature and extent of their involvement, is a crucial matter to raise and discuss initially. Creating the curriculum is mainly the province of the nursing faculty because of their work roles, knowledge, experience, and decision-making authority. Experienced faculty members offer knowledge of curriculum development, institutional policies and resources, and health care in the community; their insights can provide structure and guidance to the process. Novices can bring new ideas that are not bound by tradition and thereby help to move the group's thinking forward.

However, accountability for revising or creating a curriculum does not belong solely to faculty members who will be teaching in the redesigned curriculum. Faculty members from other programs in the school have important contributions to make and should be involved, because they can bring different perspectives of nursing and nursing education, broadening curriculum discussions. Additionally, faculty from other disciplines relevant to nursing could be invited to participate, not necessarily for the direct contributions they can make, but to build support for the curriculum through their ongoing interaction with nursing faculty and to participate in any discussion about desired changes in the non-nursing courses.

In programs with educational partners who share in offering nursing courses, it is understood that the partner faculty members are also involved, not just the nursing members of the credential-granting institution. Those who participate will likely feel most responsible and strongly invested in the curriculum and will strive to implement it in the manner envisioned.

Student participation in curriculum development is a means for students to expand their educational experience, gain valuable information about nursing education, experience colleagueship with curriculum developers, and offer ideas about the curriculum. Their experiences, perspectives, needs, and aspirations are important influences on the curriculum. Active involvement by students helps them understand the complexity of curriculum development and builds support for the curriculum. Also, periodic requests for information or reaction to proposals from student groups conveys the message that their role in shaping the curriculum is valued and that they have a professional responsibility to improve nursing education for current and future colleagues.

However, in a survey of nursing programs, less than half of respondents indicated that they partnered with students in the development of innovations (Pardue, 2006), thereby limiting the ideas that influenced the innovation. Although student participation in curriculum development can be intermittent in accordance with their schedules and priorities, inviting their participation allows them to be full participants in their education and is an expression of colleagueship, an avenue for broadening their view of future nursing careers, and a reflection of the value accorded to their ideas.

Professional practice partners are also important members of curriculum development teams, and the value of collaborative interface with colleagues from practice settings should be raised during discussion. Curriculum dialogue among clinicians, faculty, students, and administrators has been described as mutually enriching, not only to themselves, but to the curriculum and profession (Black, Morris, Harbert, & Mathias, 2008; Cambers, 2010). Service agencies are affected by the curriculum and potential faculty role changes; therefore, they are entitled to be part of the planning that will affect them. Professional practice experts and leaders can provide useful, practical input and validate suggested changes. Additionally, the involvement of colleagues from practice settings can lead to the development of collaborative projects to enhance professional practice learning environments (Palmer, Harmer Cox, Clark Callister, Johnsen, & Matsumara, 2005).

Representatives of healthcare and community agencies may not have a sustained involvement but could be included in curriculum development for particular aspects of the process. Involvement of agency personnel with responsibility for student placements is essential when professional practice experiences are being planned.

Academic administrators, in particular the school leader, participate in curriculum development through delegation of responsibilities to the curriculum leader, allocation of resources to support curriculum development, and/or by active involvement in the process. This involvement, however, will depend on other responsibilities and priorities in the school and institution, but such participation would signify the importance of curriculum development to the school and parent institution.

Active participation by institutional administrators is unlikely to occur. Yet, the idea of inviting them to events celebrating milestones in curriculum development can be proposed. If invited, their interest and support may increase.

Other stakeholders could be involved. All who have an interest in the school of nursing and its graduates could potentially be involved: program graduates, professors emeriti, healthcare leaders, educators from the school system, community leaders, clients, and members of professional bodies. Their knowledge, experience, and vested interests would contribute significantly to the creation of a curriculum that will build students' professional knowledge, skills, values, and identity, so that graduates will practice nursing professionally and competently in changing social and healthcare environments. An example is the involvement of representatives of the All-Russia Society for People with Disabilities in planning an educational program for nurse managers who would coordinate hospital and community health care for clients with disabilities (Iwasiw, personal communication, 2013). Their participation was instrumental in extending the educators' understanding of the barriers clients experienced in obtaining their needed care, and this understanding influenced curriculum goals, content, and processes. Provided in **Table 7-1** is a summary

Table 7-1   Persons Involved in Curriculum Development
Graduate and undergraduate nursing faculty
Faculty from other disciplines
Professors emeriti
Educational institution administrators
Nursing students
Program graduates
Healthcare leaders
Clinicians
Members of professional nursing associations
Community leaders
Clients
Educators from the school system

of those who could be involved in curriculum development if deemed appropriate by the faculty group.

Committee Structure, Functions, and Membership

Unless one committee is given the responsibility of completing all the work of designing a curriculum, a constellation of committees is essential. For the committees to complete the necessary work, all faculty and other stakeholders must share the work and participate in the discussion that leads to agreement and acceptance of ideas. Therefore, it is necessary for the curriculum leader, in particular, to propose which committees should be formed, their structure, and functions.

Deciding on committee structure first requires the identification of strategies to achieve the task of curriculum development expeditiously. Activities to accomplish the tasks, and the best way to use available human and material resources, should be assessed, proposed, and agreed upon. Committees, groups, and individuals, tied together horizontally and vertically through a common vision of the overall goal, possibly overlapping membership, facilitative relationships, shared communication, and information systems, will most likely be necessary to complete the activities.

A possible committee structure could be one that allows all members to function as a total faculty group, which develops and approves all curriculum proposals. This type of structure can be effective in a small school of nursing. However, in most schools, such a structure could slow curriculum development; therefore, it is more common for the total faculty group to come together to discuss and approve major aspects of the curriculum, such as the goals or outcomes. Use of a total faculty group at critical points in curriculum development can promote faculty buy-in.

A workable committee includes a curriculum committee of dedicated, knowledgeable participants who will be responsible for the overall development of the proposed curriculum. Members of the curriculum committee will become members and possibly chairs of subcommittees. Usually, the formal curriculum leader chairs the curriculum committee.

The use of subcommittees or task forces (ad hoc committees) is typical. These facilitate optimal participation of all people involved in curriculum development. Discrete tasks such as collecting contextual data or formulating the philosophical approaches are given to the subcommittees. These small groups enable each participant to contribute and appraise the work accomplished. They are transitory, task-oriented, and their dissolution is natural when the work is done. Usually, task forces do small short-term tasks, whereas subcommittees have the total ongoing responsibility of developing their portion of the curriculum and reporting back to the curriculum committee and the total faculty group.

Like subcommittees, task groups provide feedback and generate more than one alternative for every phase of their work.

In addition to subcommittees with responsibility for particular aspects of curriculum development, it is possible to have a critique committee to provide an *external* appraisal of committees' work. Members of this committee can ask questions, recommend clarification or expansion of some points, examine incongruities, suggest revision, and provide feedback, thereby adding validity to the work. Alternately, the curriculum committee might take on the responsibility of ongoing appraisal and ensure that all parts of the curriculum are consistent and unified.

The school might also enlist the help of an advisory committee, made up of members from the academic and professional communities and also consumers. These persons may be enlisted to serve on task forces or subcommittees. Advisory bodies are a useful source of information as well as a public relations mechanism to foster understanding and promotion of the curriculum.

Finally, a curriculum steering committee could be formed. This occurs most frequently when a curriculum is being planned and implemented by more than one educational institution. Committee membership can be composed of senior administrators of the institutions, formal leaders of the nursing program(s), and the curriculum committee chair(s). The number and organizational position of members from the involved institutions are usually equal. The steering committee might assume responsibilities such as:

- Offering direction to the curriculum initiative
- Ensuring that plans are in accordance with institutional policies
- Identifying needed changes in policies
- Planning for sharing of resources, if appropriate
- Liaising with institutional governing bodies and external organizations (e.g., nursing regulatory or government) as necessary

The key to successful curriculum development is a committee structure conducive to the task, yet amenable to modification if necessary. Activities of all committees and subcommittees ought to proceed in an organized fashion, be based on realistic expectations, and be supported by adequate resources. When committees are structured, important considerations are their purposes, membership, tasks to be accomplished, methods of achieving the work, and deadlines for completion.

Membership on particular curriculum committees or subcommittees is usually based on interest and expertise. Individuals can become committee members by volunteering, peer selection, appointment by the school leader (Glatthorn, Boschee, & Whitehead, 2009), or invitation by the curriculum leader or committee chair. Although all members may not fully meet the following membership criteria, the collective membership of each committee should generally have:

- A broad understanding of nursing education, the school of nursing, and the educational institution
- Knowledge of curriculum development, learning, teaching, evaluation of learning, educational and nursing philosophies, student characteristics and needs, available resources, graduation requirements, approval and/or accreditation standards, and licensing requirements
- Familiarity with health and healthcare issues and the community to be served

Recordkeeping System

Keeping a record of meetings and decisions is essential. The records need not always be formal minutes; however, they should be up to date and complete, starting with consensus agreement about values and beliefs. Copies of working papers, documents, and materials used or developed by the committee members should be dated and retained. It is important to maintain an inventory of what has been done and what has been agreed upon. These materials are a history of the development and unfolding of the curriculum, and how abstract ideas become operational.

Attached to the meeting notes or minutes should be any substantive discussion or decisions that have occurred via email between meetings. Much work is done between meetings, of course, and the email discussion among group members can easily be retained as part of the paper trail of the group's thinking and decisions. To a large extent, the emails form the notes.

Meeting notes or minutes, a record of decisions, and documents can be kept on a learning platform site. In this way, they can be accessible to everyone involved.

Communication System

The work of each task force and committee has an influence on the work of others, and decisions that have been reached will affect all subsequent work. Therefore, the curriculum leader should propose a system that will allow all curriculum developers to be informed of the work that is underway or has been approved. Information sharing can occur through regular updates from the curriculum leader via email or newsletter, and/or posting on a learning platform site. It is wise to have a central location (either virtual or real) for all approved decisions and documents. This will help to ensure that there will be no doubt about what is official and what is still being developed.

An effective communication system is more than a repository for decisions and notes. It allows opportunities for all curriculum development participants to be kept informed and provide input into subcommittees' work on an ongoing basis. This input can be verbal, via email, or through a discussion site on the learning platform.

Decision-Making and Approval Processes

Decision-making and approval processes to accomplish the work as expeditiously and smoothly as possible should be suggested and agreed upon early. These processes will likely be the ones usually employed in the school of nursing; however, explicit agreement about decision making is essential. Decisions must be made, ratified, and accepted as a basis for ongoing curriculum development.

The curriculum leader can provide suggestions about which decisions will require formal approval by the total faculty and information about those that will require institutional approval. Ideas about which aspects of curriculum development need endorsement by the total faculty will naturally lead to consideration of whether this endorsement will be gained by consensus or by voting, in formal meetings or through less formal curriculum discussions.

Creating a Critical Path

Once the proposed plan and relevant matters have been discussed, possibly modified, and agreed to, the leader has the responsibility of creating a formal critical path. This is a detailed listing of the milestones in curriculum development and will bring definition to the curriculum development process.

The critical path is a blueprint for action, specifying the steps to be completed, the deadlines, and the individuals or committees responsible for each phase of the curriculum development process. It provides a concrete means to assess whether the curriculum is being developed at a pace that will ensure implementation by the target date.

In creating the plan, the leader first places the implementation date of the first courses on the critical path, thereby giving it preeminence. The next step is to calculate back to the date the educational institution must approve the curriculum design. Then, the total time available to finalize the curriculum will be evident. Major milestones that should occur before curriculum implementation and their associated deadlines are identified. It is helpful to note which individual or committee will have responsibility for each aspect of the process, as well as the approval procedures necessary throughout curriculum development.

It is possible to make the critical path more detailed by specifying, for example, the dates for the formation of subcommittees or deadlines for preparation of materials for approval by the total faculty group. However, too much detail can be overwhelming.

The critical path is a schedule for the curriculum development process. Importantly, the overall success of a project is positively affected by the quality of the initial planning and negatively affected by constraints in the number and skills of people working on the project (Dvir & Lechler, 2004). The latter idea provides rationale for the inclusion of faculty development activities on the curriculum path and rationale for the leader to negotiate for adequate resources for curriculum work.

Table 7-2 provides an example of a critical path, beginning with the implementation date of the curriculum and working backward in time to when the curriculum development process actually begins. A 2-year period for the development of a typical 4-year undergraduate program is presented in consideration of the time needed for the change process among faculty (Mawn & Reece, 2000), various levels of approval that may exist in some institutions, and realities of faculty members' other responsibilities. Once the reverse ordering is completed, the chart can be rotated so that it starts with the most immediate activities and ends with curriculum implementation. Alternately, a Gantt chart could be devised. The advantage of the Gantt chart is that it illustrates the duration of activities to achieve each milestone. A Gantt chart to match Table 7-2 is presented in **Table 7-3**, with the shaded areas representing the time period to work on the activities necessary to achieve the milestones.

Suggesting a Faculty Development Plan

The curriculum leader could suggest a tentative plan for faculty development activities based on the overall progression of curriculum development tasks. The plan must be open to change in response to emerging needs. However, if the leader plans and schedules some initial sessions, novice curriculum developers will gain a sense of assurance in their ability to participate meaningfully in curriculum development.

Introducing the Possibility of Scholarship Projects Linked to Curriculum Work

The curriculum leader should introduce the possibility of scholarship projects arising from curriculum work and lead discussion about this. This text provides many ideas that the leader could present so that faculty members and stakeholders can consider their involvement. If there is agreement about engaging in scholarship, authorship matters should also be addressed.

Clarifying the Relationship of Curriculum Development and Implementation to Academic Freedom

The curriculum leader might clarify the relationship between curriculum development and implementation to academic freedom so that all understand that they are free to propose

Table 7-2 Example of a Critical Path for Curriculum Development

Milestones	Completion Date	Group/Individual Responsible
Implement first courses	September 2017	Course faculty
Finalize planning for first courses	May 2017	Faculty for each course
Interpret curriculum to healthcare and community partners	January–February 2017	Curriculum leader, Curriculum Committee
Achieve institutional approval	December 2016	Institutional senior academic body
Forward curriculum documents to institutional governing body for approval	October 2016	School leader, Curriculum leader
Present curriculum and policies for School of Nursing approval	October 2016	Curriculum leader
Present curriculum to Steering and/or Advisory Committee	September/October 2016	Curriculum leader
Complete all aspects of curriculum design and policy development	September 2016	Curriculum Committee, designated subcommittees
Complete course descriptions	September 2016	Course teams
Negotiate non-nursing courses	July 2016	School leader, Curriculum leader
Approve curriculum design and matrix	June 2016	Total faculty group
Complete curriculum design and matrix	May 2016	Design subcommittee
Approve philosophical and educational approaches, and goals or outcomes	April 2016	Total faculty group
Finalize philosophical and educational approaches, and goals or outcomes	March 2016	Designated subcommittees
Agree on curriculum concepts	January 2016	Total faculty group
Present contextual data	December 2015	Contextual data subgroup
Organize for curriculum development: form committees, begin faculty development	September 2015	Curriculum leader, total faculty group
Form Steering and/or Advisory Committee	September 2015	School leader

Table 7-3 Gantt Chart for Curriculum Development

Deadlines → / Milestones ↓	Sept. 2015	Oct. 2015	Nov. 2015	Dec. 2015	Jan. 2016	Feb. 2016	Mar. 2016	Apr. 2016	May 2016	June 2016	July 2016	Aug. 2016	Sept. 2016	Oct. 2016	Nov 2017	Dec. 2016	Jan. 2017	Feb. 2017	Mar. 2017	Apr. 2017	May 2017	June 2017	July 2017	Aug. 2017	Sept. 2017
Form steering and/or advisory committee(s)	■																								
Form committees		■																							
Faculty development		■	■													■	■	■	■	■	■	■	■	■	■
Collect and present contextual data			■	■																					
Agree on curriculum concepts					■																				
Finalize philosophical and educational approaches, and goals or outcomes		■	■	■	■	■	■																		
Approve philosophical and educational approaches, and goals or outcomes								■																	
Complete curriculum design and matrix								■	■	■															
Approve curriculum design and matrix										■															

Task
Negotiate regarding non-nursing courses
Complete course descriptions
Complete curriculum design and policy development
Present curriculum to steering and/ or advisory committee(s)
Approve curriculum and policies
Forward curriculum documents for institutional approval
Achieve institutional approval
Interpret curriculum to professional practice partners
Finalize planning for first courses
Implement first courses

unconventional ideas, yet are ultimately bound by the decisions of the total group. Novice faculty members might not initially realize that they need not be constrained in their curriculum suggestions by notions of what might be acceptable. Faculty committed to particular ideas may need to be reminded that the total faculty group is the ultimate authority in curriculum matters and not them alone.

Academic freedom is "the free search for truth and its free exposition" (American Association of University Professors, n.d.). This includes freedom in teaching, research, publication, and criticism of the institution. Writing about academic freedom and scientific inquiry in nursing, Kneipp, Canales, Fahrenwald, and Taylor (2007) state:

> With academic freedom comes academic duty . . . the duty to argue persuasively and logically for theoretical perspectives, areas of research and new methodological approaches, that you as a member of the scientific community, believe hold merit for advancing science in your field. (p. 8)

The same duty applies to nursing curriculum development. Each faculty member has the obligation to argue logically for preferred curricular perspectives, advance a position about the nature and content of the curriculum, and propose how the suggested perspective will advance the curriculum.

Yet, academic freedom has limits. Larson (1997) suggests that faculty sometimes perceive academic freedom as giving each nursing faculty member the right to plan courses independently, without attention to how these conform to the entire curriculum. She contends that this is not realistic nor should it be supported. "Academic freedom is a qualified right . . . a privilege enjoyed in consequence of incumbency in . . . an academic role and it is enjoyed conditionally in conformity with certain obligations to the academic institution and its rules and standards" (Shils, 1993, p. 189). The standards for the nursing curriculum are established by the nursing faculty, and each member is obligated to plan the curriculum and implement courses in accordance with those standards. Moreover, Orzeck (2012) asserts that academic freedom is not an individual right, but rather a means of self-regulation of the academic profession by professors. This means that it is the collective nursing faculty that regulate the curriculum and its implementation.

Faculty are granted freedom in the classroom in discussing their subject (American Association of University Professors, n.d.; Canadian Association of University Teachers, 2011). Yet, teaching must be undertaken "with due respect to what is thought by qualified colleagues" (Shils, 1993, p. 190). It is for this reason that curricula are created collaboratively: The curriculum represents the consensus and the self-regulation of colleagues.

There must be unity and progression within professional curricula. Therefore, creating courses in isolation from one another, or without reference to agreed-upon philosophical approaches or curriculum outcome statements, is neither acceptable nor sound. Curriculum development, however, should not be so constrained that creativity, pedagogical preferences, and expertise of faculty are stifled. There should be a balance between faculty autonomy and curriculum intent. A frank discussion among the curriculum leader, faculty members, and the school leader would ensure resolution of the latitude possible when individual courses are planned and implemented.

Finally, because the requirement to contribute to curriculum may compete with other scholarly activities, such as research, some faculty may feel their academic freedom is being restricted by an expectation that they participate in curriculum work. If this is the case, open discussion about academic rights and responsibilities is warranted. It may be reasonable for the school leader to adjust the work assignments of some faculty to accommodate individual scholarly activities during curriculum development.

Negotiating for Resources

As the overall plan for curriculum development is shaped, the necessary resources will become apparent. It is advisable for the curriculum leader to follow up preliminary discussions with the school leader and negotiate for resources to support curriculum development. The requests could include release time from teaching for key curriculum developers; a specific budget for data-collection activities, faculty development, or curriculum consultation; and secretarial support. Although alterations in work assignments may be subject to collective agreements, they are worthy of exploration, because it is primarily the faculty who must develop, accept, and implement the curriculum.

FACULTY MEMBERS' RESPONSIBILITIES IN ORGANIZING FOR CURRICULUM DEVELOPMENT

Faculty members have specific responsibilities in relation to organizing for curriculum development. Fulfilling these may require further guidance by the curriculum leader.

Participating on Committees to Complete Curriculum Development Tasks

Faculty members are obligated to join curriculum committees and to commit to achieving the committee's task. Within the committees, initial discussion may mirror the ideas described earlier, such as deciding which stakeholders to invite to join the committee, deciding on decision-making processes, and recordkeeping and communication systems. In addition, it is necessary to clarify the committee's task, schedule meetings, decide how to share the work, and complete the work assigned within the specified timeline.

Clarification of the task that each committee is to complete is usually the first matter for discussion when faculty members and other stakeholders initially meet. Although the committee responsibility would have been defined in the overall plan for committee structure, each group needs to ensure that members have a shared understanding of the task, and that the group's understanding is consistent with the intent originally conceived for it.

Regular meetings should be scheduled for participants to carefully assess, study, and create new ideas, and members should commit to being present for the meetings. If there are enough committed and qualified committee members who have expertise or who seek assistance, and who also meet on a regular basis, the goal of a developed curriculum will be achieved in a timely manner. It is neither practical nor productive to spend an extensive period of time on any one component of the curriculum. Despite the discomfort that may accompany decisions that are not firmly fixed, the group should move on to completion. As the work progresses through subsequent meetings, final decisions can be accomplished.

Curriculum development can be a slow process if groups meet infrequently. Also, the process cannot be effective if crisis-oriented approaches are used and work is begun only immediately before deadlines. Accordingly, a written, realistic timetable to guide the activities of the group is important, because it places the activity in the context of its priority and the group's commitment to the entire process. Too short a time period could be self-defeating or viewed as a lack of regard for members' time and other responsibilities. In contrast, too extended a time interval can lead to discouragement, disinterest, and disenchantment with the process and progress. A written schedule, or a detailed critical path of group activities and meetings will help to maintain participant interest and support the expectation that a revised or reconceptualized curriculum will be accomplished.

Decisions about sharing the work must be made by each committee. Inherent in all group work is the need to determine how activities will be completed. Who will do what, and to what standard? Within each committee, the matter of how to share the work will arise, and the approach is unlikely to be identical among groups. In some, all members may prefer to work together as much as possible, to explore ideas and achieve consensus before much writing is done. For others, there may be a desire to divide tasks among individuals or dyads, who would then bring back draft work to the group for discussion, revision, and consensus. Likely, some combination of these approaches will be agreed upon, depending on the nature of the task and the imminence of deadlines. Although it is beyond the scope of this text to describe all aspects of successful group functioning, some elements are worthy of review when considering how curriculum development can be accomplished:

- Agree on the goals to be achieved, including the task to be accomplished, the deadline for completion, and the standard of the work.
- Obtain commitment from each member to achieve the goals.

- Identify how much time each member can give to the task.
- Discuss how the group will work together.
- Consider the value of preparing a critical path for the group's work.

Welcoming Stakeholders

Curriculum development is accomplished through group work, and it is necessary to welcome students, clinicians, and consumers to the curriculum committees. Committee members may suggest particular individuals as possible members, or they may receive notice that some have volunteered for the committee. In either case, the stakeholders may not be familiar with the culture of nursing education and the nature of curriculum work. Therefore, it is recommended that attention be given to helping them understand the curriculum development process and making them feel they are respected members with valuable contributions to make.

Seeking Input

Faculty members working on committee tasks need to seek the input of stakeholders not represented on the committee. This can be done by inviting them to become members or to attend selected meetings, by interviews with faculty members, through survey tools for reactions to issues and ideas, and in total faculty group meetings, with materials sent out beforehand for review. Perspectives of the total student body (in addition to student representation on committees) can be obtained in a similar manner.

Considering Scholarship Projects

Finally, each group should consider the potential for a scholarship project in the work it is completing. Although this may seem daunting when the curriculum work is beginning, it is a worthwhile topic for the agenda of each committee meeting. Ideas will emerge, and possibly with the help of the curriculum leader, projects can be developed.

CORE PROCESSES OF CURRICULUM WORK

Faculty Development

Once a decision has been made to proceed with curriculum development, it would be helpful to have a faculty development session about change processes and the curriculum development process itself. Specifically, a summary of the entire process will help novices appreciate that curriculum development is an iterative process, replete with concurrent and recurrent subprocesses. However, to ensure that faculty members do not feel over-whelmed, it is wise to identify the concrete tasks that ensure timely completion of the work. The goal is for faculty to comprehend the process and believe that it is manageable. An overview of the logistics of getting organized is essential so faculty will believe that the work is achievable.

Ongoing Appraisal

Ongoing appraisal of the organizing activities occurs spontaneously as matters are being discussed. Faculty members offer ideas in response to those proposed by the curriculum leader and colleagues. These responses are a form of appraisal and will shape the final decisions about how to proceed.

To ensure that appraisal is built into the discussion, the curriculum leader might ask such questions as:

- How does that seem to you?
- Are there other possibilities that might be workable?
- Does this seem feasible?
- Can we commit to this plan?

Similarly, faculty and stakeholder members can be counted on to appraise the ideas about how to proceed within individual curriculum committees.

Scholarship

The idea of scholarship about organizing for curriculum development may seem odd, but projects, presentations, and publications about the process could be instructive for future curriculum development within the school of nursing and for colleagues elsewhere. Possible retrospective scholarship projects could be:

- Faculty, stakeholder, and curriculum leader appraisal and satisfaction with the pro-cesses undertaken to organize for curriculum development
- An analysis of the effectiveness of the committee structure, communication system, and so forth as curriculum work proceeds

A study might be undertaken to assess the pre- and post-faculty development knowl-edge, attitudes, and confidence of novice faculty members and stakeholders. This will provide insight into the effectiveness of the initial faculty development and into the areas where the curriculum leader might offer assistance through consultation with commit-tees or ongoing faculty development.

CHAPTER SUMMARY

Practical guidelines about organizing for curriculum development are the focus of this chapter. The curriculum leader is responsible for guiding faculty to consensus about values and beliefs, discussing an overall plan with faculty, creating a critical path, suggesting faculty development, introducing ideas about scholarship potential in curriculum development, and negotiating for resources. Faculty members have responsibility for participating on committees to complete curriculum development tasks, welcoming stakeholders, seeking input, and considering scholarship projects. Included are ideas about faculty development, ongoing appraisal, and scholarship related to the initial organization.

SYNTHESIS ACTIVITIES

The Sycamore University College of Nursing case includes some ideas about organizing for curriculum development. The questions that follow provide a basis for analysis of the situation. Subsequently, questions are posed that might assist readers when organizing for curriculum development in their own settings.

Sycamore University College of Nursing

The nursing curriculum at Sycamore University was developed over 3 years and has been offered in its present form for almost 10 years. One-third of current faculty members participated in the original curriculum development. Now, nursing faculty, university administrators, and alumni of Sycamore University have agreed that the current 4-year nursing curriculum warrants replacement.

Although periodic curriculum adjustments have been made in response to ongoing healthcare needs of the community, changes in nursing education, and aspirations of nursing students, it has become apparent that small changes are no longer sufficient to ensure excellence in the curriculum. In particular, many faculty members believe the curriculum's medical model is outmoded and does not allow sufficient opportunity for community nursing and the inclusion of important concepts such as *determinants of health*. Not all faculty are convinced of the need for a strong emphasis on community health, but there is consensus that after 10 years, it is time to begin the development of a new curriculum.

The school leader, Dr. Isabel Perkins, has appointed Dr. Lakeisha Williams, the current chair of the Curriculum Committee, to lead curriculum development. Dr. Perkins believes that Dr. Williams has the necessary curriculum expertise, relational skills, organizational ability, and knowledge of the university to spearhead the curriculum endeavor.

Dr. Williams meets with the Curriculum Committee to consider possible ways of organizing for the curriculum undertaking. The Committee decides that it should serve as the Steering Committee with the following responsibilities:

- Coordinating, overseeing, and supporting the work of faculty and stakeholders
- Receiving regular progress reports
- Serving as a communication link for the curriculum work

The Curriculum Committee also considers committee structure and whether it would be more advantageous to have:

- One design team to create all necessary elements of the curriculum, leaving the details of course development to the relevant faculty, *or*
- Several committees, each with defined responsibilities

Finally, committee members propose stakeholders who might be involved and, briefly, an overall timeline.

Dr. Williams informs the group that she will consolidate their ideas into an overall plan, with deadlines, and then call a meeting of faculty to present the plan and discuss organizing for curriculum development. Committee members agree that decisions will have to be made about organizational matters at that meeting so that the work of curriculum development can begin quickly.

As Dr. Williams prepares for the faculty meeting, she recognizes that whichever committee structure is decided, she will have to assist each committee or subcommittee to define the precise nature of its work and determine a critical path for completion of the work. She intends to make clear that she will do that and will assist the faculty with their work. She is also cognizant of the need for communication among working groups and will give attention to this in the faculty meeting. Dr. Williams also considers other matters to raise with faculty members, and whether or not to invite key stakeholders to the organizing meeting.

Questions and Activities for Critical Analysis of the Sycamore University College of Nursing Case

1. Assess the wisdom of the Curriculum Committee's decision to act as the Steering Committee. Consider whether the responsibilities are feasible and complete.

2. In what circumstances would it be appropriate for the Curriculum Committee to be the Steering Committee? Should other members be added? If so, who? If other members are not needed, why not?

3. Appraise the merits of the two forms of curriculum structure that were considered by the Curriculum Committee.

4. Propose committees that could be created in order to facilitate curriculum development. What purposes would they serve? Who should the members be?

5. What ideas not addressed by the Curriculum Committee will Dr. Williams have to introduce when she meets with faculty to discuss organizing for curriculum development?

6. Describe decision-making approaches that could be effective for the curriculum developers.

7. What could be the reasons for inviting key stakeholders to the organizing meeting? For not inviting them?

8. Reflect on the fact that there is consensus about the need for curriculum development, but not agreement about an emphasis on community nursing. In what ways might a discussion about values assist the faculty to work productively?

9. Explain how Dr. Williams can help faculty to view scholarship as an integral part of curriculum work.

10. Suggest faculty development activities that could be helpful as curriculum development begins.

Questions and Activities for Consideration When Organizing for Curriculum Development in Readers' Settings

1. What approaches to decision making are most commonly used in the School of Nursing? How effective are they in achieving goals? Should alternate decision-making approaches be considered?

2. When is the new curriculum to be implemented? Outline the activities necessary to develop the curriculum. What are the processes and timelines for approval within the School of Nursing and at the institutional level?

3. Determine the best way to develop a critical path. Who will assume responsibility for developing it?

4. Consider the implications curriculum development will have for the current work of faculty.

5. What committee structure(s) for curriculum development might be most efficient and successful? Who should participate on the committees and why? How will membership on committees be determined?

6. Assess the suitability of a steering committee comprised of senior administrators. Would a critique committee be advantageous? Why or why not? How could members of these committees be helpful to the curriculum development process?

7. List the agreements that should be reached within committees so members are organized to accomplish their work.

8. What would be effective recordkeeping and communication systems for curriculum development?

9. How do faculty members generally respond to faculty development activities? How are they likely to respond as they organize for curriculum development? What strategies have been most effective in moving the group forward? How can faculty development necessary to initiate curriculum development be planned?

10. Describe how the resources to support curriculum development can be discussed with the administrator.

11. How can curriculum development be achieved if resources do not exist for the appointment of a curriculum leader with teaching release time, and/or periodic release time for some faculty members?

12. What are the questions that should be asked in the ongoing appraisal of organizing for curriculum development?

13. Propose scholarship ideas related to organizing for curriculum development.

REFERENCES

American Association of University Professors. (n.d.). *1940 Statement of principles on academic freedom and tenure with 1970 interpretive comments*. Retrieved from http://www.aaup.org/report/1940-statement-principles-academic-freedom-and-tenure

Black, J., Morris, T., Harbert, A., & Mathias, C. (2008). Educational collaboration in psychiatric disability, rehabilitation, and recovery: Developing transformative solutions. *Journal of Social Work in Disability & Rehabilitation, 7*, 163–186.

Cambers, W. (2010). Collaboration and curriculum design—a stakeholder symposium. *Mental Health Nursing, 30*(2), 14–15.

Canadian Association of University Teachers. (2011). *Policy statement on academic freedom.* Retrieved from http://www.caut.ca/about-us/caut-policy/lists/caut-policy-statements/policy-statement-on-academic-freedom

Dvir, D., & Lechler, T. (2004). Plans are nothing, changing plans is everything: The impact of changes on project success. *Research Policy, 33*, 1–15.

Glatthorn, A. A., Boschee, F., & Whitehead, B. M. (2009). *Curriculum leadership: Strategies for development and implementation* (2nd ed.). Thousand Oaks, CA: Sage.

Kneipp, S. M., Canales, M. K., Fahrenwald, N., & Taylor, J. Y. (2007). Academic freedom: Protecting "liberal science" in nursing in the 21st century. *Advances in Nursing Science, 30*(1), 3–13.

Larson, E. (1997). Academic freedom amidst competing demands. *Journal of Professional Nursing, 13*, 211–216.

Mawn, B., & Reece, S. M. (2000). Reconfiguring a curriculum for the new millennium: The process of change. *Journal of Nursing Education, 39*, 101–108.

National League for Nursing. (2003). *Position statement: Innovation in nursing education: A call to reform.* Retrieved from http://www.nln.org/aboutnln/PositionStatements/innovation082203.pdf

Orzeck, R. (2012). Academic freedom, intellectual diversity, and the place of politics in geography. *Antipose, 44*, 1449–1469.

Palmer, S. P., Harmer Cox, A., Clark Callister, L., Johnsen, V., & Matsumara, G. (2005). Nursing education and service collaboration: Making a difference in the clinical learning environment. *Journal of Continuing Education in Nursing, 36*, 271–276.

Pardue, K. T. (2006). A first step toward reform: Results of the faculty survey on innovation. *Nursing Education Perspectives, 27*, 56–57.

Shils, E. (1993). Do we still need academic freedom? *American Scholar, 62*, 187–207.

PART IV

Development of an Evidence-Informed, Context-Relevant, Unified Curriculum

CHAPTER 8

Gathering Data for an Evidence-Informed, Context-Relevant, Unified Curriculum

Chapter Overview

An evidence-informed, context-relevant, unified curriculum is responsive to the educational and societal environment in which it is offered and to the environment that is expected to exist in the future. To create such a curriculum, contextual factors within and beyond the school of nursing must be investigated. The contextual factors are the forces, situations, and circumstances that curriculum developers take into account as they plan a curriculum. The typology of contextual factors presented in this chapter is a reasonable way to conceptualize them, although other categorizations are possible. Approaches to gathering data are outlined, including considerations to determine essential data and data sources to pursue. The term *gathering data* is used to differentiate the activity of obtaining information for curriculum development from the data collection of research projects. The relationship of gathering data to an evidence-informed, context-relevant, unified curriculum is explained. Additionally, the core processes of curriculum work pertinent to gathering data about contextual factors are described. Synthesis activities include a case study for analysis, and questions and activities for readers to consider when gathering contextual data.

Chapter Goals

- Identify internal and external contextual factors that influence curriculum.
- Determine essential data to gather about the contextual factors.
- Explore methods for gathering data and identify data sources relevant to curriculum development.
- Appreciate the relationship of contextual factors to an evidence-informed, context-relevant, unified curriculum.
- Consider core processes of curriculum work related to gathering data about contextual factors.

OVERVIEW OF THE CONTEXTUAL FACTORS, AND GATHERING AND INTERPRETING CONTEXTUAL DATA

The environment of the curriculum can be conceptualized as being composed of interrelated contextual factors. *Contextual factors* are those forces, situations, and circumstances that exist both within and outside the school of nursing and have the potential to influence the school and its programs. Although the factors are complex and ever changing, form and boundaries must be given to them so that the concept of contextual factors is understandable and useful for curriculum development.

For the purposes of curriculum development, internal contextual factors are those forces, situations, and circumstances that originate within the school and educational institution, that is, within the internal environment of the educational institution. External contextual factors are those forces, situations, and circumstances that originate outside the educational institution in the community, region, country, and world. A typology of internal and external contextual factors is described in subsequent sections of this chapter.

Although differentiated for the purpose of descriptive clarity, in reality, some contextual factors blend and overlap. Additionally, some factors exist in both internal and external environments. For example, culture can be seen as an internal contextual factor when described in relation to a school of nursing, and as an external contextual factor when reviewed in relation to a community.

Because the contextual factors (e.g., social, political, and economic) can be large and nebulous, an examination of the context in its totality can be complicated and overwhelming (McKeown, 2012). Therefore, curriculum developers must precisely define which data are essential to obtain about each factor. The essential data are the specific facts and information about the contextual factors deemed most likely to shape the curriculum. These data might be as subtle as nurses' attitudes toward students in one healthcare agency or as concrete as attrition rates in the nursing program. Clearly, the more definitive the data that are obtained, the stronger the basis will be for designing the curriculum.

Gathering data purposefully about the contextual factors and the subsequent analysis of the data will yield the "big picture" of the current and future environment in which the curriculum will be offered, and result in curriculum concepts that will remain relevant into the future. Thorough gathering and analysis of data are foundational to the development of an evidence-informed, context-relevant, unified nursing curriculum. The examination of the context ensures that curriculum developers do not unthinkingly react to societal events without consideration of the reasonable weighting of the events within the totality of the context, and thus within the totality of the curriculum. Events and changes in the internal and external environments may have "echo effects" (Cornbleth, 2008) within the curriculum, but a good understanding of all the relevant contextual data will lead to a curriculum echo of appropriate volume.

The emphasis on gathering and interpreting data about the contextual factors is most aligned with ideas of environmental scanning and strategic thinking, planning, and management. This approach leads to programs that are developed for current and anticipated opportunities in the external context, with careful consideration of the realities and possibilities of the internal environment (Bryson, 2011; Henry, 2011; Hunger & Wheelen, 2011). This process is not synonymous with a needs assessment, which connotes a gap between the present state and a predetermined desired state, and which could result in a curriculum with a relatively short lifespan. The approach described in this text will result in a description of the desired qualities of graduates that is deduced from contextual data. As such, the curriculum that is developed will be relevant not only for the present, but also for the future.

INTERNAL CONTEXTUAL FACTORS

As stated previously, the internal contextual factors are those forces, situations, and circumstances that originate within the school of nursing and educational institution. These include the institution's and school's mission, vision, philosophy, and goals; culture and climate; history; financial resources; programs and policies; and infrastructure.

Mission, Vision, Philosophy, and Goals

Every organization has a mission, which is a succinct statement that captures the institution's distinctive character. It is a "broadly defined and enduring statement of purpose that distinguishes an organization . . . from other organizations of its type" (Swayne, Duncan, & Ginter, 2008, p. 162). The uniqueness of the institution and the scope of its activities are evident in the mission statement. As such, the mission informs those within and outside the organization of its ultimate raison d'être. The educational institution's mission shapes the nature, scope, and boundaries of the mission, activities, and curricula of the school of nursing.

The educational institution and the school of nursing also have a vision, a mental image of what the organization will achieve when it is fully accomplishing its mission. This vision is expressed in a broad and forward-looking statement that is the organization's "hope for the future" (Swayne et al., 2008, p. 161), the goals it will strive to achieve (Harrison, 2010). As such, the vision provides direction to curriculum developers.

Institutions of higher education also have clearly articulated guiding principles, or beliefs and values, about the services offered, the community served, and the fundamental activities that take place within them. Statements about education, learning, knowledge development, scholarship, and so forth form the philosophy. In addition to understanding the institution's philosophy or guiding principles, it is important for curriculum developers to identify those that operate within the school of nursing.

The mission, vision, purpose, and values of the educational institution and school of nursing are articulated most directly in their strategic goals and strategic plans. It is advisable for curriculum developers to give these considerable attention. The long- and short-term goals, objectives, timelines, and critical outcomes for the institution and school will give insights about institutional priorities. Data from the strategic plan give direction to recommendations about the curriculum. Conversely, knowledge of the strategic plan can signal potential roadblocks to curriculum development or particular preferences about the curriculum. Because the nursing curriculum must be congruent with the educational institution's mission, vision, philosophy, and fundamental guiding principles, curriculum developers require a solid understanding of these.

Organizational Culture and Climate

Each organization has a culture or "way of being" that is unlikely to be explicitly stated, but that affects all people within the organization and those who interact with it. The culture is a pattern of shared values, assumptions, attitudes, expectations, and behaviors that are usually taught implicitly to new members. It is brought to awareness when its premises are breached, and this situation is often expressed in statements such as, "That's not the way we do things here."

Organizational climate is the shared perceptions of, and meanings attached to:

- Policies and procedures experienced by employees and others
- Observations of behaviors that are rewarded, supported, and expected (Schneider, Ehrhart, & Macey, 2013)

The concepts of organizational culture and organizational climate overlap. Therefore, adjectives or metaphors used to encapsulate prominent aspects of the culture and climate may reflect one or both concepts (e.g., progressive or traditional; friendly or hostile; bureaucratic or participatory, like a family, toxic).

Organizational culture and climate evolve over time and can be slow to change. They are formed by determinants such as the people in the organization, how these people interact and make decisions, the endeavors and decisions pursued or avoided, the consequences of these actions, and people's interpretations of all that they experience and observe. A significant aspect of the school's culture is whether change is welcomed or avoided. If a new curriculum is premised on a changed culture in the school, or will require a reallocation of resources that will alter the culture and climate, curriculum developers must strategize carefully, because a change in organizational culture and climate is difficult to accomplish.

History

Examining the institution's history will reveal past values, successes, and challenges, as well as the school's processes for curriculum development. Much can be learned about how past challenges have been met and successes achieved. This information may still be pertinent for decisions about the curriculum. For example, if the educational institution has built an international reputation, curriculum developers might examine the way this was done, and ask how the nursing curriculum could contribute to or capitalize on this renown. Answers to the following questions may provide some insight into the history of the institution and the school of nursing:

- When were the educational institution and the school of nursing founded, and why?
- Have the institution's and school's mission, vision, and purposes changed over time? If so, why and how?
- How does the school's history influence current programs and operations?
- What programs are offered? How have these evolved? Over what timeframe?
- Were programs developed for a niche market?
- What are the unique features that have developed within the institution, the school, and the programs?

When preparing a new curriculum, faculty members are shaping the future and creating the school's ongoing history. Accordingly, the processes and decisions should be recorded for future curriculum developers, so they will not be dependent on a few faculty members who are the custodians of the institutional memory, and whose recollections are lost when they leave the school.

Financial Resources

Financial resources, possibly more than any other internal contextual factor, influence the curriculum design. Knowledge of the operating costs of a school, budget planning, and budget allocation is essential. In addition, attention can be given to possible funding sources for curriculum development and innovation.

Careful analysis should be directed to the cost that would be created by a redesigned curriculum. Funding limits can constrain the curriculum design, and adequate financial resources are essential for successful implementation. For example, if there are tentative thoughts about changing from an upper division baccalaureate program to a 4-year generic program, then it is essential to ascertain what this would mean for the school's budget. Such knowledge would signal whether the idea is worthy of exploration or whether it should be abandoned.

Programs and Policies

The programs and policies of the educational institution and the school of nursing form an important aspect of the internal environment. Within the school, the type and number of programs, physical and human resources dedicated to those programs, and the relationship of the developing curriculum to other programs will influence curriculum design. For example, if caring for, and advocating with, vulnerable populations is a theme of the graduate program, it would be reasonable to expect some emphasis in this area in a redesigned undergraduate curriculum. Additionally, key features of evaluations of the current curriculum can provide ideas to curriculum developers.

The range of courses offered by other departments could be an asset to the curriculum designers or limit the scope of what they can propose. Knowledge from the physical, biological, and psychosocial sciences, as well as from the arts and humanities, contributes significantly to nursing knowledge and well-rounded graduates. Hence, courses from these disciplines are essential in a nursing curriculum. The availability of courses, prerequisites, and scheduling should be ascertained. The possibility of negotiating new non-nursing courses may exist. Although typically called *support courses*, they are called *non-nursing courses* in this text because they do not merely support the nursing curriculum; they are an integral part of it.

Additionally, programs in other health science disciplines should be surveyed. Previously unused interdisciplinary or interprofessional learning opportunities may exist, or may be negotiated if the curriculum developers consider them important.

Existing policies and guidelines are important reference points during curriculum development. Institutional and school policies and guidelines should be available and understood by the curriculum development team. It can be time consuming and complicated to gain the necessary approval for revision or addition of school policies as part of curriculum development, and any changes have to be accomplished within the context of existing institutional regulations. Requests for policy changes that might affect the educational institution are more complex and can be expected to take a longer period of time to achieve.

Infrastructure

The term *infrastructure* refers to those elements that form the structure of the educational institution and school of nursing, and serve as the foundation of educational programs. Elements of the infrastructure include human and physical resources, as well as resources to support teaching and learning. Data can be secured and scrutinized to obtain a comprehensive picture of the infrastructure.

Human Resources

Human resources form the core of the curriculum and are the most important resources of the institution. It is largely through interactions between and among students and faculty that the curriculum is experienced; therefore, people are the center of the curriculum.

Faculty are key contributors to curriculum development and implementation, and represent a vital part of the internal infrastructure. They are critical sources of insight and information about what to include in the curriculum, because they know what works, what doesn't, and why. They bring the curriculum to life, execute all its dimensions, and have a vested interest in student and curriculum success.

Information about current nursing and non-nursing faculty and the pool of potential faculty is an important determinant of curriculum development decisions. Data about areas of specialty, educational preparation, possible retirement dates, preferences for teaching area, and so forth will be valuable.

Students are an essential human resource, as important as faculty members. Schools of nursing would not exist were it not for students; without them, there is no need for curriculum. Student data form the basis of much internal contextual information critical to curriculum development, because the curriculum is designed for them. **Table 8-1** lists student data that could be obtained to enhance understanding of the internal contextual environment. Moreover, students are vital members of curriculum development teams.

The amount and nature of information that can be obtained about current and potential students and faculty are governed by institutional policies and human rights and privacy legislation. As an example, in some jurisdictions it is possible to ask about race; in others, it is not.

Stakeholders, such as adjunct faculty, guest lecturers, clinical experts, preceptors, and healthcare leaders form part of faculty resources. They need to be considered when shaping the curriculum, not only for the contributions they might make to the future curriculum, but also for the involvement and perspectives they can offer to curriculum development, implementation, and evaluation.

Support staff are another important human resource. Programs could not function without people such as secretaries, admissions officers, caretakers, information technology specialists, and others. They make possible the smooth day-to-day operations of the school. Gathering data about this group, such as numbers and skill sets, is mandatory.

Information about human resources includes details about contracts that govern the working life of faculty and staff. A review of faculty and staff collective agreements provides insights into matters such as job expectations, holiday entitlement, hours of work, and so forth. These all influence the curriculum. For example, if it is not possible to assign full-time faculty to teach on weekends, then curriculum designers would have to weigh the

Table 8-1   Student Data
Number of applicants
Number of admissions
Numbers meeting and exceeding admission requirements
Demographics: • Previous education • Age • Marital status • Number of dependents • Employment status
Catchment area
Proportion of full- and part-time students
Grade point average
Grades in nursing and non-nursing courses
Attrition rates and rationale
Success rate on registration or licensure examinations
Follow-up data about graduates: • Employment positions • Employer evaluations • Numbers admitted to graduate programs

(handwritten margin note: "9et how do we get this data?")

educational value of weekend professional practice experiences against the effects of inaccessibility of full-time faculty.

Physical Resources

Availability and quality of materials and space for classrooms, offices, and laboratories require consideration because they influence what is possible in the curriculum. Knowledge of these resources can also be a basis for negotiating for new or additional facilities to match developing ideas about curriculum design and student learning needs.

Technology is an important part of the physical resources. Availability and adequacy of office computers, student computer labs, audiovisual and clinical equipment, smart classrooms, distributed learning technology, high-fidelity mannequins, and the like should be determined. Technologies assist faculty to fulfill their roles efficiently, are necessary for effective teaching, and facilitate student learning.

Resources to Support Teaching and Learning

Resources that support teaching and learning should also be examined. Knowing what is available will assist in making curriculum decisions, planning, and negotiating for additional resources.

Library resources are essential for teaching and learning. Facilities and collections should be reviewed with respect to the strengths and gaps in the library's collection. Online databases extend the library's holdings, and their availability and ease of access have implications for curriculum and course designs, student assignments, and faculty research. Knowledge about shortcomings in library holdings provides a basis for negotiating altered or expanded materials and services.

Faculty development services are another element of the internal infrastructure. School and institution-wide programs related to teaching and research development can be sources of ideas and support for a new curriculum. If, for example, institution-wide programs for developing and enhancing online courses are provided, then curriculum developers will know that distributed learning courses could be planned or expanded. However, if there are no institution-wide programs relevant to teaching-learning or evaluation in the envisioned curriculum, then curriculum developers will have the following four choices as they plan the curriculum and its implementation:

- Create and offer the faculty development program themselves.
- Hire a consultant.
- Negotiate for an institution-wide program that will not be specific to nursing.
- Avoid particular teaching-learning and evaluation approaches in the new curriculum.

Teaching support, such as graduate teaching assistants or other university-employed or university-sponsored students, can extend faculty teaching. Typically, graduate students contribute to curriculum implementation through teaching, grading assignments, and leading tutorial sessions.

Student services related to assessment and development of academic skills, personal support, health, recreation, and financial assistance are integral aspects of the institutional infrastructure. These services can mean the difference between success and failure for many students.

An inventory of available resources, knowledge of future plans for resources and services, and the possibility of negotiating new ones are influential when shaping and bringing vitality to the curriculum. Curricularists must understand the infrastructure in which the redesigned curriculum will operate so they can plan a feasible curriculum with conviction, secure in the knowledge that the resources will be available to bring their plans to fruition.

Summary of Internal Contextual Factors

In summary, internal contextual factors are those forces, situations, and circumstances that originate within the school and educational institution and have potential to influence the curriculum. These should be examined in two ways: a macro view to capture the contextual data relevant to the institution and a micro view to focus more specifically on the school of nursing.

EXTERNAL CONTEXTUAL FACTORS

As described previously, external contextual factors are those forces, situations, and circumstances that originate outside the educational institution and also have the potential to influence curriculum. They originate in the community, region, country, and world, that is, the environment beyond the educational institution. An examination of external contextual factors is crucial to understanding the characteristics, goals, and needs of society and the nursing profession, and their application to contemporary nursing curricula. A brief survey of the most influential external contextual factors follows.

Demographics

Demography can be defined as:

> The study of human populations in terms of size, density, location, age, sex, race, occupation, and other statistics. It is also the description of the vital statistics or objective and quantifiable characteristics of an audience or population. Demographic designators include age, marital status, income, family size, occupation, and personal or household characteristics such as age, sex, income, or educational level. (Doyle, 2011)

Demographic data, which have a significant influence on healthcare delivery and nursing education, should be obtained. Information pertaining to population characteristics assists curriculum developers to know about the people who are and will be clients of the healthcare system. The nursing curriculum can then be designed to align with the attributes of those who are and will be recipients of nursing care. Local, regional, and national data can be obtained. Pertinent data include the following:

- Birth, death, and fertility rates
- Distribution according to age, sex, location, and combinations of these
- Population diversity
- Employment rates and income levels by age and sex
- Ethnicity

- Residence patterns (e.g., proportion of aged living alone, in nursing homes)
- Morbidity rates and patterns
- Family structures
- Population mobility
- Immigration and emigration patterns

Culture

Further to assessing the demographics of the human populations nurses serve, curriculum developers direct attention to the culture(s) within the external environment. *Culture of a group* refers to:

> The way of life of a people, including their attitudes, values, beliefs, arts, sciences, modes of perception, and habits of thought and activity. Cultural features of forms of life are learned but are often too pervasive to be readily noticed from within. (Blackburn, 2014)

Included in the concept are a common history; sense of destiny; value system embedded in a particular religion or mythology; and shared traditions, rituals, language with a distinctive vocabulary, and "narratives that give [express] norms, and models of behavior" (Sitelman & Sitelman, 2000, p. 12). Moreover, a culture is dynamic and experienced differently by the individuals within it (Gregory, Harrowing, Lee, Doolittle, & O'Sullivan, 2010). This multifaceted depiction of culture allows for the cultural subtleties and variations in emphases inherent in the individuals, groups, and communities that comprise the external environment in which the nursing program is situated.

Race and ethnicity are often equated with a particular culture that has its own practices, rituals, and beliefs, but this is not always the case. People of the same ethnic or racial origin may represent a unified culture, or they may have been assimilated into the dominant culture. Moreover, they can be members of more than one culture: the dominant culture and the culture of origin.

Each community has a number of subcultures that may not be immediately obvious, but which contribute to the tapestry of the community and, therefore, are relevant for curriculum planning. The cultures of youth, poverty, family violence, homelessness, gender, aging, work environments, and the culture of the healthcare system are some examples.

Respect for the traditions, shared beliefs, values, attitudes, and norms of the distinctive cultures is prerequisite when designing a curriculum. This is particularly important because migration and communication technologies bring nurses into contact with people from around the world.

The culture of the healthcare system is also worthy of note: who is entitled to health care, how and where clients receive health services, the languages in which information is available, the quality and nature of provider–client and provider–provider interactions, behavioral norms, and so forth. These influence nursing care and work life, clients' responses to healthcare providers, and consequently, the nursing curriculum.

Health and Health Care

Demographics influence the health profile of the population and health care, and are another external factor relevant for curriculum planners. The health of people clearly influences nursing care, and thus curriculum. The healthcare system is a prime determinant of the learning context for students' professional practice. The health status of the population and the nature of services may provide previously unexamined opportunities for professional practice experiences. Pertinent information related to health and the healthcare system might include the following:

- Most prevalent local and national health problems
- Nature of healthcare agencies and their services
- Nature and availability of public health and other community-based healthcare services
- Adequacy of funding for health care
- Availability of healthcare insurance
- Costs to clients and families
- Availability of healthcare resources (i.e., healthcare services, equipment, healthcare providers, health educators)
- Profile of clients receiving care
- Gaps in service

Information about health care relevant to learning opportunities for nursing students might include:

- Potential placement sites and learning experiences
- Receptiveness of healthcare agencies to students
- Willingness of healthcare providers to participate in student education
- Opportunities for professional practice education with students from other health professional programs

Curriculum developers ought to gather data pertaining to settings and opportunities for student learning experiences, as well as data about changes in prominent health problems, care services, and facilities. They should be current about healthcare delivery patterns and mindful of the needs and demands of more sophisticated healthcare consumers.

Professional Standards and Trends

Health care, nursing practice standards, and nursing education standards affect the practice and education of nurses. Accordingly, trends in these are strong influences on curriculum. Data to obtain include:

- Professional, regulatory, licensing, and accreditation requirements
- Entry-to-practice, nursing practice, legal, and ethical standards
- Self-assessment and quality assurance guidelines or requirements
- Evidence-based nursing practices and best practice guidelines
- Research on nursing education and nursing practice
- Contemporary nursing education models, frameworks, philosophies, and educational approaches
- Current and anticipated or enhanced roles and scope of practice
- Position statements from professional organizations and nursing leaders
- Reports from foundations, governmental agencies or commissions, and other groups known for making recommendations about health care, nursing practice, nursing education, and/or higher education

Educational and Healthcare Technology and Informatics

Advances in technology influence the content, teaching-learning strategies, course delivery, and course management of nursing curricula. Therefore, it is advisable to gather data about technology and informatics for education and health care, and about expected developments.

Technology is changing the nature of nursing education, and it will continue to do so. For example, web-based learning platforms are constantly evolving to make nursing education accessible to students located off campus and to enhance on-campus learning. Immersive virtual professional practice simulations (Kilmon, Brown, Ghosh, & Mikitiuk, 2010), or a virtual practicum using telehealth with real patients (Grady, 2011), could be relevant for schools with constrained placement opportunities. The use of high-fidelity mannequins, the expectation that students engage in database searching in class, and social media have changed campus-based learning and faculty-student interactions. Developments will continue faster than they are reported in the literature, and it behooves curriculum developers to be aware of learning technology available in their institutions and to lobby for those technologies that could be relevant to their curriculum.

It is neither possible nor necessary for curriculum developers to know all the technology that is used in health care. Rather, data are needed about the technologies that students will likely encounter and be expected to know during their professional practice placements. Along with this, information about electronic health record systems and healthcare agency policies about the use of electronic communication devices is important to acquire.

Environment

Environment is a broad contextual factor that refers to the atmospheric, physical, biological, and psychological milieu of a community. The influence of the environment might not be limited by geographic and political boundaries, and, therefore, must be considered in curriculum planning. For example, chemical, biological, physical, sociological, and psychological hazards and stressors can pose threats to individual, family, and community health, locally, nationally, and internationally. Data about national and international events and possible threats are important, although curriculum developers will likely focus on information about their immediate community. These data could include some or all of the following issues, in particular those that seem most relevant to the locale of the school of nursing:

- Weather patterns such as severe blizzards, extremely hot summers, tornadoes, or hurricanes
- Effects of climate change
- Air and water quality
- Presence of local industries known to produce environmental pollutants and hazards
- Environmental disasters, such as oil spills, volcanoes, forest fires
- War
- Terrorism
- Newly emerging diseases and their spread

Social, Political, and Economic Conditions

Social, political, and economic conditions form another broad contextual factor that encompasses forces, situations, or circumstances in the external environment. Because social, political, and economic events and issues are strongly interconnected, with each affecting the others, they are presented as one contextual factor. Information about this factor is important for curriculum planning.

Data about each of the previously identified external contextual factors (demographics, culture, healthcare system, professional standards and trends, technology, and environment) are related to social, political, and economic conditions, and some data pertinent to this factor may be obtained while collecting information about the others.

Information to obtain about social behaviors and issues that affect health, and thus may influence the curriculum might include:

- Illicit drug use in the community
- Unemployment rates and patterns
- Housing availability, affordability, and quality
- Nature and rate of crime in the community

Political and legislative (local, regional, provincial/state, and national) influences affect higher education, nursing education, health and social services, and eligibility for services. Pertinent data with potential curriculum implications could be:

- Support for nursing and nursing education from elected political parties, government officials, and community representatives
- Public concern about nursing shortages and access to health care
- Projections for changes to the healthcare system

Data about economic conditions that affect the curriculum may include:

- Present and projected local, provincial/state, and national economies
- Government financial support for higher education and nursing education
- Private, community, or public funding for:
  - Curriculum development
  - Faculty and student grants or scholarships

It would be advisable for curriculum stakeholders to carefully assess these and other social, political, and economic issues that can have a direct bearing on the curriculum to be developed.

Summary of External Contextual Factors

In summary, external contextual factors are those forces, situations, and circumstances that originate outside the educational institution in the community, region, country, and world. It is incumbent upon nursing curriculum developers to consider data about the external contextual factors so that a future-oriented, evidence-informed, context-relevant curriculum can be created. This type of curriculum is developed in response to demographic trends, culture, health and healthcare trends, professional standards, technology and informatics, the environment, and social, political, and economic conditions. Knowledge of these will make it possible for nurse educators to prepare professional nurses capable of caring for culturally diverse individuals, families, and groups within a dynamic society and healthcare system.

APPROACHES TO GATHERING CONTEXTUAL DATA FOR CURRICULUM DEVELOPMENT

In this text, the term *gathering data* is used rather than *data collection* to differentiate the activities of obtaining information for curriculum development purposes from the acquisition of information for research purposes. Although some of the methods may be the same, the purposes and rigor vary. Some differences are identified in **Table 8-2**.

A thorough understanding of the context in which the curriculum will be offered can be gained only through careful planning of the data to be gathered. Although some faculty members may believe that they know what the contextual situation is, and, therefore, that only a

Table 8-2   Differentiation of Gathering Data for Curriculum Development and Data Collection for Research

Characteristics	Gathering Data for Curriculum Development	Data Collection for Research
Purpose	Obtain information that will influence curriculum development	Obtain information to answer specific research questions and/or test hypothesis
Scope of information	Very broad	More limited
Procedures to obtain information	Planned, but open to change Quantitative and qualitative methods used	Formalized and limited by research design
Procedures to analyze information	Planned, but less prescribed than data analysis for research	Planned analysis, in accordance with research design
Instruments	Quantitative and qualitative instruments or guides specific to school and curriculum context Pilot-tested with convenience sample for comprehensiveness and comprehension Quantitative tools generally are not assessed for psychometric properties and may not be reused	Quantitative tools: • Psychometric testing with each use • Instruments with known psychometric characteristics and comprehension preferred Qualitative questionnaires or interview guides specific to the research project
Anonymity of data	Usually permission to reveal source required	Yes
Requirement for approval	Generally no, unless data are also being used for research purposes	Yes, by ethics review board

small amount of effort is required to gather data, this perspective is not sound. General knowledge about the context is an insufficient basis for curriculum development. The accumulation of detailed information and the curriculum decisions that flow from analysis of the information ground the curriculum in the context and ensure its relevance.

Planning this aspect of curriculum development requires agreement about the contextual factors requiring investigation, and identification of relevant data, data sources, and methods to obtain the information. The process of gathering data represents a strong public statement that a redesigned curriculum will be forthcoming, because the activities are dependent on interactions between nursing faculty and other members of the educational institution, key personnel in healthcare agencies, and community members. Although the intention to develop a curriculum is known to stakeholders involved in the planning that precedes the gathering of data, it is at this time that expectations for curriculum change are raised in the wider community. Moreover, external data gathering conveys the message that the curriculum will be relevant to its context. Because of the public nature of these activities, curriculum developers are obligated to present themselves in a credible manner, and this requires planning and organization.

The scope of data that are gathered about contextual factors and the subsequent data interpretation are foundational to the nature, relevance, and longevity of the curriculum. When deciding on the data to be collected, data sources, and methods for gathering data, curricularists strive to achieve a reasonable balance between a desire to acquire a breadth and depth of data on the one hand, and to progress in a timely manner on the other.

Deciding on Necessary Contextual Data and Data Sources

It is vital that the contextual data required for curriculum development be agreed upon so that suitable sources can be identified, and, if necessary, data-gathering tools can be developed. There should be openness to the acquisition of data that are not initially identified but subsequently recognized as important. For example, it might be decided that data about the intended programmatic directions of the major healthcare agencies in the community would be essential, that particular healthcare leaders are appropriate data sources, and that interviews would be the most expedient method of acquiring the data. If, in the course of an interview, an administrator comments that in order to introduce new programs, some clinical units will be closed for renovations, it would be prudent to ask for more information immediately, because there are clear implications for the curriculum. In making decisions about which data to collect, curriculum developers could consider the following:

- Which contextual factors seem most germane?
- What are the precise data required?
- What is the potential utility of the data for the curriculum development process?
- Which data will truly influence the curriculum?

- What is "nice to know," but not absolutely imperative for curriculum development?
- How might the data influence curriculum?
- How accessible and available are the data?
- How quickly can data be gathered?
- Is acquisition of any data so important that a delay in curriculum development is justified?
- What are the consequences of failing to gather these data?

When curriculum developers decide upon the necessary data for each contextual factor, the interrelated nature of the factors will be apparent; data gathered could be pertinent to more than one factor. It is best to record the information for all the factors to which it pertains, rather than spending time on discussions about where it belongs.

A host of individuals, groups, organizations, and documents can be used as data sources to provide information that may influence curriculum decisions. Determining which sources would be most useful is dependent on the situation within each school of nursing and the community. The decision requires judgments about information such as:

- Richness of data likely to be obtained
- Accessibility and availability of data sources
- Purpose of data gathering (solely as a basis for curriculum development or also for research)
- Resources available (time, people, finances, materials)

Methods of Gathering Data

Knowledge that shapes the curriculum is generally not obtained according to the rigorous standards of a formal research study. However, attention to institutional research ethics approval procedures is necessary if research is conducted or publications are anticipated along with curriculum development. If there is overlap or ambiguity about what is research and what is data gathering for curriculum development, it is imperative that institutional definitions of research are clarified and policies about obtaining data are heeded.

When decisions are being made about appropriate methods to gather data about the internal and external contextual factors, the main considerations are time, expertise, and resources:

- Time available for gathering data in the curriculum development plan
- Time to locate extant documents, develop interview questions and surveys, and gather and analyze data
- Expertise of curriculum developers in data-gathering and data analysis methods
- Resources to support data gathering, such as secretarial help.

Many methods could be employed to gather data about internal and external contextual factors. Those that will yield valuable data as expeditiously as possible, and for which the curriculum designers possess the required skills, are most appropriate. Frequently used methods of data-gathering for the curriculum development process are reviewed in the paragraphs that follow.

Literature Reviews and Internet Searches

Ideas about curricula, trends, philosophical approaches, and strategies for nursing education, along with significant directions for health care, can be acquired from literature reviews and Internet searches. Information about other nursing programs is available on the Internet. Knowing about the current state of nursing education beyond the local situation, and learning about the convictions and opinions of experts, will expand the views of those involved in curriculum development and provide a national and international perspective for curriculum development. Ideas from beyond national borders can furnish new and relevant insights, even though the origins of the concepts or their implementation are geographically and/or politically distant.

More specifically, published curriculum designs and examples of courses can serve as models for new curricula. Many authors provide suggestions arising from the successes and difficulties they have encountered with particular curriculum designs and implementation. Particularly valuable can be research reports about the outcomes of specific teaching-learning strategies or programs, because they provide evidence that can guide future educational practices. Authors whose ideas are particularly attractive or faculty from a school with an appealing curriculum might serve as consultants if resources permit.

Document Review

A review of existing documents can be an inexpensive means of acquiring data identified as necessary to the curriculum development process. Some documents may be readily available, such as professional practice and educational program accreditation standards or the institutional mission, vision, philosophy, and strategic plan. Conversely, others may require a more protracted effort to obtain. These might include government or healthcare agency reports. Those documents that are judged to have particular relevance for future curriculum directions should be reviewed and pertinent data extracted.

Key Informant Interviews

Key informants are people known to have information relevant to the purpose of the data gathering. Individual interviews (face-to-face, telephone, or email) can be an effective and inexpensive method to acquire pertinent data quickly. The interview questions should be carefully planned so that maximum relevant information can be acquired without unduly imposing upon an informant's time. Providing the questions in advance of the interview can help the informant prepare. It is important to record responses (usually by taking notes) so that information is not forgotten. As the interview is ending, it is wise to confirm that it would be acceptable to follow up, either in person, by telephone, or via email, if clarification or additional data are required.

Focus Group Interviews

These are planned group discussions intended to obtain information about a specified topic in a nonthreatening environment. This method of gathering data capitalizes on group inter-action to explore perceptions, attitudes, beliefs, and opinions about a particular topic or issue. Online focus group interviews are a means to expand the geographical location of participants (Kenny, 2005). The focus group typically comprises 6 to 12 individuals with a common set of interests. A facilitator whose role is to assist the group to explore the topic in depth, generally within a loose structure, guides the discussion. Although the structure is not fixed, open-ended questions are prepared in advance. According to Kreuger and Casey (2000), questions should be developed to match the following sequence of categories: *opening, introductory, transition, key*, and *ending*. Ideas are recorded (often on flipcharts in addition to audio-recording) and periodically reviewed to ensure accuracy of recording and comprehension. The goal is not consensus; rather, it is a full exploration of the topic.

A focus group interview was conducted at a holistic nursing conference as part of graduate curriculum development. Participants were asked two questions:

- "What would you identify as critical elements for curricula for graduate holistic nurse education?"
- "How should the didactic and experiential elements of curricula be determined?" (Lange & Purnell, 2011, p. 185)

The responses led to ideas that could influence curriculum development and, importantly, the realization that information from students and faculty would also be required.

Focus groups for the purpose of obtaining data for curriculum development can be used productively with faculty, students, staff nurses, and other stakeholders. The inter-view can be broad in its focus or narrow, examining one aspect of curriculum, such as the nature of professional practice learning experiences or online learning.

Surveys

Face-to-face, telephone, mail, email, or web-based surveys are used to obtain data from a large number of people in a relatively short period of time. Questionnaires require time to construct so that the items are understandable to respondents and data can be readily analyzed.

Examples of information that could be obtained with surveys are opinions about health care and curriculum directions, the nature of future nursing practice, and preferences of nurses about graduate programs.

Delphi Technique

The Delphi technique is a structured forecasting survey that provides a means of obtaining input from stakeholders who may be geographically distant and separate, but whose ideas are deemed essential. A panel of experts is asked to complete an iterative series of questionnaires that address their opinions, judgment, or predictions about a particular topic. Each set of responses is summarized and another questionnaire is sent to the same individuals for confirmation. The iterative process is repeated until consensus is achieved about the issue of interest (Polit & Beck, 2012). Selection of the experts, diminishing return rates with each round, and the total time for the process to be completed (Keeney, Hasson, & McKenna, 2006) would be of concern to curriculum developers.

An example of the use of the Delphi technique for curriculum development occurred in the determination of essential content for a dermatology nurse practitioner curriculum. Data were collected from dermatology nurse practitioners and dermatologists, who rated the importance of 91 content items related to knowledge, skills, and roles. Following two rounds of responses, consensus (defined as 70% agreement) was achieved (Bobonich & Cooper, 2012).

Consultations

Consultations with experts and/or peers at other institutions can provide valuable knowledge, insights, and guidance about particular aspects of curriculum development, future directions for nursing practice and education, and/or implementation challenges of particular curricular designs. Frequently, the counsel they offer is gained from experience that has not yet been committed to publication. The contributions of consultants and peers from other institutions can be substantial when considered within local realities. Cost is likely a factor; therefore, when a consultant is employed, it is wise to ensure that the purpose of the consultation has been explicated and that as many stakeholders as possible are able to participate in discussions.

The Work of Gathering Data

There is no formula for deciding which data to obtain about the contextual factors, data sources to contact, or data-gathering methods to employ. Rather, it is worthwhile for curriculum developers to give attention to the questions and considerations posed in the previous sections. Then, using their knowledge of the school, experience, and judgment, they can reach consensus about what is reasonable and realistic. The conclusions will likely be different for each school. A <u>worksheet could help focus thinking</u> about data gathering and, when posted, serve as a visual reminder of work to be completed.

Table 8-3 presents examples of data, data sources, and methods to gather data for the internal contextual factors of mission, vision, philosophy, and goals; culture; financial

Internal Contextual Factors	Data	Data Sources	Data-Gathering Methods
Philosophy, Vision, Mission, and Goals	Published philosophy, vision, mission, goals, strategic plan	Institutional and school documents and websites	Document review
	Values and guiding principles	Key informants, e.g., senior academics, school leader	Interviews
Culture and Climate	Organizational structure	Organizational chart	Document review
	Interaction styles Formal and informal decision-making styles Values	Key informants, e.g., faculty members, committee chairs	Interviews
Financial Resources	Institutional budget priorities	Institutional planning documents	Document review
	Current and projected school budget	School leader	Interview
History	Key features of school and institutional history	Reports Senior academics	Document review Interviews
	Factors contributing to successes		
Programs and Policies	Evaluation of current curriculum	Evaluation reports	Document review
	Curricular emphases in other school programs	Program chairs	Interviews
	Range of courses in other departments	Institutional calendar, websites	Web search Document review
	Policies regarding admission, progression, etc.	School and institution websites, calendars	Web search Document review

Table 8-3   Examples of Data, Data Sources, and Data-Gathering Methods for Internal Contextual Factors

Table 8-3   Examples of Data, Data Sources, and Data-Gathering Methods for Internal Contextual Factors (*continued*)

Internal Contextual Factors	Data	Data Sources	Data-Gathering Methods
Infrastructure			
1. Human resources	Employment agreements	Collective agreements	Document review
	Nursing Faculty		
	Number of part- and full-time faculty	School leader	
	Credentials and expertise	Faculty members	Interviews
	Expected retirements and resignations		
	Characteristics of adjunct faculty		
	Pool of potential faculty	Chair of graduate program	Interview
	Pool of potential preceptors	Healthcare agencies	Surveys, focus groups
	Non-nursing Faculty		
	Interest and availability of non-nursing faculty to develop and teach new non-nursing courses	Department chairs	Interviews
	Students		
	Applicant numbers and characteristics	Chair of admissions committee	Interview
		Admission committee reports	Document review
	Demographics of current students	School records	Document review
	Attrition, completion rates		
	Support Staff		
	Numbers, skill sets	School administrator, support staff	Interviews

(continues)

Internal Contextual Factors	Data	Data Sources	Data-Gathering Methods
2. Physical resources	Office space	Observation	Observation
	Classroom space and facilities	Physical plant documents	Document review
	Technology, including technology for distributed learning	Information technology director Department website	Interview
3. Resources to support teaching and learning	Library Holdings and services	Librarian	Interview
	Faculty Development Services Nature and availability of services	Website	
	Possibility of creating new services to support curriculum when developed	Director of institution-wide services	Interview
	Teaching Support Availability of graduate teaching assistants	Graduate program chair	Interview
	Support for distributed learning design and implementation	Director of teaching Support services for distributed learning	Interview
	Access to institutional funding for curriculum	Funding announcements	Web search
	Student Support Nature and availability of services	Student services website	Web search
	Possibility of creating new services if warranted by new curriculum	Director of student services	Interview

Table 8-3   Examples of Data, Data Sources, and Data-Gathering Methods for Internal Contextual Factors (*continued*)

resources; and infrastructure. **Table 8-4** presents similar information about the external factors of culture, healthcare systems, and professional standards and trends.

The work of gathering data may be given to a task force or shared more widely among stakeholders. Sufficient time should be allowed for this aspect of the curriculum development process to ensure that a full picture is obtained of the internal and external contexts. If the new curriculum is to endure into the future, it must be based upon accurate and comprehensive data.

Table 8-4 Examples of Data, Data Sources, and Data-Gathering Methods for External Contextual Factors

External Contextual Factors	Data	Data Sources	Data-Gathering Methods
Demographics	Population size Age and gender profile Educational levels Urban–rural ratio Income levels Birth and death rates % single or married Average number of children % with health insurance Immigration and emigration patterns	Government, business development websites	Web search
Culture	Values, beliefs, and practices of: • dominant culture • major ethnic groups • subcultures • healthcare system and providers	Key informants Publications of ethnic and cultural organizations Mission statements of healthcare agencies	Interviews Document review Document review

(continues)

Table 8-4   Examples of Data, Data Sources, and Data-Gathering Methods for External Contextual Factors (*continued*)

External Contextual Factors	Data	Data Sources	Data-Gathering Methods
Health and Health Care	Services provided by public and private organizations	Websites	Web search
	Plans for changes in services	Agency key informants Healthcare leaders	Interviews Interviews
	Gaps in services	Consumer groups Government policy statements	Interviews Document review Web search
	Ratio of professional to nonprofessional staff in major agencies	Annual reports Key informants	Document review Interview
Professional Standards and Trends	Practice regulations	Licensing bodies	Document review Web search
	Scope of practice	Legislation	Document review
	Nursing care trends	Professional bodies Nursing literature Nursing leaders Practicing nurses	Document review Literature review Interviews, focus groups Delphi technique
	Approval and accreditation standards	Approval and accreditation bodies	Document review Web search
	Nursing education trends	Nursing education leaders Nursing education literature	Survey, interviews Literature search
Technology and Informatics	Educational technology and information systems in use in educational institution	Information technology specialist Education technology specialist	Interviews
	Healthcare technology and information systems students will likely encounter	Clinical leaders Faculty engaged in professional practice and teaching	Interviews Focus groups

Table 8-4   Examples of Data, Data Sources, and Data-Gathering Methods for External Contextual Factors (*continued*)

External Contextual Factors	Data	Data Sources	Data-Gathering Methods
Environment	Recurrent environmental events, such as hurricanes	Curriculum developers' personal knowledge	Interviews
	Environmental threats	Faculty from relevant departments	
	Plausible environmental catastrophes	Government websites	Web search
Social, Political, and Economic	Governmental policies, initiatives, and funding related to higher education	Government reports	Document review Web search
	Public support for nursing	Newspaper reports Consumer groups	News review Interviews
	Grants, scholarships, and other funding for students, faculty, and the school	Alumni associations Professional bodies Foundations Government websites Student services	Document review Web search Interviews
	Regional economic situation and outlook	Government and business development websites	Web search

It is helpful to have a central repository so that data will be readily accessible for subsequent analysis. Moreover, methods that will speed analysis (such as immediate computer entry of returned questionnaire responses by an administrative or research assistant, or use of web-based questionnaires) should be employed whenever possible.

As data are gathered, ideas will arise about possible concepts, processes, or learning experiences that could be included in the curriculum. It is natural to begin to extrapolate these possibilities from the data. These ideas should be recorded with the understanding that they are only tentative and based on incomplete knowledge. It is wise to exercise caution to avoid drawing premature conclusions about what the curriculum should be like. It is only when all data are assembled, interpreted, and synthesized that evidence-informed, context-relevant, unified curriculum ideas will emerge.

RELATIONSHIP OF GATHERING CONTEXTUAL DATA TO AN EVIDENCE-INFORMED, CONTEXT-RELEVANT, UNIFIED CURRICULUM

A curriculum that is *evidence-informed* is based on systematically and purposefully gathered evidence about:

- The context in which the curriculum will be offered and graduates will practice nursing
- Students, learning, teaching, and nursing education
- Nursing practice
- Clients and their responses to health situations

Further, a curriculum that is *context-relevant* is:

- Responsive to students; current and projected societal, health, and community situations; and current and projected imperatives of the nursing profession
- Consistent with the mission, philosophy, and goals of the educational institution and school of nursing
- Feasible within the realities of the school and community

A *unified* curriculum is one that contains curricular components that are conceptually, logically, cohesively, and visibly related. In part, this means that curriculum concepts and professional abilities, derived from the contextual data, are evident in the curriculum goals and throughout the curriculum.

The creation of an evidence-informed, context-relevant, unified curriculum begins with assembling organized, comprehensive, and accurate evidence about the context in which the curriculum will be offered and in which graduates will practice nursing. This type of curriculum is defined by, and grounded in, the forces and circumstances that affect society, health care, education, recipients of nursing care, the nursing profession, and the educational institution. Context-relevant curricula have unique features reflective of local and/or regional circumstances, and these circumstance are known by gathering data about them.

Gathering data about the context is tantamount to gathering evidence for the curriculum. Therefore, it is important that the data collection be organized and comprehensive. Subsequently, the analysis of the contextual data will result in the identification of the core curriculum concepts and the key professional abilities of graduates. These will be evident throughout the curriculum and will be an important aspect of its conceptual and visual unity. Thus, the process of gathering contextual data is the basis of an evidence-informed, context-relevant, unified curriculum.

CORE PROCESSES OF CURRICULUM WORK

Faculty Development

The overall goal of faculty development in relation to gathering data about contextual factors is to expand members' appreciation and knowledge of the relationship between the contextual factors and development of an evidence-informed, context-relevant, unified curriculum. Faculty development can include a session in which internal and external contextual factors are reviewed. Discussion about which factors are significant and how these factors can influence curriculum development will help novice curriculum developers understand the importance of systematic data gathering. During such a discussion, some pertinent data, data sources, and methods to gather data can be identified, with further decisions being reserved for a task force or committee.

Attention can be given to differentiating between gathering data for curriculum development and data collection for research. It may be appropriate to include information about, and practice in, interviewing key informants if this will be a new activity for some. These faculty development activities can be readily facilitated by those members with expertise in data gathering and curriculum development.

Ongoing Appraisal

When gathering data, curriculum developers repeatedly ask themselves such questions as:

- Are we obtaining the essential data? If not, what needs to be done?
- Are there other data that would be important for curriculum development?
- Should we reconsider a decision not to gather data about particular contextual factors?
- Are we using the methods that will garner the most relevant data as expeditiously as possible?
- Are we missing any important groups, individuals, or documents with important data?
- Have we achieved the correct balance between giving the necessary time for gathering data and moving forward with curriculum development within a reasonable timeframe?

Scholarship

There is considerable opportunity for scholarship projects related to gathering data about the contextual factors. Most directly, the scholarship of teaching and learning could include presentations and manuscripts about the methods used to gather contextual data, with recommendations for future data gathering during curriculum development. A description of the context might form the basis of a manuscript, which could be completed once curriculum developers are able to explain how the context influenced the curriculum plans. Another idea that could encompass the scholarship of discovery and the scholarship of teaching and learning might be to conduct qualitative studies of the reactions of participants (those gathering and those providing data) to the process. It would be worthwhile to determine the extent to which those who provide data expect their ideas to be reflected in the curriculum.

CHAPTER SUMMARY

Gathering data about internal and external contextual factors that have the potential to influence curriculum is fundamental to the creation of an evidence-informed, context-relevant, unified curriculum. This public activity heralds a forthcoming curriculum change. Faculty members should first identify those factors that are most relevant to the school of nursing and curriculum development. Then, decisions can be made about pertinent data, data sources, and methods to gather the data. It is essential that adequate time be given to gathering data, because the strength and longevity of the revised curriculum will rest upon the quality of the data gathered and the subsequent analysis. Finally, ideas about the core processes of curriculum work are provided, including faculty development to prepare members for the decisions and activities of gathering data, questions to guide ongoing appraisal, and possible scholarship projects related to gathering data.

SYNTHESIS ACTIVITIES

The Ephesus College School of Nursing case describes preparations for gathering data for curriculum development and is followed by questions that provide a basis for consideration of the situation. Then, questions are offered that might assist readers when planning data gathering for curriculum development in their own settings.

Ephesus College School of Nursing

The Ephesus College School of Nursing has been in existence since 1945 when it first offered RN to BSN education. Since then, it has added a generic baccalaureate program and a nurse practitioner program. There is a feeling among faculty that they are overdue to offer a PhD program, but they have agreed that designing new curricula for the undergraduate programs must come first.

The curriculum leader, Dr. Marie Simone, has developed a plan for data gathering and presents it at a regular faculty meeting, asking for endorsement and for volunteers to participate. The plan entails gathering data about all the internal and external contextual factors outlined in Tables 8-3 and 8-4. She also suggests additional data sources that should be used. For example, she proposes that a survey of students be undertaken to determine their priorities for a new curriculum. This idea generates dissent from a few faculty members. They believe that data gathering will be a time-consuming process that will slow curriculum development and that students already have provided their views on the curriculum through course evaluations.

Dr. Simone also presents an overall plan whereby faculty members would be divided into small teams to gather particular data. The data would then be recorded electronically according to a format that will be useful as curriculum development proceeds. She asks for feedback about her plan. There is silence for a few moments and then comments of the following nature are made:

- It's too much work and we don't have time.
- We know most of the information you want. Is all this work really necessary? Surely our own knowledge is sufficient.
- Maybe some of it is necessary, but not all of it.
- Could we also figure out what we need to know to plan a PhD program and extend the data gathering for that purpose too?
- How many people need to be involved?
- Who is going to set up these interviews for us? Who is going to transcribe the interviews? Who is supposed to be recording the data according to the prescribed format?

Questions and Activities for Critical Analysis of the Ephesus College School of Nursing Case

1. Consider the extent to which each of the faculty comments reflects a readiness to gather data for curriculum development.
2. How could Dr. Simone respond to the comments about obtaining data from students? To the other comments?
3. Describe strategies Dr. Simone might have implemented to prepare faculty members to engage in data-gathering activities.

4. Identify the people and resources necessary to implement Dr. Simone's plans.

5. Appraise the merits of gathering data in preparation for curriculum development for both undergraduate and PhD programs at the same time.

Questions and Activities for Consideration When Gathering Contextual Data in Readers' Settings

1. Consider a way to explain that gathering contextual data for curriculum development is important.

2. Develop criteria to determine the contextual data essential for curriculum development.

3. Apply the criteria to decide whether it is necessary to gather data about all internal and external contextual factors.

4. What would be the important sources for the data deemed essential for curriculum development?

5. Decide how the data could best be obtained. Will data-gathering tools be necessary? If so, who will design them?

6. How could the work of gathering data be organized?

7. Create a detailed plan for gathering data that includes people to be involved, resources, and a timeline.

8. Identify resources necessary to expedite the work of gathering and recording data. What resources are available? How can the gathering and recording of data be accomplished if resources are limited?

9. Establish a central repository for data.

10. Determine the faculty development activities about gathering data for curriculum development that might be necessary.

11. Propose a plan for incorporating ongoing appraisal into the processes of gathering and recording data.

12. How can scholarship projects become part of the processes of gathering and recording data? Suggest some suitable and feasible scholarship projects.

REFERENCES

Blackburn, S. (Ed.). (2014). *The Oxford Dictionary of Philosophy* (2nd revised ed.). Oxford Reference Online. New York: Oxford University Press. Retrieved from http://www.oxfordreference.com.proxy1.lib.uwo.ca/view/10.1093/acref/9780199541430.001.0001/acref-9780199541430-e-800?rskey=OpkUdt&result=1

Bobonich, M. A., & Cooper, K. D. (2012). A core curriculum for dermatology nurse-practitioners. *Journal of the Dermatology Nurses' Association, 4,* 108–120.

Bryson, J. M. (2011). *Strategic planning for public and nonprofit organizations: A guide to strengthening and sustaining organizational achievement* (4th ed.). San Francisco: Jossey-Bass.

Cornbleth, C. (2008). Echo effects and curriculum change. *Teachers College Record, 110,* 2148–2171.

Doyle, C. (2011). *A dictionary of marketing* (3rd ed.). New York: Oxford University Press. Retrieved from http://www.oxfordreference.com/view/10.1093/acref/9780199590230.001.0001/acref-9780199590230-e-0532?rskey=aKsY4L&result=6&q=demography

Grady, J. L. (2011). The virtual clinical practicum: An innovative telehealth model for clinical nursing education. *Nursing Education Perspectives, 32,* 189–194.

Gregory, D., Harrowing, J., Lee, B., Doolittle, L., & O'Sullivan, P. (2010). Pedagogy as influencing nursing students' essentialized understanding of culture. *International Journal of Nursing Education Scholarship, 7*(1).

Harrison, J. P. (2010). *Essentials of strategic planning in healthcare.* Chicago: Health Administration Press.

Henry, A. E. (2011). *Understanding strategic management* (2nd ed.). New York: Oxford University Press.

Hunger, J. D., & Wheelen, T. L. (2011). *Essentials of strategic management* (5th ed.). Upper Saddle River, NJ: Prentice Hall.

Keeney, S., Hasson, F., & McKenna, H. (2006). Consulting the oracle: Ten lessons from using the Delphi technique in nursing research. *Journal of Advanced Nursing, 50,* 205–212.

Kenny, A. J. (2005). Interaction in cyberspace: An online focus group. *Journal of Advanced Nursing, 49,* 414–422.

Kilmon, C. A., Brown, L., Ghosh, S., & Mikitiuk, A. (2010). Immersive virtual reality simulations in nursing education. *Nursing Education Perspectives, 31,* 314–317.

Kreuger, R. A., & Casey, M. A. (2000). *Focus groups: A practical guide for applied research* (3rd ed.). Newbury Park, CA: Sage.

Lange, B., & Purnell, M. J. (2011). Curriculum as environment: A focus group study. *Holistic Nursing Practice, 25,* 184–191.

McKeown, M. (2012). *The strategy book.* Harlow, England: Pearson Education.

Polit, D. F., & Beck, C. T. (2012). *Nursing research: Generating and assessing evidence for nursing practice* (9th ed.). Philadelphia: Wolters Kluwer/Lippincott Williams & Wilkins.

Schneider, B., Ehrhart, M. G., & Macey, W. H. (2013). Organizational climate and culture. *Annual Review of Psychology, 64,* 361–388.

Sitelman, F. G., & Sitelman, R. (2000). Ethics and culture: From the claim that God is dead, it does not follow that everything is permitted. In M. L. Kelley & V. M. Fitzsimons (Eds.), *Understanding cultural diversity: Culture, curriculum and community in nursing* (pp. 11–21). Sudbury, MA: Jones and Bartlett.

Swayne, L. E., Duncan, J. W., & Ginter, P. M. (2008). *Strategic management of health care organizations* (6th ed.). San Francisco: Jossey-Bass.

CHAPTER 9

Analyzing and Interpreting Contextual Data for an Evidence-Informed, Context-Relevant, Unified Curriculum

Chapter Overview

Once data have been gathered about the internal and external contexts and recorded in an organized manner, it is time to integrate the information and determine its meaning for the curriculum. The contextual data become the basis from which curriculum concepts and professional abilities are derived, curriculum possibilities become evident, and an evidence-informed, context-relevant, unified curriculum begins to take shape.

Following definitions of terms is a description of the cognitive processes involved in the analysis and interpretation of contextual data. These processes include integrating data, inferring curriculum concepts and professional abilities that program graduates will require, proposing curriculum possibilities, deducing curriculum limitations, and identifying administrative issues that affect curriculum design. Also discussed is the determination of core curriculum concepts and key professional abilities through syntheses of ideas generated from the contextual data. To enhance clarity, the thinking processes that bridge data gathering and the emerging curriculum are presented in a procedural fashion. However, the processes are iterative and integrative in nature, with all ideas influencing previous and subsequent thinking. The relationship between the analysis of contextual data and an evidence-informed, context-relevant, unified curriculum is explained. The core processes of curriculum work are addressed. After the chapter summary, an extended case is presented to illustrate the main ideas. Questions to guide consideration of the case are included, as well as questions to stimulate thinking about analyzing and interpreting contextual data in readers' settings.

Chapter Goals

- Appreciate the multiple cognitive processes inherent in analysis and interpretation of contextual data.
- Gain insight into how core curriculum concepts and key professional abilities of graduates are derived from analysis and interpretation of internal and external contextual data and subsequent synthesis of ideas.
- Understand the relationship of the analysis and interpretation of contextual data to an evidence-informed, context-relevant, unified curriculum.
- Consider the core processes of curriculum work related to analyzing and interpreting contextual data.

DEFINITION OF TERMS

A number of terms are introduced and defined. They are presented in a conceptually logical order that matches the order of their full explication in the chapter, rather than in a more conventional alphabetical sequence.

Curriculum concepts are abstract ideas that form the substance of the curriculum. The core curriculum concepts are derived from the contextual data and are essential for graduates to know and use in the context in which they will practice nursing. These concepts permeate the curriculum and contribute to the curriculum's uniqueness, evidence base, and unity.

Professional abilities are the capabilities necessary for nursing practice. The professional abilities include, but are not limited to:

- Cognitive skills, such as use of theory in practice, problem solving, critical thinking, and clinical reasoning
- Affective skills, including caring, empathy, and professional comportment
- Technical skills related to the execution of healthcare procedures and use of health and information technologies
- Interpersonal skills, such as communicating effectively, collaborating, leading, and delegating
- Ethical decision making and comportment
- Professional judgment, that is, the integration and judicious use of the aforementioned skills and behaviors within the context of nursing

The key professional abilities are essential for nursing practice and are derived from the contextual data. They form the basis of curriculum goals or outcomes, are emphasized throughout the curriculum, and contribute to the curriculum's uniqueness, evidence base, and unity. Knowledge is prerequisite to all professional abilities.

Curriculum foundations are those ideas that underpin the entire curriculum. They are the essence of the curriculum, and continuous attention to them is essential to ensure curriculum unity in further curriculum development, implementation, and evaluation. The foundations are composed of the core curriculum concepts, key professional abilities, and philosophical and educational approaches.

Curriculum possibilities are imaginative ideas about potential teaching-learning experiences, curriculum design options, courses, and content areas.

Curriculum limitations are restrictions or constraints on teaching-learning experiences, curriculum design options, or potential content areas.

Administrative issues are those logistical, personnel, and/or budgetary matters that are beyond the authority of faculty members to resolve, but which can significantly affect the curriculum design.

ANALYSIS AND INTERPRETATION OF CONTEXTUAL DATA

Analysis (determining essential elements), interpretation (deriving meaning), and synthesis (combining parts to form a whole) of the contextual data are necessary to arrive at the core curriculum concepts and key professional abilities. These iterative and interactive processes require logical and reflective thought, an open mind, and free communication. Despite the fact that these are clearly nonlinear processes, they are deliberately presented separately in this chapter. This presentation facilitates explanation and may further understanding of curriculum development processes by making apparent how an evidence-informed, context-relevant, unified curriculum is derived from contextual data.

Analyzing data about contextual factors and deriving meaning to reach conclusions about the curriculum entail a confluence of examination, integration, interpretation, reflection, and inference-making about curriculum concepts and professional abilities; generation of curriculum possibilities and recognition of contextual limitations; identification of administrative issues; and decision making. These deliberations occur in collaboration with colleagues whose perspectives, conclusions, and values may be divergent. Therefore, group discussion and consensus are essential.

The following five processes are described as part of the analysis and interpretation of contextual data:

1. Examining and integrating contextual data to identify patterns and trends
2. Inferring curriculum concepts and professional abilities
3. Proposing curriculum possibilities
4. Deducing curriculum limitations
5. Identifying administrative issues

Although presented separately, these processes occur almost simultaneously, because ideas about curriculum are generated through free-flowing discussion. Ideas relevant to all aspects of the processes arise concurrently, with one thought sparking many others.

Examining and Integrating Contextual Data

Examining and integrating data are activities for the total faculty group. All those who develop and eventually implement a new curriculum must understand the context in which the curriculum will be operationalized and in which graduates will work. Therefore, individual members should review the data about the contextual factors, determine the influence factors have upon one another, and generate ideas about trends. Individual or small-group reviews form the basis for discussion by the total faculty group. Collectively, members discuss the ideas that were generated and identify patterns or trends. Data, patterns, and/or trends will reveal the current state of affairs and form the basis of an evidence-informed, context-relevant, unified curriculum. Curriculum developers can ask two questions:

- What data are available about this contextual factor?
- What patterns and/or trends emerge from the data about this one factor?

Review and discussion about data and trends for individual contextual factors will make apparent the overlap and connections among contextual data for several factors, and how data and trends about one contextual factor influence, and are influenced by, data and trends of other factors. The overall goal of reviewing contextual data and identifying trends is to achieve an integrated view of the data and a shared understanding of the big picture of the context in which the curriculum will be operationalized and graduates will practice nursing. Some of the questions that might be considered include the following:

- How do data or trends about one particular factor affect trends in other contextual factors? For example, how might changes to legislation about health insurance, or benefits to people with disabilities, influence the wellbeing of those affected?
- If these or any other trends continue, what might the consequences be for other contextual factors? For instance, what might nursing shortages mean for publicly funded hospitals?
- What are the dominant features of the context in which graduates will practice nursing?

Predicting possible futures in response to these and similar questions helps curriculum developers anticipate the context for which the curriculum will be developed and in which it will be implemented. In understanding the big picture, curricularists also come to agreement about which contextual factors should be most important in influencing curriculum. More important factors may be readily apparent and agreed upon; less important ones might require discussion and consensus. There is no need to reach quantitative conclusions about the relative importance of each factor. Instead, faculty members need to reach accord with respect to the comparative weight of all contextual factors so that the most, more, and less important ones are determined. In this way, the curriculum becomes responsive to the predominant aspects of the context.

Inferring Curriculum Concepts and Professional Abilities

Review of contextual data, trends, and patterns will lead to insights about curriculum concepts, which are abstract ideas that form the substance of the curriculum. Further, professional abilities essential for nursing practice can be inferred. The professional abilities, as noted previously, include, but are not limited to, cognitive, affective, technical, and interpersonal skills; ethical comportment; and professional judgment.

Curriculum concepts and professional abilities are inferred mainly from the external contextual factors, although some may also be evident from internal factors. Furthermore, additional ideas are stimulated about these curriculum concepts and professional abilities by those already suggested. The generation of these ideas occurs concurrently, not sequentially. Curriculum developers can ask the following questions:

- What inferences about important curriculum concepts that graduates should know and apply in nursing practice can be made from the contextual data and from patterns and trends?
- What inferences about professional abilities can be made from the contextual data, from patterns and trends, and from curriculum concepts?
- What additional ideas about relevant curriculum concepts arise from the professional abilities that have been suggested?
- What additional ideas about professional abilities arise from the curriculum concepts that have been suggested?

The intent is to record all the ideas that arise from brainstorming, without censor or concern about the format in which they are expressed.

Proposing Curriculum Possibilities

From ideas about curriculum concepts and professional abilities, thoughts about curriculum possibilities flow spontaneously. Curriculum possibilities (i.e., imaginative ideas about potential teaching-learning experiences, curriculum design options, courses, and content areas) result from creative thinking, unfettered by consideration of logistics. To determine the curriculum possibilities of the contextual data, curriculum concepts, and professional abilities, this question could be posed: What possibilities arise from the contextual data, patterns, trends, curriculum concepts, and professional abilities about:

- Curriculum design options?
- Courses?
- Potential fit with content areas?
- Educational processes and experiences?

Ideas about curriculum possibilities can be drawn directly from data, trends, curriculum concepts, professional abilities, or from a combination of these. If, for instance, the data include a growing trend toward home health care, then a possibility might be to develop or expand professional practice placements with agencies providing nursing services in people's homes. If, as another example, the curriculum concept of professional responsibility and the professional abilities of critical thinking and political action are determined, then experience with the political action committee of a professional organization might be proposed as a curriculum possibility.

The intent is to generate many ideas about curriculum possibilities. Some may seem ridiculous or bizarre, and others more conventional. The apparently outlandish possibilities may be appealing, but impractical. However, with subsequent application of pragmatic and logical thinking, these might later be modified into innovative and feasible suggestions.

Inferences about curriculum concepts and professional abilities, and proposals about curriculum possibilities, could lead to considerable discussion and debate, even when only a single contextual factor is being examined. For instance, some faculty may interpret a low fertility rate in the community as signaling the necessity for a curricular emphasis on prenatal assessment and health promotion, while others may conclude that maternal-infant health requires little attention. Some ideas, such as health promotion, could be considered a concept, professional ability, and/or a potential content area. It is unnecessary to decide which category it fits best. Rather, it should be recorded in every applicable category. Repeated recording of the same idea in several categories signifies its importance to the curriculum.

It is useful to record all thoughts that occur, and at this stage to avoid debate about suitability, categorization, inclusions, or exclusions. Such decisions will be made in subsequent integrative discussions about curriculum and course design. The reason for producing and recording as many ideas as possible is that they naturally arise from an examination of the contextual data and help curriculum developers move forward. The ideas being recorded are tentative and should be retained for detailed curriculum and course design. They may be accepted, modified, or eliminated as curriculum development proceeds.

Identifying Curriculum Limitations

In contrast to curriculum possibilities, curriculum limitations are restrictions or constraints on teaching-learning experiences, curriculum design options, or potential content areas. These are derived from a pragmatic or logical interpretation of the contextual data, trends and patterns, curriculum concepts, professional abilities, and curriculum possibilities. Curriculum builders might ask the following questions:

- How do internal and external contextual data and trends constrain what might be possible in the curriculum?
- What restrictions do curriculum concepts and/or professional abilities place on curriculum possibilities?

Both internal and external contextual data can point to curriculum limitations that warrant serious attention by the curriculum team. For example, a faculty group whose nursing practice expertise lies mainly in acute care might identify the faculty profile as a limitation, if community-based professional practice experiences have been proposed as a curriculum possibility. Another example could be that particular professional practice experiences are constrained by limited availability of student placements.

Importantly, some of the curriculum possibilities and limitations can lead to actions that could profoundly change the school and the curriculum. For example, data about the nursing profession likely include a statement describing the current and projected worldwide shortages of nursing faculty. This fact could limit the likelihood of successfully implementing a small-group, case- or problem-based curriculum, which would require relatively large numbers of faculty. Alternatively, it could spur faculty to lobby senior administrators to initiate vigorous faculty recruitment and retention efforts, or to enlist clinicians with adjunct university appointments to lead the small groups.

Deducing Administrative Issues

Invariably, administrative issues that might affect the curriculum will become apparent as contextual data are analyzed and curriculum possibilities and limitations are identified. Administrative issues (i.e., those logistical, personnel, and/or budgetary matters that are beyond the authority of faculty members to resolve) can significantly affect the new curriculum. The question to be answered is: What logistical, personnel, and/or budgetary issues should be raised with the school leader?

It is worthwhile to note administrative issues and bring them to the attention of the school leader, specifying the effects they could have on the curriculum and the desired resolution. Then, with the school leader's support, guidance, and action, strategies can be developed and implemented to address the issues. Indeed, the curriculum design will likely be dependent on the resolution of some administrative matters.

Summary of Processes

Several processes have been described to illuminate the thinking that emanates from the contextual data: examining and integrating contextual data, inferring curriculum concepts and professional abilities, proposing curriculum possibilities, identifying curriculum limitations, and deducing administrative issues. Although delineated separately, the processes are interactive and occur almost concurrently, with each idea influencing others.

The processes involved in analyzing and interpreting contextual data are illustrated in **Table 9-1** and **Table 9-2**. Table 9-1 includes data about internal contextual factors for Golden Wheatfields University School of Nursing, which is described in the Synthesis Activities section at the end of this chapter. The internal factors typically yield relatively few ideas about curriculum concepts and abilities but may point to curriculum limitations and administrative issues that influence the curriculum design. Some of the same limitations and administrative issues may be identified once again as external data are analyzed, thereby highlighting their importance. Table 9-2 is an example of how data about the external contextual factors, also for Golden Wheatfields University School of Nursing, could be analyzed. Included in both tables are highly abbreviated sets of contextual data and the patterns and trends arising from the data. Curriculum concepts, professional abilities, curriculum possibilities and limitations, and administrative issues are suggested. The columns in the tables provide a convenient and organized method of recording ideas but are not meant to connote sequential or segmented thinking.

DETERMINING THE CORE CURRICULUM CONCEPTS AND KEY PROFESSIONAL ABILITIES

Descriptions of the core curriculum concepts and key professional abilities are presented, along with the processes to derive them. These form some of the curriculum foundations (along with the philosophical and educational approaches) that give clear direction for further curriculum development and that ensure curriculum unity. Therefore, confirmation of the core curriculum concepts and key professional abilities is prerequisite to further curriculum development.

Table 9-1 Analysis of Internal Contextual Data for Golden Wheatfields University

Data	Patterns and Trends	Philosophy, Mission, and Goals				
		Curriculum Concepts	Professional Abilities	Curriculum Possibilities	Curriculum Limitations	Administrative Issues
Publicly funded university supports diversity, competency-based education, accountability, development of knowledgeable citizens.	Increasing emphasis on measurable outcomes			Development of a competency-based curriculum		Need to involve faculty expert in evaluation to ensure that curriculum and its outcomes conform to accountability measures
Increased research activity and funding are strategic goals for the university.		Evidence-informed nursing practice Knowledge generation	Evidence-informed nursing practice	Student involvement in faculty research		
School philosophy emphasizes student-centeredness, respect for differences, ethical behavior, importance of nursing to society.		All concepts that form the school's philosophy	Provide care in accordance with philosophy			Competing requirements for school's success: faculty involvement in curriculum development vs. research productivity

(continues)

			Culture			
Data	Patterns and Trends	Curriculum Concepts	Professional Abilities	Curriculum Possibilities	Curriculum Limitations	Administrative Issues
University is changing from centralized to more decentralized authority for academic programs.	Speed of program modification increased	Leadership, decision making	Leadership	Course devoted to leadership; Leadership experiences in healthcare agencies, nursing organizations; analysis of leadership behaviors in different contexts		No faculty expertise in interprofessional teams; Need to plan interprofessional practice with other disciplines and agencies
Much interdisciplinary research		Interdisciplinary multidisciplinary interprofessional	Work collaboratively with members of other disciplines and interprofessional healthcare teams	Course, experience, and/or analysis of healthcare teams	No provision for interprofessional practice experiences in agency contracts	
Although outwardly respectful to each other, different priorities are held by those with a strong research focus and those with a strong teaching focus.		Values; Professional career paths; Nursing role; Respect, civility, team-building				
All appreciate the school leader, who has a goal of developing a more unified faculty group.						

History

Data	Patterns and Trends	Curriculum Concepts	Professional Abilities	Curriculum Possibilities	Curriculum Limitations	Administrative Issues
Good relationships with healthcare agencies		Change	Work effectively in changing healthcare and social environment	Incorporate community health and health promotion concepts more fully into all nursing courses		Reluctance of faculty nearing retirement to make significant changes in teaching emphasis
Curricular emphases have been rural health, community health	Curriculum has changed in response to societal and healthcare trends	Social determinants of health				

Financial Resources

Data	Patterns and Trends	Curriculum Concepts	Professional Abilities	Curriculum Possibilities	Curriculum Limitations	Administrative Issues
University budget dependent on government allocation; economic downturn constrains government funding allocation	Budget constraints will continue			Reduced professional practice time to limit costs	Purchase of resources limited	No hiring of additional tenure-track faculty
"Tight" school budget but meeting present needs				Coursework only in year 1 with no professional practice		Funds for faculty and curriculum development

(continues)

Table 9-1 Analysis of Internal Contextual Data for Golden Wheatfields University (continued)

Programs and Policies

Data	Patterns and Trends	Curriculum Concepts	Professional Abilities	Curriculum Possibilities	Curriculum Limitations	Administrative Issues
MSN, PhD programs in school University policies regarding undergraduate degree requirements School can create policies for nursing program		Lifelong learning Career planning	Engage in ongoing learning, value education	Undergraduate students work on faculty-supervised research with graduate students	Disproportionate numbers of undergraduate and graduate students	

Infrastructure

Data	Patterns and Trends	Curriculum Concepts	Professional Abilities	Curriculum Possibilities	Curriculum Limitations	Administrative Issues
Human Resources						
28 tenure or tenure-track faculty 18 contract faculty 100 part-time 5 secretarial and clerical staff	Increasing number of non-tenure-track faculty over past 5 years; Constantly changing part-time contingent				Many who will implement curriculum are not involved in its development Nonresearchers may not be able to teach meaningfully about evidence-informed practice	Need to stabilize part-time faculty contingent Faculty development regarding new curriculum for all members
900 undergraduate students 220 graduate students Almost all students employed in positions ranging from half-time to full-time Student population is mainly local	Increasingly fewer are truly full-time students			Curriculum design to include a path for part-time students		

Physical Resources

All classrooms wired	University ensures current technology for teaching	In-class data searching		Faculty development regarding simulation needed
Nursing skills and simulation labs in school		Increased reliance on simulation	Few faculty knowledgeable about simulation development and teaching	
Computer labs for students on campus				
Inadequate office space for part-time faculty; little privacy for professional practice evaluation meetings with students		Online professional practice evaluation		

Resources to support teaching and learning

Library

Subscription to wide range of journal databases	Continuous investment in library by university	Greater involvement of nursing librarian in teaching literature-searching, citing and referencing, etc.		
Librarian dedicated to nursing programs				
Open 18 hours/day				

(continues)

Table 9-1 Analysis of Internal Contextual Data for Golden Wheatfields University (*continued*)

Data	Patterns and Trends	Curriculum Concepts	Infrastructure				Administrative Issues
			Professional Abilities	Curriculum Possibilities	Curriculum Limitations		
Faculty development							
University-wide teaching centre with ongoing programs to improve teaching and research into teaching-learning				Involvement of teaching centre personnel in new teaching approaches			Ensure all faculty are aware of teaching centre and its services
Student services							
Wide range of services: academic and personal counselling, financial aid, chaplains, health services, recreational services, gym membership, bus passes Computer labs open 18 hours/day				Rigorous curriculum			Ensure all faculty are aware of resources to support student success

Table 9-2   Analysis of External Contextual Data for Golden Wheatfields University

				Demographics			
Data	**Patterns and Trends**	**Curriculum Concepts**	**Professional Abilities**	**Curriculum Possibilities**	**Curriculum Limitations**	**Administrative Issues**
Life expectancy: Females 81.1 yrs Males 75.9 yrs	Greater numbers and percentages of seniors and the "old-old"	Aging Aging in place Healthy aging Health promotion	Health promotion Care of individuals with chronic illness(es)	Course on gerontological nursing or interprofessional course on aging		No faculty expert in gerontological nursing
Age profile: <5 yrs 5.6% 6–18 yrs 14.4% 19–64 yrs 61.4% >64 yrs 17.6%	Declining birth rate overall	Social support Health and health promotion and maintenance throughout the lifespan Evidence-informed practice	Care of elders with concurrent acute and chronic illness Provision of care in institutions and community Retrieve, critique, and use evidence Use information technologies	Health promotion and maintenance throughout the lifespan Professional practice experiences in community, long-term care, and acute care agencies		
	More home deliveries by midwives; students not welcome Increasing teen pregnancy rate					
Fertility rate 1.52	Increasing rate of illicit drug use among pregnant teens	Maternal–infant health	Health promotion from pre-conception to post-natal Care of women during labour and delivery	Community-based experiences to promote healthy child growth and development Involvement in prenatal classes at public health unit	Limited student placements on labour and delivery units	Need to establish relationships and placement agreements with midwives

(continues)

Table 9-2   Analysis of External Contextual Data for Golden Wheatfields University (continued)

| Data | Demographics | | | | |
	Curriculum Concepts	Professional Abilities	Curriculum Possibilities	Curriculum Limitations	Administrative Issues
	Physiological, psychological, and social aspects of teen pregnancy and child-rearing Effects of noxious substances on foetus, newborn Family and social support Evidence-informed practice Social support	Care of the neonate Referral to social agencies	Health promotion with pregnant teens in schools, community centers Theory course re maternal and child health Traditional labor and delivery practice placements Labor and delivery simulations		
1 in 5 are foreign-born Population growth through immigration Immigrants' regions of origin: Asia and Middle East	Culture Cultural safety	Cultural competence Communication enhancers and inhibitors	Health promotion sessions (e.g., BP, diabetes prevention clinics) with particular ethnic or cultural groups Attention to culture in all classes and professional practice experiences	Difficulty negotiating access to some cultural groups	

(continues)

Culture

Data	Patterns and Trends	Curriculum Concepts	Professional Abilities	Curriculum Possibilities	Curriculum Limitations	Administrative Issues
Western European/North American culture dominates.		Cultural norms, values, traditions, beliefs	Entering and working effectively in different cultures	Raise issues of ethnicity and culture in classroom and professional practice experiences	Caution not to teach stereotyped images of cultures	Identify and build relationships with cultural groups in the community
Asia and Middle East are main sources of immigrants.	Immigrant generation rooted in culture of origin; North American–born generation caught between cultures; third generation assimilated	Cultural safety / Diversity	Cultural competence		Most faculty are of Western or Central European origin with few links to other groups	
Chinese, Indian, and Thai grocery stores and restaurants are becoming more evident.		Intercultural stress	Recognizing situations of family stress	Cultural competence training		
		Intergenerational family stress	Working with community leaders and members / Adapting health promotion and caring strategies to diverse cultural groups	Health promotion activity with seniors or school children of particular ethnic or cultural groups / Written assignment about health beliefs of several cultures, including student's own culture		

Table 9-2   Analysis of External Contextual Data for Golden Wheatfields University (*continued*)

Health and Health Care

Data	Patterns and Trends	Curriculum Concepts	Professional Abilities	Curriculum Possibilities	Curriculum Limitations	Administrative Issues
Heart disease, cancer, stroke, chronic lung disease, accidents, and diabetes are the major causes of death and chronic illness	Incidence of diabetes, obesity increasing among all age groups	Perceptions and meanings of health and illness	Provision of care during preventative, acute, and rehabilitation phases	Traditional acute care placements	Many health science students (nursing, OT, PT, medical, etc.) exhaust patients	Need to negotiate new placements with home health and public health unit (possibly immunization clinics, prenatal classes)
25% with mental illness	Smoking rates increasing among teen girls	Specific physiologic concepts (e.g., oxygenation, perfusion, elimination, hormonal regulation)	Use of knowledge in care	Placements with home health nurses, outpatient clinics		
1 in 5 emergency admissions are related to mental health	Association between mental illness and homelessness	Pathophysiology	Rapid decision making	Separate course on mental health/ psychiatric nursing *or* integrate relevant concepts throughout the curriculum		
5 acute-care centers	Emphasis on safety	Mental health and illness	Health promotion	Professional practice experiences in many settings		
2 rehabilitation centers	Shorter hospital stays; more emphasis on home care	Marginalization	Culture of mental illness, street people			
1 psychiatric hospital with outreach teams	Individuals awaiting long-term care placement or rehabilitation sometimes take up acute care beds	Stigmatization	Retrieve, critique, and use evidence	In class: case studies requiring students to seek evidence in real time		
Public health unit focuses on maternal-child health, prevention and control of infectious diseases		Health promotion	Use information technologies			
		Culture of safety	Use relevant health technology			
		Evidence-informed care in all settings	Provision of safe, competent care			

Case managers in coordinating centre for homecare services arrange home care by contracting services	Shorter stays in psychiatric hospitals; more community-based services	Personal safety in community settings	Assessment, intervention, and reflection on care in all settings.
		Social support	
Community hospitals outside the city have been downsizing or closing over the past 10 years.	New focus on maternal-child services with immigrant groups	Determinants of health	Health promotion in all settings
		Professional boundaries	Delegating
		Cultural competence	Advocacy
Nursing shortage in local hospitals	Shortage is expected to worsen	Epidemiology, infection control	Interprofessional collaboration
		Delegation	Assessing
Home healthcare agencies	Many patients are distant from home community while receiving care in the city	Social support	Making clinical decisions and judgments
		Navigating the healthcare system	
		Assessment	
		Decision making	
		Clinical judgment	

(continues)

Table 9-2 Analysis of External Contextual Data for Golden Wheatfields University (*continued*)

			Professional Standards and Trends			
Data	**Patterns and Trends**	**Curriculum Concepts**	**Professional Abilities**	**Curriculum Possibilities**	**Curriculum Limitations**	**Administrative Issues**
Approval and accreditation standards for nursing programs	Emphasis on accountability, evidence-informed practice, safety, ongoing professional development, interprofessional collaboration	Regulation of the nursing profession	Commitment to maintenance of professional standards and comportment	Inclusion of approval and accreditation elements in curriculum	Interprofessional practice opportunities	Negotiation regarding interprofessional course(s) and practice experiences
Practice standards		Role of professional associations	Competence in all aspects of practice in all settings	Course on professionalism	Creation of valid and reliable evaluation methods	
Licensure or registration requirements		Professional roles, responsibilities, competence	Evidence-informed practice	Inclusion of all concepts regarding professionalism in all nursing courses		
Nature and structure of NCLEX	Growing backlash against competency-based education	Codes of ethics	Retrieval, critique, and use of evidence	Interprofessional course(s) and practice experiences		
Eclectic philosophies in nursing programs		Reasoned thinking	Enactment of relationships consistent with philosophical approaches	Formal testing regarding key nursing competencies		
Emphasis on student-centered teaching	Desire for seamless nursing education with ease of progression in the acquisition of higher credentials	Evidence-informed practice		Evaluation of relationship building in theory and practice courses		
Competency-based education		Career possibilities and trajectories				
Movement to baccalaureate as the entry to practice requirement in developed countries		Links between school's philosophical approaches and professional relationships (nurse–client, nurse–nurse, and interprofessional)				

Technology and Informatics

Electronic health care record (EHR) introduced throughout the city	Increasing dependence on electronic devices at point of care	Relationship of EHR and other documentation formats to culture of safety Confidentiality, accountability regarding EHR	Accurate and timely documentation Retrieval, critique, and use of data	Dedicated time regarding use of EHR Incorporation of real-time evidence retrieval in classes	No EHR in the school, restrictions regarding student use in some agencies Faculty discomfort with students being online in class	Negotiate for student access to EHRs in all settings Negotiate with vendor regarding EHRs in school Decisions regarding purchase of point-of-care technology
Wireless data retrieval possible from most locations		Criteria for evaluation of online sources				Faculty development in online data retrieval
Use of simulated patient scenarios (low, medium, and high fidelity) to replace or augment practice experiences		Value and purpose of simulated experiences				Faculty development in creation of scenarios, teaching or coaching, debriefing

Environment

Annual tornados, summer heat waves, and severe winter storms with loss of electrical power	Generally, more intense weather with global climate change	Disaster planning and response Care of individuals and groups in extreme situations or needing shelter Stress Community support Rapid assessment, triage, and intervention	Care of individuals and groups in extreme situations or needing shelter	Course related to disaster situations, governmental, and nursing responses; could include disaster response officials in planning and delivering parts of the course Could expand the above course to be interprofessional	No faculty member seems qualified to teach this course
Safe water supply except with loss of electricity					

(continues)

Table 9-2 Analysis of External Contextual Data for Golden Wheatfields University (*continued*)

			Professional Standards and Trends			
Data	Patterns and Trends	Curriculum Concepts	Professional Abilities	Curriculum Possibilities	Curriculum Limitations	Administrative Issues
		Social, Political, and Economic				
Local unemployment rate: 9.8%	Slow economic growth predicted	Family interactions, stress	Assessment of family functioning in all settings	Family health course		
Unemployment rate of 18–15 year old age group: 20%	Growing rates of crime, particularly violent crime	Domestic violence and safety	Screening for family violence	Visiting families in the community		
		Social determinants of health	Referring to social agencies	Workshops regarding domestic violence screening		
		Community resources to assist families in distress		Group assignment regarding learning about community resources		
		Health care for underinsured or uninsured				
		Ethical dilemmas regarding care	Contributing to resolution of ethical dilemmas related to health and care	Course on ethics (could be interprofessional)		Negotiation regarding interprofessional ethics course

Synthesizing Core Curriculum Concepts

Curriculum concepts are abstract ideas that form the substance of the curriculum. These are concepts that are essential for graduates to know and use in the context in which they will practice nursing. The curriculum concepts represent one aspect of an evidence-informed curriculum, because they are derived from contextual data. They permeate the curriculum, contributing to its unity and uniqueness.

The process for identifying the core curriculum concepts involves integration and synthesis. First, the curriculum concepts derived from the most important contextual factors are reviewed, and commonalities are integrated. Then, the same process is followed separately for the more important and less important contextual factors. The three sets of curriculum concepts that emerge are synthesized, with attention to the factors' relative importance. Concepts not integrated are reexamined to ensure that relevant ones are not omitted. There may be agreement to delete or modify some concepts, or it might seem more suitable to consider such decisions later when more detailed curriculum planning occurs.

Simultaneously with analysis of the contextual data, curriculum developers will be identifying the philosophical and educational approaches for the curriculum. The predominant ideas from these also contribute to the core curriculum concepts.

Synthesis and integration of the curriculum concepts and incorporation of the philosophical and educational approaches lead to identification of the core curriculum concepts. The core curriculum concepts:

- Are overriding ideas nurses should know
- Shape students' views about clients and how nurses think and behave
- Permeate and are prominent throughout the curriculum
- Are part of the curriculum content and structure used to organize content
- Reflect an integrated analysis of contextual data

Questions to guide synthesis of the core curriculum concepts are suggested in **Figure 9-1**.

Synthesizing Key Professional Abilities

Professional abilities are the capabilities necessary for nursing practice. These include, but are not limited to, cognitive, affective, technical, and interpersonal skills; ethical decision making; and professional judgment. The key professional abilities are essential for nursing practice. Like the core concepts, the key abilities represent one aspect of an evidence-informed curriculum, because they are derived from contextual data. These abilities permeate the curriculum, contributing to its unity and uniqueness.

Figure 9-1   Questions to guide synthesis of curriculum concepts.
Reproduced from Iwasiw, C., Goldenberg, D., & Andrusyszyn, M. A. (2009). *Curriculum development in nursing education* (2nd ed.). Sudbury, MA: Jones and Bartlett.

- What are the commonalities among curriculum concepts inferred from each of the *most important, more important,* and *less important* contextual factors?
- Can curriculum concepts inferred from the *more* and *less important* contextual factors be integrated with those of the *most important* contextual factors?
- Of those curriculum concepts that have not been integrated, which should be included in the curriculum?
- Does the synthesis reflect the relative weighting assigned to the contextual factors?
- Are there ideas evident from the combination and inter-relationships of contextual factors that have not been identified?
- Which concepts from the philosophical approaches should also be included?
- Does the synthesis truly encapsulate the important ideas that are essential for graduates to know and use, so they can practice successfully within present and future societal and healthcare contexts?

The professional abilities identified for each factor are synthesized in the same fashion as the curriculum concepts. The synthesized professional abilities lead to identification of the key professional abilities. Questions to guide the synthesis of professional abilities are included in **Figure 9-2**. Further, the philosophical approaches influence these key professional abilities.

Figure 9-2   Questions to guide synthesis of professional abilities.
© C. L. Iwasiw.

- What are the commonalities among the professional abilities inferred from each of the *most important, more important,* and *less important* contextual factors?
- Can the professional abilities inferred from the *more* and *less important* contextual factors be integrated with those of the *most important* contextual factors?
- Of the professional abilities that have not been integrated, which should be included in the curriculum?
- Does the synthesis reflect the relative weighting assigned to the contextual factors?
- Are there ideas about professional abilities evident from the combination and inter-relationships of contextual factors that have not been identified?
- Should abilities deduced from the philosophical approaches also be included?
- Does the synthesis truly encapsulate the important professional abilities that are essential for graduates to practice successfully within present and future societal and healthcare contexts?

The key professional abilities serve a similar function in the curriculum as the core curriculum concepts. The key professional abilities:

- Are overriding professional abilities that nurses utilize in all practice contexts
- Shape students' thinking about the nature of nursing practice
- Permeate and are emphasized throughout the curriculum
- Form part of the curriculum content
- Are evident in professional practice experiences
- Reflect an integrated analysis of contextual data

Confirming Core Curriculum Concepts and Key Professional Abilities

Finally, the curriculum team must employ its professional judgment about the core curriculum concepts and key professional abilities that have been derived. Members will want to review all completed work before committing themselves to these curriculum foundations.

To reach agreement, considerable discussion could be necessary. Understandably, decisions can be fraught with conflict if aspects of the current curriculum valued by particular faculty members are likely to be excluded or reduced in prominence. It is natural for faculty to use the current curriculum and personal teaching experience as a frame of reference for discussion. If consensus is difficult to reach, it would be wise to review the reasons for curriculum redesign, the data about the most important contextual factors, and values held by faculty. This reexamination could lend objectivity to the discussion.

It is vital that the total faculty group achieve resolution. Confirmation is essential, because a successful curriculum is dependent on total support. Final decisions about the core curriculum concepts and key professional abilities should be clearly justifiable by the constellation of contextual data and responsive to the reasons that led to curriculum development in the first place. Only then can curriculum developers be assured that they are building the foundation of a unified curriculum that will be evidence informed and relevant for its present and future contexts. Following confirmation of the core curriculum concepts and key professional abilities, in combination with philosophical and educational approaches, goals are formulated, and curriculum design is created.

RELATIONSHIP OF ANALYSIS AND INTERPRETATION OF CONTEXTUAL DATA TO AN EVIDENCE-INFORMED, CONTEXT-RELEVANT, UNIFIED CURRICULUM

The contextual data provide evidence upon which a curriculum can be designed. The derivation of core curriculum concepts and key professional abilities from the contextual data ensures that these two aspects of the curriculum foundations are evidence-informed and context relevant. Moreover, the core concepts and key abilities will be prominent throughout the curriculum and will be an important part of the unity within the curriculum. Identification of curriculum limitations and administrative issues, and subsequent attention to these in curriculum planning, grounds the curriculum in the feasible realities of the context. Finally, creative ideas about curriculum possibilities provide a basis for further thinking as curriculum design proceeds. The curriculum possibilities will be assessed in relation to their congruence with the curriculum foundations and the curriculum context. The ideas that are accepted will further contribute to creation of an evidence-informed, context-relevant, unified curriculum context.

CORE PROCESSES OF CURRICULUM WORK

Faculty Development

The goal of faculty development in relation to analysis and interpretation of contextual data is to expand appreciation and understanding of the processes involved in deriving the core curriculum concepts and key professional abilities, and how the processes relate to curriculum development. Participants require knowledge of the process, because decisions based on the contextual data will determine part of the curriculum foundations and thus shape the school's activities for a number of years.

Faculty development, in workshop format, can be focused on the processes that will move faculty and other stakeholders from contextual data to curriculum foundations and should be based on contextual data that have been obtained. In this way, faculty development is integrated into the work that will lead to a completed curriculum.

First, participants could discuss the contextual data to gain a common understanding of the environment. Then, they might divide into groups to derive curriculum concepts, professional abilities, curriculum possibilities and limitations, and administrative issues for one contextual factor. In this way, all could have experience in the analysis of the same contextual factor, so that differing perspectives would be evident and discussed. The remaining contextual factors could be divided among groups, with each group to consider a different factor, thereby expediting the curriculum development process. Practice with the process should promote understanding. Presentation of the subgroups' work could lead to synthesis of the concepts and professional abilities derived, to determine the core concepts and key professional abilities. This will likely entail further discussion about the processes and the decisions achieved and could require some values clarification. These activities can be facilitated by those members with experience in this aspect of curriculum development, or if appropriate, by an outside expert.

Ongoing Appraisal

Ongoing appraisal is an inherent part of the discussions that result in identification of the core curriculum concepts and key professional abilities. During discussion, curriculum developers should ask the following:

- Do the curriculum concepts and professional abilities flow logically from the contextual data? Are they really appropriate for the context?
- What alternative interpretations could be considered?
- Are we identifying concepts and abilities at a suitable level of abstraction or synthesis?
- Have we missed anything important?
- Are there other core curriculum concepts and key professional abilities that should be discussed?
- Are our conclusions likely to be supported? Why or why not?

Scholarship

There are many possibilities for scholarship projects related to analyzing and interpreting contextual data. A relatively straightforward project would be to describe the processes and discussion that lead to consensus about core curriculum concepts and key professional abilities, and then to offer suggestions about the process. A more ambitious project could be to compare the conclusions reached by groups of curriculum development participants who have examined the same contextual data independently, offer explanations for similarities and differences in their conclusions, and propose the curriculum implications of the differences. As in all phases of curriculum development, a study could be undertaken to examine participants' perspectives. In this case, it would be perspectives about engaging in the process of analyzing and interpreting contextual data and the contribution of the activity to their understanding of nursing curriculum development.

CHAPTER SUMMARY

In this chapter, a further step in the curriculum development process is described, namely the analysis and interpretation of contextual data to derive the core curriculum concepts and key professional abilities. The processes of analyzing and interpreting contextual data and synthesizing ideas generated from the analysis are emphasized as being iterative and nonlinear, although a procedural approach is described for explanatory purposes. Questions are provided to assist in integrating data, inferring curriculum concepts and professional abilities, proposing curriculum possibilities, identifying curriculum limitations, and deducing administrative issues. Confirming the core curriculum concepts and key professional abilities can involve emotions and values. Therefore, open communication, values clarification, and rigorous intellectual discussion are essential to achieve acceptable foundations for an evidence-informed, context-relevant, unified curriculum. Ideas for faculty development activities, ongoing appraisal, and scholarship are proposed.

SYNTHESIS ACTIVITIES

In the Golden Wheatfields University School of Nursing case, a description is given about how the curriculum developers came to consensus about core curriculum concepts and key professional abilities that were derived from contextual data in Tables 9-1 and 9-2. The data in the tables form part of the case. These data are significantly abbreviated from what would normally be gathered but should be sufficient to illustrate the processes described in the chapter. The case is followed by questions and activities that provide a basis for examining the case. Then, ideas are offered that might assist readers when analyzing and interpreting contextual data in their own settings.

Golden Wheatfields University School of Nursing

Golden Wheatfields University has its origins in Golden Wheatfields primary school, a one-room school built in 1847 in response to a growing movement for mandatory education for children until the age of 12. Over time, as immigration grew, the local residents saw the value of education for their children, first to be "one step above" the immigrants, and then to help immigrant children learn to adapt to community values. With growth in the community, education became valued as a means for children to better themselves and "get ahead." From these beginnings, the school grew in size to offer Grades 1–12. In the mid 1920s, in response to the increased economic importance of the local farming community, the government voted to build and support a small university dedicated to science, agriculture, and domestic science. Since then, the publicly funded university has developed a wide range of programs and research centers. The farming community has become a city of 750,000 with five acute-care hospitals, two rehabilitation hospitals, one psychiatric facility, a regional public health unit, and a coordinating agency for homecare services.

The School of Nursing was founded in 1937, in response to Canada's anticipated involvement in the forthcoming war in Europe and the expected need for nursing leadership in the armed forces. First there was a 1-year program in hospital supervision and administration for registered nurses, and this was quickly followed in 1940 by a 3+1 bachelor of science in nursing (BScN) program for students with no preparation in nursing. The 3+1 program was comprised of 3 years in a hospital diploma nursing program followed by 1 year of university courses, which included nursing leadership and sciences pertinent to surgical field hospitals. In 1948 when the war ended, the arrangements with local diploma nursing programs were phased out and the School of Nursing introduced an integrated, 4-year BScN curriculum.

Over the years, there have been many curriculum changes in response to trends in nursing education and provincial health and healthcare initiatives. Through all these changes, the School of Nursing has remained steadfast in its commitment to a 4-year integrated nursing program.

The School of Nursing is currently comprised of 900 undergraduate students and 220 graduate students in master's and PhD programs. There are 42 full-time faculty members, 28 of whom are tenured or on the tenure track. The remaining 18 have contracts of 2, 3, or 5 years, with an emphasis on teaching and a small research commitment. Research areas include rural health and rural nursing, community health and community nursing, and acute care nursing. More than 100 clinicians are employed on a part-time basis for professional practice teaching. Community health is a strong feature of the present program.

The School of Nursing is now developing a new curriculum. Although the original intent was "curriculum renewal," it became apparent that a new curriculum with new ideas was needed. Accordingly, faculty members have engaged in extensive data gathering and are now ready to interpret the contextual data. The curriculum leader, Dr. Yana Palamarchuk has convened a 1-day retreat of faculty and stakeholders to link the contextual data to curriculum.

The group had previously attended a short faculty development workshop about analyzing contextual data. They now feel ready for the work. Faculty and other stakeholders are committed to the ideas of inferring curriculum concepts and professional abilities, proposing curriculum possibilities, and deducing curriculum limitations. Many members are not convinced of the need to identify administrative issues. They believe they already know what the administrative issues are: not enough faculty and a budget that is too small.

In preparation for the retreat, data had been organized for each contextual factor on a chart, and hard copies had been distributed. The chart was loaded onto laptop computers so ideas could be immediately recorded and preserved. The total group was divided into subgroups, each to examine all the data to get a sense of the complete context in which the curriculum would be offered and graduates would practice.

The group first examined all the data to determine their meaning and the interrelationships among the contextual factors. They also addressed curriculum concepts, professional abilities, and curriculum possibilities without labeling the ideas in this way. They raised such ideas as:

- What the aging population might mean for healthcare and nursing services
- Whether the nursing shortage might mean that they should plan for increased enrollment
- How government healthcare priorities would influence healthcare services, and, in turn, student placement opportunities
- Growing reliance on point-of-care health technology and employers' expectations that graduates know the technology

In trying to reach a shared understanding of the context in which the curriculum would be implemented and graduates would practice nursing, several integrated summaries were offered. Each resulted in some disagreement. Finally, the group agreed that the environment could be described as one in which:

- There will be less institutionalized health care and growing emphasis on community-based care.
- Independent decision making and supervision of nonprofessional healthcare providers will become a stronger feature of baccalaureate nursing practice.
- Vulnerable groups in the community may grow in size.
- The proportion of aged people in the community will increase.
- Ethnic diversity will become more apparent.

Dr. Palamarchuk asked the group to consider which factors should be most influential in shaping the curriculum. Initially, there was a strong sentiment that all contextual factors were of equal weight, apart from the internal factors of history, philosophy, mission, goals, and culture, all of which seemed less important. With further discussion, the group considered whether it was the recipients of nursing services (demographics), the nature of nursing (professional standards and trends), or the location and nature of health services (health care) that was most important. Finally, they agreed that most important were the people being served, and, therefore, demographics and external culture would be most significant in determining the curriculum concepts and professional abilities. History was immediately labeled as being of least importance. Eventually, there was consensus about the ordering of contextual factors:

1. Demographics, external culture
2. Health care, professional standards, and trends; infrastructure
3. Social, political, and economic conditions
4. Technology
5. Environment; philosophy, mission, and goals of the university and school of nursing; internal culture; and history

Small groups were formed. Each group was assigned two internal and two external contextual factors from which to derive concepts and professional abilities and to propose curriculum concepts, professional abilities, curriculum possibilities, curriculum limitations, and administrative issues.

In reviewing the contextual data, members recognized that curriculum concepts, professional abilities, and curriculum possibilities and limitations did not necessarily arise from each internal factor. However, they noted that the data about some of the factors could ultimately influence decisions about curriculum, either limiting or propelling the curriculum design. For example, when examining the school's infrastructure, they recognized that the existence of wired classrooms meant that in-class database searching was a possibility in all courses, whereas the school budget and faculty numbers could constrain the curriculum design. Accordingly, they reaffirmed their intention to identify the curriculum possibilities and limitations as they examined each contextual factor. As the groups worked, they recognized again that the contextual factors do not operate in isolation and that their ideas reflected the interrelated nature of the internal and external contexts. The ideas arising from the internal and external contextual data were recorded. See Tables 9-1 and 9-2 for the analyses.

Questions and Activities for Critical Analysis of the Golden Wheatfields University School of Nursing Case

1. Explain why the ordering of the contextual factors does (or does not) seem reasonable. Compare the ordering completed by the Golden Wheatfields faculty with the ordering that might be proposed for your school of nursing. Consider why there might be similarities or differences.

2. Review Tables 9-1 and 9-2. What missing data would be important to include?

3. Examine Tables 9-1 and 9-2. Propose other interpretations of the data, concepts, professional abilities, curriculum limitations and possibilities, and administrative issues.

4. Based on the analyses in Tables 9-1 and 9-2, complete the synthesis of the curriculum concepts and professional abilities to determine the core curriculum concepts and key professional abilities.

5. Critique the processes used by the Golden Wheatfields School of Nursing to analyze the contextual data.

6. Discuss how ongoing appraisal might have been deliberately included in the processes followed by Golden Wheatfields' faculty and stakeholders.

Questions and Activities for Consideration When Analyzing and Interpreting Contextual Data in Readers' Settings

1. How can faculty development be planned to prepare for analyzing and interpreting contextual data?

2. Who should be involved in the analysis and interpretation of contextual data?

3. In what way can the contextual data be organized and displayed in a manner that will be helpful for analysis?

4. Describe approaches that could be useful for achieving a common understanding of the contextual data.

5. Devise procedures that could be used for analyzing and interpreting the contextual data in a manner that balances expediency with faculty and stakeholder involvement.

6. Suggest a feasible plan for recording the analysis of contextual data.

7. Propose a procedure to determine the relative weighting of the contextual factors.

8. Determine how curriculum concepts and professional abilities can be synthesized. How can consensus be achieved?

9. What is a reasonable timeframe in which to accomplish this work?

10. Propose ideas about how divergent viewpoints might be addressed constructively.

11. Create a faculty development plan and a means to incorporate ongoing appraisal into the analysis and interpretation of contextual data.

12. Suggest some desirable and feasible scholarship projects.

CHAPTER 10

Establishing Philosophical and Educational Approaches for an Evidence-Informed, Context-Relevant, Unified Curriculum

Chapter Overview

In this chapter, philosophy is introduced with definitions and purposes. These are presented from the perspectives of general education and nursing education. Traditional philosophies are considered first. Then, ideas about teaching and learning include information about learning theories and the science of learning. Brief descriptions are given of some educational theories, frameworks, and pedagogies, with specific reference to their use in nursing curricula. This is followed by the authors' conceptualization of *philosophical and educational approaches* for curriculum development, including their development and relationship to an evidence-informed, context-relevant, unified curriculum.

  The core processes of curriculum work are addressed: faculty development, ongoing appraisal, and scholarship. After the chapter summary, a case illustrates the main ideas of the chapter. Questions to guide consideration of the case are included, followed by questions to stimulate thinking about developing philosophical and educational approaches in readers' settings.

Chapter Goals

- Understand the purposes of *philosophical* and *educational approaches* in curriculum development.
- Gain insight into some theories, research, frameworks, and pedagogies relevant for philosophical and educational approaches.
- Consider processes for developing philosophical and educational approaches.
- Appreciate the relationship of philosophical and educational approaches to an evidence-informed, context-relevant, unified curriculum.
- Reflect on the core processes of curriculum work in relation to establishing philosophical and educational approaches.

CURRICULUM PHILOSOPHY

Philosophy is the:

> study of the most general and abstract features of the world and categories with which we think: mind, matter, reason, proof, truth, etc. In philosophy, the concepts with which we approach the world themselves become the topic of enquiry. A philosophy of a discipline . . . seeks to study. . . . the concepts that structure such thinking, and to lay bare their foundations and presuppositions. In this sense philosophy is what happens when a practice becomes self-conscious. (Blackburn, 2014)

In general education, philosophy statements include assumptions about human nature; the purpose and goals of education, instruction, and learning; and the roles of teachers, students, and programs. John Dewey, a renowned American educator, interpreted philosophy as a "general theory of educating," whereas one of his students, Boyd Bode, viewed it as a "source of reflective consideration" (Wiles & Bondi, 2011, p. 35).

A curriculum philosophy is part of the curriculum foundation. It is a statement of carefully examined beliefs about the purpose and nature of education and learning, as well as beliefs about students, faculty members, and teaching-learning processes. More expansively, Valiga (2012) described curriculum philosophy as a:

> way of framing questions . . . [about] what is presupposed, perceived, intuited, believed, and known. It is a way of contemplating, or thinking about what is taken to be significant, valuable, or worthy of commitment . . . of becoming self-aware and thinking of the everyday as "problematic" so that questions are posed [about what, how, and why things are done].

A curriculum philosophy provides a basis for:

- Curriculum development, implementation, and evaluation—that is, determination of goals or outcomes, subjects and content to include, methods and materials to use, organization of content, teaching-learning processes, activities and experiences to emphasize, and what and how to evaluate (Orstein & Hunkins, as cited in Oliva, 2009; Wiles & Bondi, 2011)
- Shaping students' ideas about clients, nursing, and health care; thinking processes in nursing; knowledge acquisition, development, and creation
- Discussions about curriculum practices and preferences
- Professional development (Petress, 2003)
- Decision making for the profession (White & Brockett, 1987)

Curriculum Philosophy in Nursing Education

In nursing education, the curriculum philosophy is a description of the value system that grounds the curriculum; thus it includes ideas about education and nursing. Ideas that might be included in a philosophy of nursing education or a curriculum philosophy could be beliefs about:

- The nature of learning
- Purposes of the curriculum
- Roles of faculty and students
- The nature of faculty–student interactions
- Other values, such as social justice, diversity, service

Because an important part of the mission of all undergraduate schools of nursing is to prepare nurses for practice, the curriculum philosophy also includes reference to the metaparadigm of nursing (nature and goals of nursing, role of nurses in society and health-care systems, persons, rights and obligations for health, and environment). Although the components of the metaparadigm may be described in greater detail in a separate document, these beliefs form an essential part of the curriculum philosophy. Within the description of nursing are concepts and abilities drawn from the analysis of contextual data.

Traditional Curriculum Philosophies

Although classical philosophies date back some 2,500 years to Greek scholars of the 6th century BCE, differences in the philosophical bases of various disciplines began only in the last two centuries (Uys & Smit, 1994). It was not until late into the 1800s that the first well-rounded philosophy about nursing education was developed by Florence Nightingale (Csokasy, 2005). Since Nightingales' time, traditional curriculum philosophies have been seen in nursing curricula. These philosophies include idealism, realism, perennialism, essentialism, progressivism, and reconstructionism (Oliva, 2009; Wiles & Bondi, 2011).

Idealism

According to this philosophy, truth is universal, values are unchanging, and individuals desire to live in a perfect world of high ideals, beauty, and art. The curriculum is built on humanism, liberal arts education, and promotion of intellectual growth. Teachers serve as role models for students, who are encouraged to think and expand their minds by applying knowledge to life. Ideas of social justice and service learning in nursing curricula are rooted in idealism.

Realism

The main tenet of realism is that natural laws compose the world and regulate all of nature. The curriculum is structured to present and reflect these universal laws, and is organized around content. Teachers provide information sequentially in an efficient, simple-to-complex manner. Students are motivated to learn through positive reinforcement, and they are rewarded for learning basic skills and responding to new experiences with scientific objectivity and analysis. Nursing curricula that are content driven and in which testing is mainly by means of multiple-choice examinations reflect some element of the philosophy of realism.

Perennialism

According to this philosophy, the aims of education are the disciplining of the mind, development of reasoning ability, and pursuit of truth that is unchanging. Emphasis is placed on logic and classical literature. A nod to perennialism is given in nursing curricula in which students are taught to think like a nurse, using cognitive processes essential to the discipline. However, the idea of unchanging truths that can be absolutely known is not consistent with science and contemporary health care.

Essentialism

This philosophy is built on the idea that cultural heritage must be preserved and that it is the role of education to do so. Similar to perennialism, the aims of education within an essentialist philosophy are intellectual development, with curricula built around subjects essential to a field of study. This idea persists in nursing curricula with required subjects such as physiology or psychology, both of which are viewed as essential bases for nursing practice. Behaviorist learning theories are associated with essentialism.

Progressivism

This orientation to education holds that the growth of students should be the centre of educational activities and not the subject matter. Because the world is constantly changing, students must learn to think (Kilpatrick, 2010). Thus, education is not subject matter to be mastered, but a lifelong process of learning. According to this philosophy, students should be actively engaged in experiences that build their mental, emotional, physical, spiritual, social, and cultural capacities. The scientific method, humanism, gestalt psychology, cognitive constructivism, and critical inquiry are consistent with progressivism in that individual capacities are developed through activities that invoke student involvement in problem solving, shared decision making, logical and creative thinking, reflection, and divergent thinking. Nursing curricula in which students are engaged in active learning and exploration of a wide range of human and nursing experiences reflect ideas of progressivism.

Reconstructionism

This school of thought holds that the purpose of education is to improve society; therefore, students are exposed to controversial social problems, study them, and reach solutions through consensus. Reconstructionism is evident in nursing courses in which students address social, healthcare, and professional situations where inequities or questionable practices exist. The goal of reconstructing a situation is at the root of questions such as: *How can you address this in your role as a student? What can you do when you are a practicing nurse? How can/should the profession take this matter in hand?*

IDEAS ABOUT TEACHING AND LEARNING AS PART OF CURRICULUM PHILOSOPHY

Ideas about learning and teaching, that is, the educational approaches, form part of the curriculum foundations, along with the core curriculum concepts, key professional abilities, and the curriculum's philosophical approaches. They might be described separately from the curriculum philosophy or be incorporated into it. The educational approaches can be based on a single learning theory or framework, or a combination of ideas about learning and teaching. As with other aspects of the curriculum, there must be logical consistency among the ideas selected.

Learning Theories

There are hosts of theories that explain learning and that have been grouped in many ways. Broad categories of theories evident in nursing education curricula are behaviorist, cognitive, humanist, social and situational, and, more recently, integrated theories of learning.

Behaviorist Theories

Behaviorist theories, espoused by theorists such as Pavlov, Watson, and Skinner, define learning as a change in behavior. Learning is stimulated by events in the external environment. The educator's role is to arrange the environment to stimulate a desired response. Behaviorism is evident in the use of behavioral objectives, psychomotor skill development, and competency-based education.

Cognitive Theories

Cognitive theories focus on internal mental processes such as information processing, memory, and perception. Learning is cognitive structuring or restructuring. Accordingly, educators have a responsibility to structure learning activities whose purpose includes student development of the skills and capacity to learn better. Problem-based learning is an example of the use of cognitive theory. Cognitive theorists are Piaget, Ausubel, Bruner, Gagné, and Vygotsky.

Humanist Theories

Humanist theories of learning are premised on the belief that individuals strive to reach their full potential, and, thus, learning is a personal act designed to meet this goal. Because learning is viewed as both affective and cognitive, the educator's role is to facilitate development of the whole person. Maslow, Rogers, and Mezirow are the theorists most associated with humanist theories of learning.

Social and Situational Theories

Social and situational theories of learning combine ideas about cognitive, affective, and situational factors in learning. The premise is that learning occurs in social contexts in which individuals observe their own behavior and that of others, experience and observe the affective and behavioral consequences of actions, mentally process observations and experiences, and reach conclusions about themselves. Educators using these theories provide opportunities for individuals to have relevant experiences and build self-confidence. The most researched example of a social and situational learning theory is Bandura's (1977) Social Learning Theory.

Integrated Theories

Integrated theories take into account internal psychological processes such as managing the learning content and directing the mental energy to run the process, as well as an individual's personal situation, external conditions, and the resultant learning. The interactions among the components are dynamic. These theories incorporate aspects of cognitive theories and social and situational theories, and also give attention to an individual's psychology. Illeris (2009) notes that four types of learning can result: *cumulative* or mechanical learning, *assimilative* learning (by addition), *accommodative* or transcendent learning, and significant or *transformative* learning. Jarvis (2009) gives attention to the whole person (body and mind), an individual's psychology, and society. In education, it is expected that programs are seen by students to be relevant, challenging, and aligned with their personal needs. Therefore, it is incumbent on educators to make evident the value of the educational event for students' identity and goals.

Science of Learning (Brain-Based Learning)

Research findings from neuroscience, education, psychology, and neuroeducation have led to conclusions about learning and conditions for learning. As cognitive neuroscience continues to provide insights into mental processes and neural systems, teaching will become more science-based, more "brain-based" (Van Dam, 2013).

According to Tokuhama-Espinosa (2010), there are five firmly established facts about the brain:

- Each brain is unique.
- Brains are highly plastic (i.e., neural connections can grow and change throughout life).
- All brains are not equal in problem-solving ability.
- The brain connects new information to old.
- The brain is changed by experience.

Probably true, but not definitively so, are findings about the impact of emotions, and physiological processes on teaching and learning (Tokuhama-Espinosa, 2010). Specific concepts, principles, and teaching guidelines have been identified and extrapolated from the definite and probable conclusions. These instructional guidelines are summarized as follows:

- Good learning environments have physical and mental security, respect, intellectual freedom, and self-regulation.
- Learning should be put into the context of the learner's world, with attention to prior learning and transfer.
- Teachers ought to attend to auditory, visual, and kinesthetic neural pathways, and plan for individual and group work to improve recall.
- A change in the style of interaction, pace, and/or topic is necessary about every 20 minutes.
- Learners require opportunities for peer interaction in order to develop and test ideas.
- Class scheduling should accommodate students' need for rest and nutrition.
- Activities and interactions should be planned to allow students to develop their own understandings.
- Significant learning activities are necessary for students to be active learners.
- Time and opportunity are required for student reflection and metacognition.
- Teachers are obligated to learn about skill development at different life stages and plan appropriately, while recognizing that learning is lifelong (Tokuhama-Espinosa, 2010).

Similarly, Straumanis (2012) has summarized research findings from six Science of Learning Centers in the United States about conditions that promote robust learning. *Robust learning* entails (1) long-term retention, (2) preparation for further or deeper learning and application, and (3) transfer of knowledge to new situations. The conditions for robust learning are:

- Engagement of the brain's motivational and reward systems. The intrinsic rewards of engaging in learning activities should compete successfully with distracters such as online social sites.
- Plenty of social interaction.
- Use of multimodal forms of input, such as adding music to cognitive content. When more than one part of the brain is engaged, the neural systems reinforce one another, particularly if the pleasure center of the hippocampus is stimulated.
- Sufficient sleep to consolidate memory. Different types of learning are reinforced by different sleep phases.
- Management of the timing of practice and reinforcement. Learning performance plotted against assistance yields a U-shaped curve. For each task there is a time when assistance is most effective. Also, the longer the interval between reinforcement sessions, the longer the retention.
- Engagement through active learning such as short writing breaks, self- and peer explanations, problem solving, and discussion (Straumanis, 2012).

Other ideas about brain-based learning and teaching include the following:

- Focused attention is fundamental to acquiring new knowledge.
- Multitasking slows down learning (Thomson, 2012; Van Dam, 2013).
- Emotions play an important role in learning (McGinty, Radin, & Kaminski, 2013).

Research findings and subsequent extrapolations about brain-based teaching do not constitute a philosophy themselves. However, if faculty members attend to research findings about learning and effective teaching, appraise their soundness and utility, and institute practices stemming from the research, they are reflecting a commitment to active learning by students and evidence-informed teaching. This commitment ought to be evident in the philosophical statements of the curriculum.

Learning Theories, Educational Frameworks, and Pedagogies

One or more learning theory, educational framework, or pedagogy can be used as part of the philosophical base and learning orientation of the nursing curriculum. It is important that those selected are reflective of faculty views about learning, teaching, student characteristics, and the educational environment. They should also be consistent with descriptions of nursing in the school's philosophy and with the educational institution's philosophy. For example, if clients of nursing services are viewed as active participants in their care, it would be logically consistent to view students as active participants in their education.

The following alphabetical listing of current nursing curriculum philosophies, frameworks, and pedagogies, albeit merely highlighted, evidence some differences, but also commonalities. As can be detected, there is a blending of philosophy and learning theory or framework, as well as an intermingling of beliefs, values, and teaching and learning applications.

Adult Learning (Andragogy)

This framework is premised on the belief that adults are self-directed, goal oriented, and motivated to learn in response to real-life problems or situations that require knowledge and/or skills they lack. Adults are oriented to relevancy and practicality in their learning, which is influenced by their life experiences. Adults are seen as being able to structure their learning experiences, that is, to identify their learning needs and goals, resources to meet those goals, and criteria for assessing their success. They are also capable of evaluating their achievement against the self-defined criteria. Respect for learners and their experiences and preservation of their self-esteem are important in learning situations (Knowles & Associates, 1984; Knowles, Holton, & Swanson, 1998).

Apprenticeship

Cognitive apprenticeship is a teaching-learning approach in which students participate with experts in a community of practice to learn expert knowledge, physical skills, procedures, thinking processes, and the culture of the field. Students observe, participate, and discover expert practice through teaching strategies such as modeling, coaching, scaffolding (hints, directions, reminders, physical assistance), and learning strategies such as articulation, reflection, and exploration (Taylor & Care, 1999). In accordance with ideas about cognitive apprenticeship, Reutter and colleagues (2010) have described a research apprenticeship in which nursing students in a 4-year honors bachelor of science in nursing program are paired with experienced researchers for the length of the program, the culmination being the development of students' own research projects.

More broadly than the previous descriptions, Benner, Sutphen, Leonard, and Day (2010) have advanced the idea of three "high-end" apprenticeships that encompass the whole range of professional practice, in which students learn nursing knowledge and science, skilled knowhow and clinical reasoning, and ethical comportment and formation. The apprenticeship involves integrative learning experiences that make visible key aspects of practice, supervision of student practice, coaching to help students articulate and examine their practice, attention to the salient features of a situation, and reflection on practice.

Cognitive Constructivism

This learning theory is based in cognitive psychology, particularly understandings of how memory works and how ideas are linked and transformed in an iterative fashion. The theory holds that people build knowledge, in contrast to merely acquiring it. Preeminence is given to students' construction of concepts and the relationship of new understandings to previous learning, with each individual developing his or her own meanings. Thus, learning occurs in a spiral fashion, with new ideas influencing previous conceptions and being understood within each person's mental framework (Brandon & All, 2010). Curricula are characterized by active, student-centered learning that allows students to develop deep knowledge and meanings. Factual information emerges from preparatory reading, experience, and discussion. Emphases are on students' ability to build and link concepts, construct meanings, and use those understandings in analysis and professional practice (Biggs & Tang, as cited in Joseph & Juwah, 2012; Richardson, 2003). Students are active learners who are responsible for organizing and using knowledge.

Critical Social Theory

This theory is concerned with justice, equality, and freedom. Maintained is that knowledge as truth is socially constructed, and facts are relevant only in the lived experiences of persons (Duchscher, 2000). The premise is that all meanings and truths are created and interpreted in the context of social history (Henderson, 1995). Understanding patterns of human behavior involves knowledge of existing social structures and the communication processes that define them. Critical social theory enables students and faculty to share a revisioning and reconstruction of former potentially oppressive and coercive cultural, political, and social ideologies and practices. Empathy and confidence in interpersonal relationships develop through critical self-reflection, self-transformation, discussion, and dialogue (Duchscher, 2000). With this action-oriented theory, students examine health care and other structures (including their own role in oppressive practices), and advocate for changes in the situations that create oppression and influence health (Mohammed, 2006).

A belief in social justice stems from critical social theory, and social justice has been proposed as a framework for curricula (Boutain, 2005, 2008). A desire to enact ideas of social justice has led to the inclusion of service-learning in many schools of nursing, with an emphasis on service to those in socially disadvantaged positions. One example is a service-learning project to enhance access to cardiac health screening. Participation in the service project, journaling, and critical discussion led to students' recognition of health and health service inequities and to creation of strategies to produce change through empowerment of community members (Gillis & MacLellan, 2013).

Deep Learning

Deep learning is characterized by:

> intrinsic motivation, engagement with the subject matter, and a desire to know everything about a given topic. Conversely, students who opt for a surface approach to learning are not interested in the task per se, but aim at learning the minimum amount of material required to pass [the course]. (Chamorro-Premuzic, as cited in Dinsmore & Alexander, 2012)

Deep learning is seen as a process of exploration, discovery, and growth in which students invest themselves (Platow, Mavor, & Grace, 2013). It involves critical analysis of new ideas, linking them to previously known concepts and principles. The result is understanding and long-term retention so concepts can subsequently be used for problem solving in unfamiliar contexts. To achieve deep learning, students must make connections among concepts and experiences within and beyond course content. Therefore, within an educational stance that values deep learning, covering content is not a focus. Rather, students are expected to be self-motivated, interested in the topics, and willing to do the necessary intellectual work to achieve understanding of the relationships between and among concepts and topics. Faculty are facilitators of intellectual exploration, critical analysis, and the creation of connections to previous learning.

Epistemology

An epistemological philosophy emphasizes the relationship between persons and knowledge. It is recognized that much significant learning occurs apart from formal educational experiences and that informal and incidental learning from lived experiences account for most learning. Because students shape learning through experience, intuition, intellect, and practice (Heron, 1992), value is given to all these ways of knowing. A belief in epistemology leads to use of patterns of knowing (Carper, 1978; Chinn & Kramer, 2011) in nursing curricula.

Feminism and Feminist Pedagogy

Feminism is an ideology originally premised on values and beliefs about women, and relationships of gender, specifically that gender is "a difference that makes a difference" (di Stefano, as cited in Tong, 2007). Although there are many forms of feminism (e.g., liberal, radical, Marxist-socialist, multicultural, global, postmodern, third-wave), they all share the view that women are disadvantaged. Based in feminism, feminist pedagogy serves as a means for educational development and social change to meet educational needs of women. More broadly interpreted, feminism and feminist pedagogy value persons regardless of gender, with the goal of ending previous dehumanizing polarizations.

Feminism provides a framework that promotes development of intellectual growth and activism, and incorporates professional nursing values such as self-awareness, independence, empowerment, caring, and nursing's patterns of knowing. Students question, reflect, and challenge values and assumptions of nursing practice. Together with faculty, they co-construct meaning from life experiences. Students are empowered and test ideas through critical thinking, analysis, synthesis, and self-evaluation.

Humanism

A philosophy of humanism is concerned with rights, autonomy, and dignity of human beings, and a belief that learning is motivated by a desire for personal growth and fulfillment. In a humanistic-existentialist curriculum, the focus is on personal meaning in human existence (Csokasy, 2005). Faculty question the need for outcome assessment and rely instead on students' critical thinking, application of knowledge, and interpretation of learning experiences. The role of the teacher is to motivate and encourage experiential learning and facilitate students to establish and attain their own goals.

Based in part on ideas of humanism, feminism, and personal freedom, Bevis and Watson (2000) spearheaded ideas of the *caring curriculum*. Although no longer a predominant framework in nursing education, ideas prominent in this approach, such as *praxis*, continue. Moreover, the ideas have been extended by Hills and Watson (2011) to the creation of a Caring-Human Science curriculum. In this curriculum, the teaching-learning approaches of the humanistic caring curriculum are followed and tenets from a number of nurse theorists are integrated.

Learner-Centeredness (Student-Centeredness)

A learner-centered approach is premised on the idea that learners and the learning process are paramount in teaching-learning encounters, not the faculty member. The environment of learning contexts is termed *safe*, that is, students are supported in their learning efforts, free to explore ideas without criticism. Students take greater responsibility for their learning and classroom processes, and thus they are motivated and empowered to learn. Student experiences and knowledge are valued in learning that is relevant to their lives and goals (Colley, 2012). Teaching-learning strategies include problem-based learning, discovery learning, self-directed learning, case-based learning, choices of assignments, and other activities that engage students.

Although the preceding description is the general understanding in nursing education, Neuman (2013) comments that the term *student-centered* has several meanings and is often used without clear explication of what is intended. From his analysis of the literature, he proposes three "relational contours," or learning contexts. The teaching-learning relationship may center *in* students: Students control what and how they learn. The relationship may center *on* students: They are allowed choices and flexibility within a framework established by a faculty member. The third relationship is *with students.* This is a partnership, reflective of reciprocal planning and learning with decreased relational distance and in which the partners co-create the curriculum. In nursing education, faculty members generally create the educational framework and experiences, thereby adhering to a focus *on* students. However, with the course framework, many nursing faculty members give considerable attention to the other two relationships.

Narrative Pedagogy

Narrative pedagogy is a humanistic educational approach (Brown, Kirkpatrick, Mangum, & Avery, 2008) that has a significant basis in interpretative phenomenology. It allows for conventional, alternate, and new approaches to converge (Diekelmann, 2001). It relies on the lived experience of faculty, students, clients, and clinicians as the basis of student learning. The multiple perspectives of those involved in narratives are explored, so that students gain many views about the meaning of experiences and nursing. Public sharing and collective interpretation of narratives enrich learning and make the learning memorable. In this student-centered approach, "thinking is an experience of participative and interpretative practices that attend not only to issues of content (what is known and not known), but also to multi-perspectival issues of significance" (Ironside, 2005, p. 447).

Phenomenology

Phenomenology is an orientation and research method that focuses on lived experience and personal meaning. It emphasizes that people are always situated within a context, that there are multiple realities, and that people's perception of their experiences are valid. In nursing education, consideration is given to the experience of the individual (student, client, teacher). Learning experiences and the curriculum are framed in relation to these experiences.

Postmodernism

A postmodern orientation focuses on knowledge and meaning as opposed to prediction, control, rational analysis, and predetermined outcomes. This approach involves the inclusion of varying perspectives on complex problems. The intent is to "open up possibilities and provide a different way of theorising, structuring, and organising that could generate new understandings and offer emancipatory potential by acknowledging the importance of disparate . . . narratives in the co-creation of reality" (Gilligan, 2012, p. 461). Absolute truth, authority, and hegemony are rejected in favor of the creation of shared meaning and understanding. Deconstruction of established ideas and systems is an important activity of those espousing postmodernism, and this includes attention to how matters of race, age, gender, colonialism, and so forth influence and are influenced by social systems. Within this philosophy, the goals of education are the inclusion of marginalized people and the creation of a citizen with a full social identity. Students and faculty work together to construct knowledge and "a conception of knowledge which is academic, practical, and critical" (Nguyen, 2010, p. 96). The knowledge and the conception of knowledge are constantly questioned and transformed.

Pragmatism

Central to pragmatism is the testing of ideas, a combination of idealism and realism. Pragmatism in education is based on the idea that change is constant (Henson, 2010), and students need to experience the world. Therefore, they are actively engaged in learning and exploring, laboratory work, simulations, field trips, and social and community activities. They are encouraged to take in new information, interpret it, and apply it to previous learning and current client experiences (Csokasy, 2002). Learning outcomes are assessed through examinations and observation of students interacting with clients.

Transformative Learning

Mezirow (2000, 2009) proposes that adults have a frame of reference, their own perspective with which they view and interpret the world. The perspective is developed from experiences, the emotions associated with experiences, prior learning, unexamined instincts, and habits of the mind. When confronted with events or ideas that do not conform to their perspective, people may discount the event, or experience a disorienting dilemma. The disorientation can lead to critical reflection on their beliefs and possibly a perspective transformation. A transformation in perspective is a 10-step process that begins with recognition of a situation inconsistent with present beliefs; leads to self-examination, reflection, and development and testing of new ideas and skills; and culminates in the establishment of a new perspective. Morris and Faulk (2012) have proposed that transformative learning theory can be a basis for nursing curricula and for ongoing development throughout nurses' personal and professional lives. Within the curriculum there is emphasis on critical reflection, critical self-reflection, and critical dialogue.

In summation, the preceding descriptions of learning theories, educational frameworks, and pedagogies are merely an overview, because it is beyond the scope of this text to provide a comprehensive description of educational ideas. The theories, frameworks, and pedagogies lead to ideas about faculty and student responsibilities. Implications of some educational approaches are summarized in **Table 10-1**.

Table 10-1   Implications of Selected Philosophical and Educational Approaches for Nursing Curricula

Educational Approach	Key Ideas	Implications for Faculty	Implications for Students
Adult learning	Adults are self-directed learners with experiences that affect their learning. They are motivated to learn in response to real-life situations. They are capable of setting their learning goals and evaluating their success. Emotional climate is important.	Guide students toward greater self-direction. Emphasize the relevancy of learning. Draw on and respect students' experiences. Participatory decision making and interaction are important.	Take responsibility for learning. Identify learning goals, resources, and criteria for evaluation. Contribute relevant experiences to discussion. Strive to extend theory base of actions.
Apprenticeship	In a master–apprentice relationship, the novice learns from the master. The apprenticeship can encompass nursing knowledge and science, skilled knowhow, clinical reasoning, and ethical comportment.	Pair students with master nurses who can articulate their practice, coach, and supervise students, focusing on many aspects of nursing practice and students' integrative thinking.	Learn by example. Be receptive to coaching and motivated to question observed practice to further understanding.
Brain-based learning	Learning is continually possible and is influenced by individuals' emotional and physiological state. Individuals have different capacities. Frequent changes in focus, pace, and style of interaction are required to maintain student motivation.	Plan meaningful learning activities that are intrinsically rewarding. Plan for student–student interaction. Use multimodal methods. Space learning, review, and reinforcement sessions.	Take care of needs for food, hydration, and rest. Engage fully in learning activities. Attend to learning task. Pair learning and study with nonintrusive pleasant stimuli to build neural pathways.
Cognitive constructivism	Knowledge is constructed, linked to previous knowledge, and transformed iteratively in response to new experiences. Constructions of knowledge are individual and facilitated by interaction with others.	Use high-level questioning to facilitate idea creation and linking, critical analysis, deep thinking, reasoning, collaboration, and the co-construction of meaning.	Do preparatory reading. Articulate understandings and discuss with peers. Be willing to do intellectual work and use new understandings in analysis and professional practice.

(continues)

Table 10-1   Implications of Selected Philosophical and Educational Approaches for Nursing Curricula (*continued*)

Educational Approach	Key Ideas	Implications for Faculty	Implications for Students
Critical Social Theory	Meanings and reality are interpreted in the context of social history. Self and experience are examined through critical self-reflection. Autonomy, empowerment, emancipation, and self-responsibility are goals.	Assist students to identify inequitable situations. Pose questions and problems to simulate analysis, critical self-reflection, and intention to create change. Arrange service-learning experiences.	Share in revisioning and reconstructing oppressive and inequitable practices. Develop empathy, confidence, and competence in human relations. Advocate for change.
Deep learning	Learning is a process of exploration, discovery, and growth in which students invest themselves.	Facilitate intellectual depth through questioning, problem posing, allowing time for exploration of concepts, and stimulating students to make connections in their learning.	Be self-motivated and make time to explore a topic in depth. Make connections among concepts and experiences within and beyond course content.
Epistemology	The relationship between learner and knowledge is emphasized. Most learning is informal and incidental, resulting from lived experience.	Value all ways of knowing. Plan learning activities that engage more than one way of knowing. Attend to multiple ways of knowledge development in nursing.	Identify own and clients' ways of knowing. Engage in learning activities to develop multiple ways of knowing. Identify sources of knowledge.
Feminist pedagogy	People in all circumstances are valued. Lived experiences, creative and critical thinking, and empowerment are means to advance learning and emancipation. It incorporates self-awareness, independence, empowerment, caring, and patterns of knowing.	Facilitate student empowerment through democratic practices, discussion of power relationships, and questions that stimulate analysis of values and assumptions.	Question, reflect, and challenge values and assumptions. Co-construct meaning from experience.

Table 10-1 Implications of Selected Philosophical and Educational Approaches for Nursing Curricula (*continued*)			
Educational Approach	**Key Ideas**	**Implications for Faculty**	**Implications for Students**
Humanism	Learning is motivated by a desire for personal growth. Personal meaning is a focus.	Encourage experiential learning and facilitate students to establish and attain their own goals. Be a co-learner with students. Focus on interpretation, critique, and reflection.	Establish own goals and strategies to achieve them. Identify own values. Be a co-learner with peers and faculty. Engage in active learning.
Learner-centeredness	Student learning processes, not the faculty member, are the focus. Students are motivated to learn in safe environments where they have some control over activities and where their knowledge and experiences are valued. Student engagement in active learning is important.	Be willing to give up lecturing and control of ideas. Give students choices and support their learning efforts. Plan learning sessions that require active learning such as case study analysis, problem-based learning.	Participate actively in learning sessions. Be willing to share ideas with peers. Take responsibility for learning and do not expect that all that should be learned will be "covered" in the classroom.
Narrative pedagogy	Based in interpretative phenomenology. Public sharing and interpretation of the lived experience of faculty, students, clients, and clinicians are the bases of student learning.	Invite story telling by individuals relevant to class focus. Use literature and film to convey stories of human experience. Facilitate the interpretation and connections to theory.	Share own perspective and appreciate perspectives of others. Participate in interpretation of stories. Journal to capture own stories. Connect theory and develop concepts and generalizations from stories.
Transformative learning	Individual perspectives can be transformed by disorienting dilemmas and critical reflection.	Foster critical reflection, critical self-reflection, and critical dialogue. Facilitate identification of values and assumptions.	Identify personal perspectives and challenges to them. Engage in critical reflection, critical self-reflection, and critical dialogue.

PHILOSOPHICAL AND EDUCATIONAL APPROACHES

It is important that the curriculum be built on an explicated and coherent philosophical base that is then embodied and evident throughout the curriculum. Because most, if not all, nursing education curricula are based on blended ideas drawn from nursing theorists, concepts derived from analysis of contextual data, philosophies, and ideas about teaching and learning, the term *philosophical and educational approaches* is more fitting than *philosophy*. This conceptualization can encompass eclecticism, pluralism, assumptions, beliefs, and values. Some latitude in thoughts, views, values, assumptions, principles, and beliefs is thus possible. There must, however, be logical consistency among the ideas and the curriculum foundations, and consistency with the values of faculty and the educational institution.

Developing Philosophical and Educational Approaches

A sound beginning in the development of a statement of philosophical and educational approaches is for a subcommittee to create a draft document. The group might decide to divide the task so that one subgroup initially works on philosophical approaches and the other works on educational approaches, while keeping in touch to share resources and ensure that there is some consistency in their thinking. They will eventually need to merge their results as they prepare an overall draft statement.

One step is to conduct a literature search about curriculum and nursing education philosophies; learning science, theories, and frameworks; and nursing curricula. Because of the blending of nursing education philosophies and educational approaches, there could be considerable overlap in the literature that is accessed by each subgroup. Therefore, sharing the literature will speed the work. In addition, a review of the statements of philosophical and educational approaches of other schools of nursing would be beneficial, if these are posted on websites. The literature and Internet searches will assist the subcommittee members to:

- Appreciate the range of philosophical and educational ideas that could influence nursing curricula
- Identify ideas that resonate with them
- Assess the style in which statements of philosophical and educational approaches are expressed in other schools of nursing

The subcommittee has a responsibility to understand the beliefs and values of colleagues, because all faculty will be implementing the curriculum. One strategy could be to summarize the main precepts of several philosophies and educational theories, frameworks, and pedagogies gleaned from the literature and request that curriculum development participants indicate those that best fit their ideas. Alternately, a template could be given to faculty and other stakeholders, with a request that they write their beliefs about matters such as teaching and learning, the nature and purpose of student–faculty and nurse–client relationships, health, and so forth. Common ideas within the responses could be the basis of the curriculum's philosophical and educational approaches. A third activity might be to delineate the teaching and learning implications of several philosophical approaches and seek information about participants' preferences.

Furthermore, it is necessary for the subcommittee to keep in touch regarding the analysis of contextual data, which may be happening simultaneously. The ideas that emerge about major concepts for the curriculum and key abilities of nurses will affect the statement of philosophical and educational approaches.

Once information is obtained from faculty and stakeholders, literature, websites, and the contextual analysis, a draft of the statement of philosophical and educational approaches for the curriculum can be prepared and distributed with a request for feedback. This might generate considerable discussion, because differing beliefs will have to be reviewed, examined, and reconciled. Several drafts are generally required before agreement is reached.

The following questions could be considered when developing the philosophical and educational approaches for the nursing curriculum:

- How can we become more knowledgeable about philosophical and educational approaches in general education and nursing education?
- Should value statements, assumptions, or a single, pluralistic, or eclectic approach be used for the curriculum? What are the advantages and disadvantages of each?
- How can faculty members' and stakeholders' views be determined in a reasonable time period?
- Which philosophical and educational approaches seem most consistent with the beliefs and values of curriculum participants and the educational institution?
- What are the curriculum implications of the philosophical and educational approaches we prefer?

Confirming Philosophical and Educational Approaches

The importance of consensus among the total faculty group about the philosophical and educational approaches cannot be overemphasized. These approaches form part of the curriculum foundations. Therefore, agreement and a common understanding about philosophical and educational approaches are essential before subsequent curriculum work is undertaken. The chosen approaches are the basis of further curriculum development.

Time spent on reaching a shared understanding and agreement by the total faculty group is time well spent. Once this is achieved, the subcommittee can attend to perfecting the written statement.

RELATIONSHIP OF PHILOSOPHICAL AND EDUCATIONAL APPROACHES TO AN EVIDENCE-INFORMED, CONTEXT-RELEVANT, UNIFIED CURRICULUM

The philosophical and educational approaches are statements of the value orientation of faculty. They represent carefully examined ideas about nursing and education and a promise about the tone and enactment of the curriculum. The philosophical and educational approaches, along with the core curriculum concepts and key professional abilities, form the foundations of the nursing curriculum.

Ideas derived from the analysis of the contextual data and reading about educational and philosophical approaches ensure that the curriculum foundations are context-relevant and evidence-informed. Information about present and potential students and faculty and their values, as well as abilities needed by graduates, provide a basis for evidence-informed decision making about philosophical and educational approaches.

The inclusion of major curriculum concepts and key professional abilities in the statement of philosophical and educational approaches adds to the conceptual and visual unity of the curriculum. Furthermore, preliminary ideas about teaching and learning developed in the analysis of the contextual data will subsequently be confirmed, modified, or rejected on the basis of the chosen educational approaches. The subsequent selection of learning experiences and evaluation methods, stemming from the philosophical and educational approaches, will be important in the operational unity of the curriculum.

Development of the statement of philosophical and educational approaches is a basis for identifying:

- Curriculum concepts and professional abilities that may not have been identified in the analysis of the contextual data
- Theories, teaching methods, and learning experiences (Bevis, 1986; Clayton, 1989; Keating, 2011; Yura, 1974)
- Desired patterns of thought and conduct within a nursing program (Lawrence & Lawrence, 1983)

Although statements of philosophical and educational approaches have the potential to be prepared and forgotten, they are meant to be part of the living curriculum, to underpin and direct it. When based in the best evidence for the curriculum context and adhered to faithfully, the statements of philosophical and educational approaches contribute importantly to unity within the curriculum. These statements are simultaneously the guide for the curriculum and the substance of the curriculum.

CORE PROCESSES OF CURRICULUM WORK

Faculty Development

Faculty development can focus on the purpose and importance of agreed-upon philosophical and educational approaches in the curriculum. Values and beliefs about nursing, education, persons, learning, and so forth should be discussed. This discussion can serve to clarify and examine beliefs, and can be used as a source of information for the subcommittee drafting the statements of philosophical and educational approaches. Information about philosophies and educational theories, frameworks, science, and pedagogies could be presented and their curriculum implications discussed. Sample statements of philosophical and educational approaches might be circulated to help those in attendance see what others have developed. The drafting of beginning belief and value statements could occur in a faculty development session. There is value in having some practice with writing these statements, particularly if the format of the statements is changing from an existing one.

Ongoing Appraisal

Ongoing appraisal is an inherent part of the discussions that result in a statement of philosophical and educational approaches. During discussion, curriculum developers might ask some or all of the following questions:

- What would these ideas mean for us? How would we enact these ideas?
- How will our curriculum look if we adopted this philosophical or educational approach? What will teaching be like? What would be expected of students? What would be the nature of faculty–student interactions? What types of evaluation of learning will be consistent?
- Is it possible for the ideas to be applied consistently in all teaching-learning contexts? How can they be applied to student and faculty interactions with clients?
- Do we have sufficient knowledge about the use of these ideas in other schools of nursing?
- In what ways are the ideas that we favor consistent with the curriculum concepts and key professional abilities that have been identified? In what ways are the ideas aligned with faculty, student, and stakeholder values and preferences?
- If we are to use blended approaches, is there logical consistency among them?

- Are we satisfied that we have sufficient evidence to support the appropriateness of these ideas for our context?
- Are our conclusions likely to be supported? How do we know?
- How can we ensure that our written statement of philosophical and educational approaches is clear, complete, and understandable?

Scholarship

There are many possibilities for scholarship projects related to the development of philosophical and educational approaches. A description of processes and discussions undertaken to develop the statements of faculty members and to achieve consensus about them could be instructive to faculty at other schools. It would also be valuable to design a research project in which faculty members from one school, or several schools, describe their involvement in the decisions about philosophical and educational approaches, and their subsequent degree of commitment to the decisions. A final suggestion is to conduct a survey of schools of nursing to determine the philosophical and educational approaches currently in use and/or planned.

CHAPTER SUMMARY

The philosophical and educational approaches of the nursing curriculum reflect the beliefs, values, and convictions of faculty members. These approaches should be congruent with the philosophy of the educational institution and be enacted throughout the entire curriculum.

In this chapter, the conceptualization and purposes of a curriculum philosophy are presented. Some traditional curriculum philosophies are briefly described. Ideas about teaching and learning that could form part of a nursing curriculum philosophy are also presented. The authors' view of philosophical and educational approaches is explained, and ideas about how to develop these approaches for the curriculum are offered. Suggestions about faculty development, ongoing appraisal, and scholarship in relation to philosophical and educational approaches precede the chapter summary and synthesis activities.

SYNTHESIS ACTIVITIES

The case of Mountain Peaks College of Nursing is presented for review, analysis, and discussion. It includes some ideas about philosophical and educational approaches that are under consideration by faculty. Questions are offered to stimulate examination of the case. Then, questions and activities are suggested about developing philosophical and educational approaches for the curriculum in readers' settings.

Mountain Peaks College of Nursing

The faculty members at Mountain Peaks College of Nursing are engaged in curriculum development. After nearly 20 years with a caring humanistic curriculum, they recognized that considerable deviation from the original curriculum intent has occurred, and that newer ideas have necessitated the development of a reconceptualized curriculum. Analysis of contextual data is occurring simultaneously with the work of the six-member subcommittee responsible for formulating a draft statement of philosophical and educational approaches.

The subcommittee engaged in their work with enthusiasm. The members reviewed literature and the websites of prominent nursing schools in North America to expand their knowledge of curriculum philosophy, learning science, theories, and frameworks, as well as nursing theories and frameworks. Mindful that they were not developing a statement solely for themselves, they surveyed faculty members, asking about their beliefs and values related to person, health, nursing, nurse, nursing education, and learning. They created a chart of the findings from the literature and the predominant ideas from the faculty. The chart was circulated with a request for faculty to rate the items on a 5-point scale with 1 being *do not agree at all,* 2 *disagree somewhat,* 3 *neutral,* 4 *agree somewhat*, and 5 *strongly agree.*

There was considerable agreement about several ideas, with a majority of faculty completing the rating. Items rated as 4 or 5 are listed as follows, with concepts and professional abilities from the contextual data analysis in bold type:

- People are self-actualizing, continually developing, and striving to achieve their full potential.
- All people have inherent worth and dignity.
- Nursing's role is to assist clients (individuals, families, communities) to **promote and maintain their health** (physical, social, emotional, spiritual) and to support efforts to achieve individual potential.
- Although nurses may sometimes do *for* clients, the overarching perspective should be to **work with** clients, with client **empowerment** as a goal.
- **Collaboration** with clients, other nurses, and **interprofessional** team members is essential.

- **Health** is a basic human right and nurses must strive to uphold this right.
- **Social justice** is an important goal for the profession.
- Lifelong learning is essential for professional nurses.
- Students are responsible for their own learning.
- Client **safety** cannot be compromised by student learning.

Each of the following ideas had moderate support, with mean ratings ranging from 3.25 to 4:

- Feminism is an important foundation of nursing education and practice.
- Cognitive constructivism is a good basis for our curriculum.
- Brain-based learning is a good basis for our curriculum.
- Some aspects of nursing courses (or some courses) are best taught by lecture.
- Teaching approaches such as discussion, exploration of concepts, and problem posing result in learning relevant to nursing.
- Political action is an important part of nursing.
- Students need to learn the comportment of the profession.
- Knowledge of disease processes is important for students to learn.
- Faculty should ensure that students are adequately prepared for professional practice.

Items that yielded means of 3 or less were:

- Experience in hospital-based professional practice should be emphasized over other types of professional practice experiences.
- Students should participate actively in course planning and execution.
- Narrative pedagogy is a good basis for our curriculum.

The subcommittee convened a meeting of faculty to discuss the results prior to drafting a statement of philosophical and educational approaches.

Questions and Activities for Critical Analysis of the Mountain Peaks College of Nursing Case

1. Assess the items that were included in the survey. What other items might have been included?
2. What types of activities might the committee have undertaken in advance of surveying faculty?

3. Do the results seem logically consistent or inconsistent? Offer the rationale for your response.

4. Propose the goals of a meeting with faculty. Plan the meeting.

5. Decide if the survey information is sufficient for drafting a statement of philosophical and education approaches. Explain your response.

Questions and Activities for Consideration When Developing Philosophical and Educational Approaches in Readers' Settings

1. Who should be involved in the development of a statement of philosophical and educational approaches? How should development of the statement proceed?

2. Describe what ought to be included in a statement of philosophical and educational approaches.

3. Which curriculum concepts and key professional abilities derived from the analysis of contextual data should be evident in the statement?

4. Identify philosophical approaches and educational approaches that are consistent with the ideas, beliefs, convictions, and values of faculty and other stakeholders. What can be done to ensure that those ideas, beliefs, convictions, and values are brought to awareness?

5. Is consensus possible if there is inconsistency or conflict among strongly held convictions, values, and beliefs about philosophical and educational approaches for the curriculum? Describe strategies for achieving consensus in this situation.

6. Determine if eclecticism or pluralism might be appropriate.

7. In what ways are the developing ideas about philosophical and educational approaches consistent with the institutional stance?

8. What resources and how much time will be required to complete the work of developing philosophical and educational approaches? Propose a plan to ensure that the work will be completed in a thorough, yet expeditious manner so that other curriculum work can proceed.

9. Describe faculty development activities that could help in the development of educational and philosophical approaches.

10. Formulate ongoing appraisal questions that could be asked as a statement of educational and philosophical approaches is prepared.

11. Outline scholarship activities that should be considered and undertaken.

REFERENCES

Bandura, A. (1977). *Social learning theory*. Englewood Cliffs, NJ: Prentice Hall.

Benner, P., Sutphen, M., Leonard, V., & Day, L. (2010). *Educating nurses: A call for radical transformation*. San Francisco: Jossey-Bass.

Bevis, E. O. (1986). *Curriculum building in nursing: A process* (3rd ed.). St. Louis, MO: Mosby.

Bevis, E. O., & Watson, J. (2000). *Toward a caring curriculum: A new pedagogy for nursing*. Sudbury, MA: Jones and Bartlett.

Blackburn, S. (2014). Philosophy overview. *The Oxford dictionary of philosophy* (2nd rev. ed.). Oxford Reference Online. New York: Oxford University Press. Retrieved from http://www.oxfordreference.com/view/10.1093/acref/9780199541430.001.0001/acref-9780199541430

Boutain, D. (2005). Social justice as a framework for professional nursing. *Journal of Nursing Education, 44*, 404–407.

Boutain, D. (2008). Social justice as a framework for undergraduate community health clinical experiences in the United States. *International Journal of Nursing Education Scholarship, 5*(1), 1–12. doi:10.2202/1548–923X.1419

Brandon, A. F., & All, A. C. (2010). Constructivism theory analysis and application to curricula. *Nursing Education Perspectives, 3*, 89–92.

Brown, S. T., Kirkpatrick, M. K., Mangum, D., & Avery, J. (2008). A review of narrative pedagogy strategies to transform traditional nursing education. *Journal of Nursing Education, 47*, 283–286.

Carper, B. A. (1978). Fundamental patterns of knowing in nursing. *Advances in Nursing Science 1*, 13–23.

Chinn, P. L., & Kramer, M. K. (2011). *Integrated theory and knowledge development in nursing* (8th ed.). St. Louis, MO: Elsevier Mosby.

Clayton, G. M. (1989). Curriculum revolution: Defining the concepts. *Journal of Professional Nursing, 5*(1), 6, 55.

Colley, S. L. (2012). Implementing a change to learner-centered philosophy in a school of nursing: Faculty perceptions. *Nursing Education Perspectives, 33*, 229–233.

Csokasy, J. (2002). A congruent curriculum: Philosophical integrity from philosophy to outcomes. *Journal of Nursing Education, 41*(1), 32–33.

Csokasy, J. (2005). Philosophical foundations of the curriculum. In D. Billings & J. Halstead (Eds.), *Teaching in nursing: A guide for faculty* (2nd ed., pp. 125–143). St. Louis, MO: Elsevier Saunders.

Diekelmann, N. (2001). Heideggerian hermeneutical analyses of lived experiences of students, teachers, and clinicians. *Advances in Nursing Science, 23*(3), 53–71.

Dinsmore, D. L., & Alexander, P. A. (2012). A critical discussion of deep and surface processing: What it means, how it is measured, the role of context, and model specification. *Educational Psychology Review, 24*, 499–567.

Duchscher, J. E. B. (2000). Bending a habit: Critical social theory as a framework for humanistic nursing education. *Nurse Education Today, 20*(6), 453–462.

Gilligan, C. (2012, June). Can post-modernism contribute to saving the world? *European Conference on Research Methodology for Business and Management Studies*, 461–471. Kidmore End, UK: Academic Conferences International Limited.

Gillis, A., & Mac Lellan, M. A. (2013). Critical service learning in community health nursing: Enhancing access to cardiac health screening. *International Journal of Nursing Education Scholarship, 10*, 31.

Henderson, D. J. (1995). Consciousness-raising in participatory research: Method and methodology for emancipatory inquiry. *Advances in Nursing Science, 17*, 58–69.

Henson, K. T. (2010). *Curriculum planning: Integrating multiculturalism, constructivism, and education reform* (4th ed.). Long Grove, IL: Waveland Press.

Heron, J. (1992). *Feeling and personhood: Psychology in another key*. Newbury Park, CA: Sage.

Hills, M., & Watson, J. (2011). *Creating a caring science curriculum: An emancipatory pedagogy for nursing*. New York: Springer.

Illeris, K. (2009). A comprehensive understanding of human learning. In K. Illeris (Ed.), *Contemporary theories of learning* (pp. 7–20). New York: Routledge.

Ironside, P. (2005). Teaching thinking and reaching the limits of memorization: Enacting new pedagogies. *Journal of Nursing Education, 44*(10), 441–449.

Jarvis, P. (2009). Learning to be a person in society: Learning to be me. In K. Illeris (Ed.), *Contemporary theories of learning* (pp. 21–34). New York: Routledge.

Joseph, S., & Juwah, C. (2012). Using constructive alignment theory to develop nursing skills curricula. *Nurse Education in Practice, 12*, 52–59.

Keating, S. B. (2011). The components of the curriculum. In S. B. Keating (Ed.), *Curriculum development and evaluation in nursing* (2nd ed., pp. 149–194). New York: Springer.

Kilpatrick, W. H. (2010). The case for progressivism in education. In F. W. Parkay, E. J. Anctil, & G. Hass (Eds.), *Curriculum leadership: Readings for developing quality educational programs* (pp. 36–39). Boston: Allyn & Bacon.

Knowles, M. S., & Associates. (1984). *Andragogy in action: Applying modern principles of adult learning*. San Francisco: Jossey-Bass.

Knowles, M. S., Holton, E. F., & Swanson, R. A. (1998). *The adult learner* (5th ed.). Houston, TX: Gulf.

Lawrence, S. A., & Lawrence, R. M. (1983). Curriculum development: Philosophy, objectives, and conceptual framework. *Nursing Outlook, 3*(3), 160–163.

McGinty, J., Radin, J., & Kaminski, K. (2013). Brain-friendly teaching supports learning transfer. *New Directions for Adult and Continuing Education, 137*, 49–59.

Mezirow, J. (2000). *Learning as transformation: Critical perspective on a theory in progress*. San Francisco: Jossey-Bass.

Mezirow, J. (2009). An overview on transformative learning. In K. Illeris (Ed.), *Contemporary theories of learning* (pp. 90–105). New York: Routledge.

Mohammed, S. A. (2006). (Re)Examining health disparities: Critical social theory in pediatric nursing. *Journal for Specialists in Pediatric Nursing, 11*, 68–71.

Morris, A. H., & Faulk, D. R. (2012). *Transformative learning in nursing*. New York: Springer.

Neuman, J. W. (2013). Developing a new framework for conceptualizing "student-centered learning". *The Educational Forum, 77*, 161–175.

Nguyen, C. H. (2010). The changing postmodern university. *International Education Studies, 3*(3), 88–99.

Oliva, P. F. (2009). *Developing the curriculum* (7th ed.). Boston: Pearson Education.

Petress, K. (2003). An educational philosophy guides the pedagogical process. *College Student Journal, 37*(1), 128–135.

Platow, M. J., Mavor, K. I., & Grace, D. M. (2013). On the role of discipline-related self-concept in deep and surface approaches to learning among university students. *Instructional Science, 41*, 271–285.

Reutter, L., Paul, P., Sales, A., Jerke, H., Lee, A., McColl, M., . . . Visram, A. (2010). Incorporating a research apprenticeship model in a Canadian honors program. *Nurse Education Today, 30*, 562–567.

Richardson, V. (2003). Constructivist pedagogy. *Teachers College Record, 105*, 1623–1640.

Straumanis, J. (2012). What we're learning about learning (and what we need to forget). *Planning for Higher Education, 40*(3), 6–11. Retrieved from http://www.scup.org/asset/62115/PHEV40N4 _Article_What-Were-Learning-About-Learning.pdf

Taylor, K. L., & Care, D. W. (1999). Nursing education as cognitive apprenticeship. *Nurse Educator, 24*(4), 31–36.

Thomson, J. (2012). The neuroscience of making learning stick. *Training and Development, 39*(3), 18–20.

Tokuhama-Espinosa, T. (2010). *The new science of teaching and learning: Using the best of mind, brain, and education science in the classroom.* New York: Teachers College Press.

Tong, R. (2007). Feminist thought in transition: Never a dull moment. *Social Science Journal, 44*(1), 23–39.

Uys, L. R., & Smit, J. H. (1994). Writing a philosophy of nursing. *Journal of Advanced Nursing, 20*(2), 239–244.

Valiga, T. M. (2012). Philosophical foundations of the curriculum. In D. Billings & J. Halstead (Eds.), *Teaching in nursing: A guide for faculty* (2nd ed., pp. 125–143). St. Louis, MO: Elsevier Saunders.

Van Dam, N. (2013). Inside the learning brain. *T and D, 67*(4), 30–35.

White, B., & Brockett, R. (1987). Putting philosophy into practice. *Journal of Extension, 25*(2). Retrieved from http://joe.org/joe/1987summer/a3.html

Wiles, J., & Bondi, J. (2011). *Curriculum development: A guide to practice* (8th ed.). Boston: Pearson Education.

Yura, H. (1974). Curriculum development process. In *Faculty curriculum development: Part 1: The process of curriculum development.* New York: National League for Nursing.

CHAPTER 11

Formulating Curriculum Goals or Outcomes for an Evidence-Informed, Context-Relevant, Unified Curriculum

Chapter Overview

In this chapter, attention is given to the formulation of curriculum goals or outcomes. First, taxonomies of thinking and performance are described, followed by clarification and comparison of the terms *objectives*, *goals*, *outcomes*, and *competencies*. The purposes of goal or outcome statements in curriculum development are then described. Formulating curriculum goals and outcomes is presented next. The relationship of curriculum goals or outcomes to an evidence-informed, context-relevant, unified curriculum is explained. The core processes of curriculum work are considered, followed by a chapter summary. Finally, synthesis activities conclude the chapter.

Chapter Goals

- Appraise the use of the educational taxonomies as a basis for curriculum goal or outcome development.
- Understand various terms used to describe the intended achievement of students in a nursing curriculum.
- Recognize the purposes of curriculum goal or outcome statements for various stakeholders.
- Consider processes for formulating curriculum goals or outcomes.
- Appreciate the relationship of curriculum goals to an evidence-informed, context-relevant, unified curriculum.
- Reflect on the core processes of curriculum work in relation to formulating curriculum goals or outcomes.

TAXONOMIES OF THINKING AND PERFORMANCE: BASES FOR DESCRIBING THE EDUCATIONAL DESTINATION

The educational destination of a nursing curriculum is the desired knowledge, abilities, values, and comportment of graduates. These are described in the curriculum goals or outcomes, along with an indication of the context in which the abilities are enacted. Similarly, course goals (or objectives) or competencies describe the expectations of students completing individual courses.

In education, three realms of thinking and performance are used to describe learning and the intended educational destination: the cognitive (thinking), affective (values), and psychomotor (movement) domains. Taxonomies of learning have been developed to specify expectations of students in these three domains. The taxonomies have been a boon to educators, enabling them to describe precisely what is expected of students.

A *taxonomy* is a classification of ideas that specifies the relationship among them. Therefore, within each of the three learning domains, several levels or categories of thinking or performance are defined. Further, there are subcategories that describe student behaviors reflective of each category or level.

The original taxonomies of cognitive and affective learning were developed by Benjamin Bloom and his associates from an analysis of learning objectives written by educators in the 1940s and 1950s. Each domain has been categorized into a hierarchical taxonomy, with every level reflecting greater difficulty or complexity than the preceding level. The aim of Dr. Bloom and his students was not to describe all types of learning that could occur but rather to codify the expectations teachers had for students at that time (Gander, 2006). Thus, the cognitive and affective taxonomies are named *Taxonomy of Educational Objectives,* although the cognitive taxonomy is commonly referred to as *Bloom's Taxonomy.*

Several taxonomies of psychomotor objectives were developed and published in the 1970s. The two used most frequently in nursing curricula are presented in the sections that follow. Although the taxonomies were developed to classify educational objectives, they are understood to be taxonomies of learning. Hence, they are a basis for describing educational endpoints and students' achievement.

The Cognitive Domain of Learning

Bloom's Taxonomy

The taxonomy of the cognitive (understanding and thinking) domain, as initially conceived, has six categories or levels of achievement: *knowledge, comprehension, application, analysis, synthesis*, and *evaluation* (Bloom, Englehart, Furst, Hill, & Krathwohl, 1956). With the exception of *application,* each is divided into subcategories. The categories are ordered from simple to complex and from concrete to abstract. Mastery of each level is assumed to be necessary for advancement to the successive level.

The original Bloom's Taxonomy was revised by Anderson and colleagues (2001). All categories were named with a verb to reflect cognitive processes: *remember, understand, apply, analyze, evaluate,* and *create.* The order of the original *synthesis* and *evaluation* was reversed. Also, a second dimension, the *knowledge domain* was included. Four types of knowledge were identified:

- *Factual*: "basic elements a student must know to be acquainted with a discipline or solve problems in it" (Anderson et al., 2001, p. 29)
- *Conceptual*: "interrelationships among the basic elements within a larger structure that enable them to function together" (Anderson et al., 2001, p. 29)
- *Procedural*: "how to do something, methods of inquiry, and criteria for using skills, algorithms, techniques, and methods" (Anderson et al., 2001, p. 29)
- *Metacognitive knowledge*: "knowledge of cognition in general [and] awareness and knowledge of one's own cognition" (Anderson et al., p. 29)

All cognitive processes (remember, understand, apply, analyze, evaluate, and create) can operate with each of the four types of knowledge.

In **Table 11-1** is a summary of the cognitive processes of the revised taxonomy, and selected associated verbs that reflect each category and include the subcategories of each level. Although the six main categories are generally referenced in the original and revised cognitive taxonomies, their richness and utility lie in the delineation of the subcategories.

New Taxonomy of Educational Objectives

Marzano and Kendall (2007, 2008) have developed *The New Taxonomy of Educational Objectives* that emphasizes cognition and metacognition. They assert that the difficulty of mental processes cannot be ordered in a hierarchical manner. Rather, they believe that mental processes can be ordered in relation to control: some processes control other processes. Six levels of mental processing are described. The first four levels are the processes of the cognitive system. Level 5 is the *metacognitive system*, and Level 6 is the *self-system*:

- The *self-system* makes a judgment about: the importance of a new learning task or endeavor, efficacy beliefs about own ability to improve or understand, emotions associated with the task, and motivation to proceed with the task.

Table 11-1   Cognitive Process Dimension of the Revised Cognitive Taxonomy and Selected Associated Verbs

Categories	Associated Verbs
Remember: retrieve information from long-term memory	Define, describe, identify, list, name, recall, recognize, select, state
Understand: determine the meaning	Classify, compare, explain, exemplify, extend, infer, interpret, paraphrase, summarize
Apply: carry out or use a procedure or concept in a given situation	Apply, change, execute, implement, modify, predict, prepare, relate, solve, use
Analyze: separate material or concepts into component parts and determine the relationships among the parts and to the overall structure	Attribute, analyze, break down, compare, contrast, differentiate, discriminate, deduce, infer, relate, separate
Evaluate: make judgments based on criteria	Appraise, check, critique, defend, judge, evaluate, justify
Create: build something new from diverse elements	Compose, create, design, develop, generate, organize, plan, produce, reconstruct

Source: Some data from Anderson, L. W., Krathwohl, D. R., Airasian, P. W., Cruikshank, K. A., Mayer, R. E., Pintrich, P. R., . . . Wittrock, M. C. (Eds.). (2001). *A taxonomy for learning, teaching, and assessing: A revision of Bloom's taxonomy of educational objectives.* New York: Longman; Bloom, B. S., Englehart, M. D., Furst, E. J., Hill, W. H., & Krathwohl, D. R. (1956). *Taxonomy of educational objectives. The classification of educational goals: Handbook 1: Cognitive domain.* New York: David McKay.

- The *metacognitive system* is activated if a task is selected. This system sets goals about the task and strategies to achieve the goals. It then monitors progress toward the goal, clarity of understanding, and accuracy.
- The *cognitive system* then processes relevant information for the task. These processes are retrieval, comprehension, analysis, and knowledge utilization.

This taxonomy has two dimensions: levels of processing and *knowledge*. All the levels of mental processing operate within the three domains of knowledge: *psychomotor procedures*, *mental procedures*, and *information.*

The Affective Domain of Learning

The affective domain relates to the development of values, attitudes, and beliefs. The levels of the affective taxonomy are *receiving, responding, valuing, organizing,* and *characterization by a value* (Krathwohl, Bloom, & Masia, 1964). This taxonomy describes a

Table 11-2 Affective Domain Levels and Selected Associated Verbs for Learning Objectives

Level	Associated Verbs
Receiving: aware, willing to hear, sensitive to ideas	Accept, ask, listen (for), recognize
Responding: attending and reacting to a particular situation	Answer, comply, conform, discuss, examine, respond
Valuing: attaching worth to particular ideas, phenomena, or behaviors	Choose, demonstrate, explain, initiate, justify, support
Organization: organizing values into priorities by contrasting different values, resolving conflicts between them, and creating a unique value system	Adhere, balance, arrange, display, defend, formulate, generalize, integrate
Characterization by a value set: having a value system that consistently controls own behavior	Act, display, internalize, perform, practice, question, resolve, verify

Source: Some data from Krathwohl, D. R., Bloom, B. S., & Masia, B. B. (1964). *Taxonomy of educational objectives: Handbook II: Affective domain*. New York: David McKay; Oermann, M. H., & Gaberson, K. B. (2014). *Evaluation and testing in nursing education* (4th ed.). New York: Springer Publishing Company.

progression from simple awareness of a value or belief to internalization of the value such that it is a consistent basis for behavior. In **Table 11-2** are descriptions of the taxonomy levels and related verbs for each level of the affective domain.

The Psychomotor Domain of Learning

The psychomotor domain describes behaviors related to physical movement and proficiency in execution of manual tasks. Like Bloom's taxonomies, the categories are listed from the simplest behavior to the most complex. Although other psychomotor taxonomies have been created, the two that have had the most acceptance in nursing education are those developed by Simpson (1972) and Dave (1970) (as cited in Oermann & Gaberson, 2014). Simpson (1972) describes seven categories of psychomotor performance:

- *Perception*: noticing sensory cues to guide motor activity
- *Set*: being ready to act, including physical, mental, and emotional dispositions
- *Guided response*: completing a task with guidance or instruction
- *Mechanism*: performing a complex skill at an intermediate stage, with some confidence and proficiency

- *Complex or overt response*: performing complex motor acts automatically, quickly, accurately, and with a high degree of coordination
- *Adaptation*: adapting a skill in novel situations
- *Origination*: creating new movement patterns to fit a particular situation or problem

The first two categories of Simpson's taxonomy are not observable and therefore are difficult to evaluate. In contrast, all categories of Dave's 1970 taxonomy of the psychomotor domain (*imitation, manipulation, precision, articulation,* and *naturalization)* as cited in Oermann & Gaberson, 2014) are observable and amenable to evaluation. This taxonomy has been modified to change the names of each category to verbs: *imitate, manipulate, perfect, articulate,* and *embody* (Atkinson, 2012). A brief description of the original and revised categories, along with some associated verbs, is presented in **Table 11-3**.

Table 11-3   Psychomotor Domain Levels and Selected Associated Verbs for Learning Objectives

Dave's Levels	Atkinson's Levels	Associated Verbs
Imitation: observing and patterning behavior after someone else	**Imitate**: copy; replicate the actions of others following observation	Copy, follow, mimic, imitate, repeat
Manipulation: performing certain actions by memory or following instructions	**Manipulate**: repeat or reproduce actions to prescribed standard from memory or instructions	Complete, demonstrate, follow, perform, manipulate
Precision: performing a skill with control and independently of instruction	**Perfect**: perform with expertise and without intervention; and demonstrate and explain to others	Be precise, demonstrate, perform (accurately, smoothly)
Articulation: coordinating and adapting a series of actions in an appropriate sequence to achieve harmony and internal consistency	**Articulate**: adapt existing skills in a nonstandard way, in different contexts, using alternative tools and instruments to satisfy need	Adapt, construct, develop, modify, revise
Naturalization: mastering a high-level performance until it becomes second nature, without needing to think much about it	**Embody**: perform actions in an automatic, intuitive, or unconscious way appropriate to the context	Alter, create, change, design, execute (effortlessly), invent

Source: Some data from Atkinson, S. P. (2012). *Updated: Taxonomy circles—visualizations of educational domains.* Retrieved from http://spatkinson.wordpress.com/2012/11/13/updated-taxonomy-circles-visualisations-of-educational-domains/; Oermann, M. H., & Gaberson, K. B. (2014). *Evaluation and testing in nursing education* (4th ed.). New York: Springer Publishing Company.

Interrelationships Among the Learning Domains

Bloom's cognitive taxonomy (original and revised), the affective taxonomy, and psychomotor taxonomies can be interpreted to mean that learning in each domain is compartmentalized, separate, and unconnected to learning in the other domains. Nurse educators, and, indeed, all educators, have always known this to be untrue. The domains of learning do not operate in three separate vacuums. Each domain is intimately interconnected with the others. For example, the manual execution of a nursing skill requires cognitive processing. Students should understand and apply knowledge of concepts, principles, and procedures as they carry out a psychomotor task. In addition, continuous cognitive evaluation of the precision of performance is an inherent component of providing physical care. Moreover, all aspects of nursing care are based on knowledge and judgment and are expressed through a set of values and beliefs, which themselves first require knowledge, evaluation, and internalization, processes associated with the cognitive and the affective domains.

CURRICULUM GOALS AND OUTCOMES

Many terms are used to describe the knowledge, skills, and attitudes that students are expected to attain in educational programs: *objectives*, *goals*, *competencies*, and *outcomes*. The terms are all meant to convey the educational destination that students are required to attain by the end of a unit of learning or curriculum. Each term connotes a slightly different idea from the others, although all are written to be meaningful to several curriculum audiences.

The educational destination that students are expected to reach at the end of the nursing program must be specified, because this description becomes the basis for subsequent curriculum decisions. The discussion in this chapter is restricted to identifying and articulating what students should accomplish, and not the development of teaching or instructional goals or objectives.

Clarification of Terms

Learning Objectives

Learning objectives are descriptions of what a student should be like after successful completion of a learning experience (Mager, 1997). Learning objectives are based on the work of Ralph Tyler (1949), who was interested in broad goals. However, Tyler's format of goals has changed to align with behaviorism. Behavioral objectives each describe only one specific behavior from one domain of learning and are created from the taxonomies of learning. The objectives should state the criteria for successful achievement, be attainable within a particular timeframe and/or context, and be measurable.

As conceived, behavioral objectives are far too specific to describe the endpoint of a curriculum, because an endless list would be necessary and the complexities of integrated thinking and acting would likely not be evident. Yet, some nursing programs continue to use the term *objectives*, even though the curriculum objectives are multidimensional. These statements are generally more akin to goals. In general, programs with curriculum goals will have level or year goals and course goals or objectives.

Learning Goals

Learning goals are student-focused, broad statements that describe the educational destination to be reached by students. A goal can encompass several objectives, or it can stand alone if objectives are not specified. Goals can incorporate cognitive, affective, interpersonal, ethical, and/or psychomotor dimensions; that is, they can integrate multi-domain behaviors. Unlike learning objectives, goals do not contain criteria for achievement (Oliva, 2009). In the Model of Evidence-Informed, Context-Relevant, Unified Curriculum Development, the goal statements are student-focused, and they are derived from and incorporate the philosophical and educational approaches, core curriculum concepts, and key professional abilities (the latter two being derived from the analysis of contextual data) in a comprehensive, holistic fashion. The context of goal achievement is specified.

Learning Outcomes

Learning outcomes are written statements of the professional abilities students are projected to attain as the result of an educational program. The outcome statements focus on students and what they should be able to demonstrate at the completion of a process of learning (Kennedy, Hyland, & Ryan, 2007). This includes knowledge, attitudes, and skills. More specifically, within nursing curricula, they are practice-oriented statements, integrating several domains of knowledge so that higher level functions, such as nursing care, can be performed. The focus is on a pattern and complexity of knowledge domains pertinent to, and evident in, professional practice. Outcomes are assessable (Glennon, 2006). The curriculum outcomes incorporate the core characteristics required by graduates and the context in which the attributes will be enacted (Boland, 2012).

In nursing education literature, the term *outcomes* has been used with two connotations. First, the term is employed to describe the intended or expected cognitive processes and practice behaviors that students will exhibit at program completion. Although generally termed *outcomes*, it is really the *outcome statements* that embody the anticipated professional abilities of graduates and to which curriculum writers give attention. Secondly, the term *outcomes* has been used to describe the actual cognitive processes and practice behaviors of graduates. These actual outcomes can be known only through evaluation at program completion and follow-up studies of graduates. Therefore, the curriculum outcome statements should be written in a manner that will provide direction to these studies.

Competencies

Competencies are the knowledge, skills, and attitudes that students need to develop in order to accomplish the outcomes. They are behaviorally based, although not limited to one behavior as behavioral objectives are. They are focused on the student, specify the type and level of behavior, and include the context in which the behavior is to occur. The competencies are the prerequisites to achieving the outcomes.

Comparison of Goals and Outcomes

There is considerable overlap in the descriptions of learning goals, outcomes, objectives, and competencies. All are intended to describe an endpoint of a period of learning, are focused on the student, and describe an integration of knowledge, attitude, and skills. They are projections or expectations of what students will accomplish. Goals and outcomes elucidate the ends, but not the means by which students will achieve the ends.

Goals and objectives have their genesis in the work of Ralph Tyler and behaviorist educators who were influential from approximately 1950 to 1990. Although objectives and goals are often described as *teacher centered*, this is not necessarily so in their modern use. Student-centered outcomes and competencies arise from outcome-based education that began in the 1980s (Wittman-Price & Fasolka, 2010) and that also has its roots in behavioral objectives (Kennedy et al., 2007).

Goals, as conceived in the Model of Evidence-Informed, Context-Relevant, Unified Curriculum Development, and curriculum outcomes are both derived from an assessment of the context. Outcomes are derived from the practice context. Goals, on the other hand, are derived from a broader assessment of the total environment of the school of nursing, of which the healthcare environment is an important component. Evident in the goals are the philosophical and educational approaches, the core curriculum concepts, and key professional abilities in a comprehensive, holistic fashion. The philosophical approaches may not be evident in the outcomes, and unless the curriculum is concept based, significant curriculum concepts are likely absent.

"Outcomes are practice oriented and should make sense to practicing professionals, as well as academic professionals" (Glennon, 2006, p. 56). This practice orientation makes them understandable and appealing to students. In contrast, as traditionally written, goals may not be directly connected to practice. However, in the model proposed in this text, curriculum goals are generally practice oriented.

The identification of the educational endpoint (abilities or characteristics of graduates) requires the determination of the constituent abilities to achieve the goals or outcomes. Constituent objectives are derived from learning goals, and constituent competencies are derived from learning outcomes, and these provide a roadmap for students. Therefore, the progression toward the endpoint should be evident in both approaches. Writers of competencies and objectives look to the learning taxonomies to identify the nature and level of learning that they want students to achieve. Like the original format of objectives, outcome and competency statements should include a description of the context in which the desired behavior will be demonstrated (Wittman-Price & Fasolka, 2010). There is variation in authors' views about whether or not criteria are included in the outcomes. It seems reasonable to think that if criteria are included, they would be present in the outcomes of small units of learning, and not the final curriculum outcomes. Goals generally include the context in which the learning is to be expressed.

The orientation of course and curriculum endpoints can influence students' ease in articulating what they can offer to employers. Outcome statements allow graduates to answer the question: *What can you* do *now that you have obtained your degree?* Although students graduating from a curriculum with goal statements could respond to this question in the same way, they may be more likely to describe what they *did* to achieve the degree (Purser, Council of Europe, as cited by Kennedy et al., 2007).

An important distinction is in the connotation of the words themselves. The term *outcomes* is confident, definite, and firm. Therefore, outcome statements are a declarative description of achievement. In contrast, the term *goals* conveys a tone of hope and aspiration, something to strive for, but not necessarily to achieve.

Examples of a curriculum goal and a curriculum outcome are presented to illustrate the similarities and differences between them. A curriculum goal is: *Graduates will be able to practice ethical, evidence-informed nursing from a holistic, health promotion and caring perspective in a variety of settings and contexts with diverse client groups across the lifespan* (Western-Fanshawe Collaborative BScN Program, 2013). Evident in this goal are:

- *Key professional abilities*: practice ethical, evidence-informed nursing
- *Aspects of the philosophical approach*: caring, clients as partners (practice *with*), holism
- *Curriculum concepts*: evidence-informed, caring, health promotion, culture, and context
- *Context where behavior will be demonstrated*: variety of settings and contexts, with diverse clients across the lifespan.

An example of a curriculum outcome is: *The graduate is a critical, reflective thinker who provides holistic nursing care to individuals and families in institutional and community settings.* This is shorter than the goal statement and incorporates:

- *The attribute of the graduate*: critical, reflective thinker
- *An action verb specifying what the graduate will do*: provide holistic care
- *The context*: to individuals and families in institutional and community settings

In summary, outcomes and competencies, or goals and objectives, describe the intended accomplishments of students. Both are a foundation for ongoing curriculum development. See **Table 11-4** for a comparison of behavioral objectives; goal statements as conceived in the Model of Evidence-Informed, Context-Relevant, Unified Curriculum Development; and curriculum outcomes. Behavioral objectives are included in this table, because they are the root of goals and outcomes.

Purposes of Goal or Outcome Statements

The curriculum goal or outcome statements, which ultimately appear in published descriptions of the curriculum, are of interest to many groups. Each reads them for a different purpose.

Curriculum Developers

Curriculum developers use the goal or outcome statements as a source of direction for all subsequent aspects of curriculum planning, implementation, and evaluation. This means that the curriculum design, level and course goals or competencies, learning activities, course requirements, evaluation of learning, and curriculum evaluation all derive their focus and intent from the curriculum goal or outcome statements. Curriculum developers are obligated to create and sequence learning experiences that will allow motivated and capable students to achieve the intended curriculum goals or outcomes.

Faculty designing individual courses turn to curriculum goals or outcomes (from which more specific level expectations emanate) as their reference point for course development, including course goals or competencies, strategies to ignite learning, and assessments of student learning. The curriculum goals or outcomes and level expectations specify what students are to achieve and are the touchstone against which faculty members assess the suitability of their course development and implementation.

Current Students

Students enrolled in a school of nursing look to curriculum goal or outcome statements as the target they should reach by graduation and to course goals or competencies as targets

Table 11-4   Comparison of Behavioral Objectives; Curriculum Goals in the Model of Evidence-Informed, Context-Relevant, Unified Curriculum Development; and Curriculum Outcomes

Characteristic	Behavioral Objectives	Goals	Outcomes
Purpose	Specify what students should achieve	Describe what students are expected to achieve	Describe what graduates can do
Evidence base	Not described	Analysis of deliberatively gathered contextual data, including population characteristics, healthcare system, professional practice competencies, health policy, governmental health priorities, trends, etc.	Interpretation of nursing practice requirements
Contextual relevance	Dependent on individual school's connection with community and individual faculty members' knowledge	Strong	Dependent on individual school's connection with community and individual faculty members' knowledge
Student-centered	Possibly	Yes	Yes
Describes integrated, multi-domain behaviors	No	Yes	Yes
Practice-oriented	Possibly, but typically mainly in professional practice courses	Yes	Yes
Major curriculum concepts evident	No	Yes	No
Philosophical bases of curriculum evident	No	Yes	No
Includes context where behavior is demonstrated	Yes	Yes	Yes
Includes criterion/criteria for success	Yes	No	Possibly
Assessable	Yes	Yes	Yes
Content-focused	Yes	No	No
Provides a basis for curriculum unity	No	Yes	Possibly

for smaller units of learning. To make the destination statements meaningful to students, faculty should refer to them frequently, identifying how particular learning activities contribute to achievement of the goals or outcomes. In this way, the statements have an educational value to students and are not merely rhetoric that seems unrelated to courses. Additionally, frequent and explicit reference to curriculum goals or outcomes, and to course goals or competencies, helps students articulate their professional abilities and achievements.

Prospective Students

Potential applicants can review the goal or outcome statements to determine if the curriculum will match their view of nursing, personal expectations, and philosophical orientation. The statements can attract applicants whose interests are aligned with the curriculum purposes and processes.

Clinicians and Potential Employers

These groups can use the published statements to understand what students are expected to accomplish and what professional abilities they will have at graduation. Reference to curriculum goal or outcome statements by faculty can be effective in helping clinicians appreciate why the nursing curriculum may not be organized in the manner some clinicians might prefer. Similarly, statements that indicate curriculum concepts and key professional abilities such as clinical reasoning, reflective and collaborative practice, or leadership could assist employers to recognize the value graduates can bring to organizations.

Other Members of the Educational Institution

Faculty teaching non-nursing courses, chairs of institution-wide committees concerned with curricula and standards, and administrators are interested in whether the nursing curriculum goal or outcome statements are congruent with the mission and values of the parent institution. If institution-wide expectations have been delineated for programs, these should be apparent in the nursing curriculum goals or outcomes, although presented within the context of nursing.

Representatives of Accrediting Organizations, State Boards of Nursing, and Provincial Licensing Bodies

Representatives of organizations concerned with nursing education and nursing practice standards also have a legitimate interest in the curriculum goal or outcome statements. They want to be assured that graduates' abilities match the expectations for the program level (practical nursing, associate degree, diploma, baccalaureate, or graduate) and are congruent with established standards. Additionally, curriculum goal or outcome statements, among other information, are evaluated when graduates seek licensure in jurisdictions other than where they were originally licensed.

Members of Professional Nursing Organizations

These persons review nursing curriculum goals or outcomes to keep abreast of educational expectations and professional abilities of new graduates. Furthermore, the statements could signal the type of student placement experiences that the school of nursing might request within professional organizations. Also, the statements may contribute to the rationale used to substantiate recommendations to legislators about nursing practice and healthcare policy.

Members of the Public

Healthcare recipients generally read curriculum goal or outcome statements only when they encounter a problem in nursing practice. In those instances, if a complaint to a licensing body or a lawsuit is considered, members of the public and/or their legal representatives may want to determine the curriculum goals or outcomes graduates should have achieved.

FORMULATING CURRICULUM GOAL OR OUTCOME STATEMENTS

A first decision in formulating goal or outcome statements is which to develop: goals or outcomes? If curriculum developers have an option, they should consider carefully the purpose and format of each, and which is more aligned with their own perspectives. However, the decision may not rest with nursing faculty. Rather, it may be a reflection of institutional practices.

There could be considerable similarity in the curriculum goal statements or outcome statements of many schools of nursing because curriculum developers are guided by similar contextual influences, such as nursing practice or performance standards; codes of ethics; licensure and accreditation requirements; provincial, state, or national positions on higher education; and prevailing educational philosophies. Yet, as much as possible, the statements should give an indication of the uniqueness of each school's curriculum.

When writing the statements, it would be wise for curriculum developers to remain mindful of the intended audiences and ensure that the terminology is understandable. Attention to the taxonomies of learning, synthetic thinking, artful writing, and ongoing discussion among faculty is required for the creation of goal or outcome statements that reflect the intent of the curriculum.

Curriculum Goal Statements

In the Model for Evidence-Informed, Context-Relevant, Unified Curriculum Development, goal statements are developed from the agreed-upon philosophical and educational approaches, core curriculum concepts, and key professional abilities. It is recognized that congruency of the goal statements with the mission, vision, and goals of the school of nursing and educational institution is essential.

The language and format of the curriculum goal statements must be consistent with the philosophical and educational approaches, and incorporate the key professional abilities and core curriculum concepts. The statements are to be comprehensive, yet concrete enough to be meaningful. They are also to be sufficiently broad to allow for ongoing curriculum refinement.

It is advisable that the subcommittee preparing the goal statements be immersed in the philosophical approaches, core curriculum concepts, key professional abilities, nursing education standards, entry to practice requirements, and other relevant information assembled as part of the contextual data. Goal statements from other schools may provide useful ideas.

Goal statements are composed of four parts:

- Key professional abilities, expressed in an action verb that incorporates a constellation of behaviors from more than one taxonomy of learning
- Aspects of the philosophical approach
- Curriculum concepts
- Context in which the action will be demonstrated

Curriculum Outcome Statements

Curriculum outcome statements, as presently conceived in the nursing education literature, are relatively brief statements that describe the program graduates. They are made up of three parts:

- An attribute
- An action verb that reflects a synthesis of several behaviors, usually from more than one taxonomy
- The context in which the behavior will be demonstrated

Outcome statements are based on an understanding of current and anticipated realities of nursing practice. The statements address the attributes of a graduate in relation to nursing practice. **Table 11-5** includes some questions that curriculum developers might ask themselves as they formulate curriculum goals or outcomes.

Table 11-5 Questions to Guide the Development of Curriculum Goals and Outcomes	
Curriculum Goals	**Curriculum Outcomes**
From a review of the analysis of contextual data, which are key professional abilities to be included in the goal statements?	From a review of the current and anticipated practice environments, what are the attributes necessary for graduates to practice nursing successfully?
From a review of the analysis of contextual data, which are the major curriculum concepts to be included in the goal statements?	N/A
From a review of the analysis of contextual data, which contexts of nursing practice are to be included in the goal statements?	In what contexts should the attributes be demonstrated?
How can the philosophical approaches of the curriculum be made evident in the goal statements?	N/A

Formulating Statements of Level Expectations

Once the educational destination has been determined, it is necessary to identify the constituent abilities students will need to develop in order to achieve the final destination. These abilities are deduced from the endpoint by answering the question: *What goals or competencies will students need to achieve at preceding levels of the curriculum in order to reach the endpoint successfully?* In other words, this answer is reached by identifying the prerequisite goals or competencies, and these become the Level 3 expectations. The goals or competencies prerequisite to Level 3 become the Level 2 expectations, and so forth. **Figure 11-1** illustrates this process and contrasts it with the process experienced by students in the curriculum. **Table 11-6** lists examples of leveled goals, and **Table 11-7** is an example of an outcome with leveled competencies. Typically, the curriculum goals or outcomes are the expectations for the final level of the program.

Confirming Curriculum Goals or Outcomes and Level Expectations

Faculty members are rightfully concerned about accuracy, reasonableness, and comprehensiveness in the goal or outcome statements and, therefore, discussion about both the substance and phraseology can be anticipated before approval by the total faculty group

Figure 11-1 Processes of curriculum development and student experience in relation to curriculum goals or outcomes.
© C. L. Iwasiw.

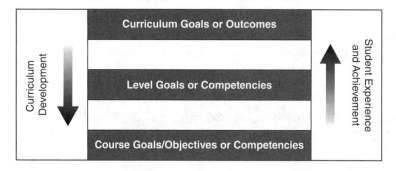

Table 11-6	Examples of Leveled Goals
Year 4:	Collaborate with others, in professional and public contexts, for optimal health for all within the global society.
Year 3:	Advocate with others in professional contexts for public policy that will address health and social justice locally, nationally, and internationally.
Year 2:	Analyze and critique local, national, and international situations of health and social inequity and propose solutions in classroom contexts.
Year 1:	Explain, in classroom contexts, the social determinants of health, nursing's legacy of social justice, and the roles of individual nurses, and the nursing profession as advocates and partners for health.

Source: Modified from Western-Fanshawe Collaborative BScN Program. (2013). *Western-Fanshawe Collaborative BScN Program Guide*. London: ON: Author. Used with permission.

Table 11-7	Example of Outcome and Leveled Competencies
Outcome:	The graduate is a skilled communicator who participates in collaborative decision making with clients and other health professionals.
Level 3 Competency:	Contributes to interprofessional discussion and decisions
Level 2 Competency:	Analyzes care situations with clients and healthcare team members
Level 1 Competency:	Demonstrates active listening skills and problem exploration with standardized patients

© C. L. Iwasiw.

is achieved. It is prudent to allow sufficient time for review and discussion of the curriculum and level expectations before proceeding with other aspects of curriculum development. The outcome or goal statements are a declaration of what students can expect to achieve and constitute a public promise of what successful students will be like. Therefore, faculty need to feel satisfied with these statements before they can commit to further curriculum development and adherence to the curriculum intent during implementation.

RELATIONSHIP OF CURRICULUM GOALS AND OUTCOMES TO AN EVIDENCE-INFORMED, CONTEXT-RELEVANT, UNIFIED CURRICULUM

In the Model of Evidence-Informed, Context-Relevant, Unified Curriculum Development, goals embody the educational destination, and this destination includes the key professional abilities that graduates will demonstrate, the major concepts that will influence their nursing practice, and the philosophical underpinnings of the practice. The concepts and professional abilities are derived from the analysis of contextual data; therefore, the goals are evidence informed. Furthermore, their relevance to the context in which graduates will practice nursing is ensured. The philosophical approaches are developed with a view to what is relevant in the current and anticipated healthcare and social context, and permeate the curriculum. The inclusion of some elements of the philosophical approaches in the goals creates a foundation for ongoing attention to the philosophy throughout the curriculum.

Moreover, the presence of the key abilities, major concepts, and philosophical approaches contributes to the unity of the curriculum. From the curriculum goals, the level goals are derived, and from the level goals, the course goals. In this way, the elements of the overall curriculum goals are present in goals throughout the curriculum, and this contributes to operational, conceptual, and visual unity.

The curriculum goal statements arise from the context and lead to the next phases of curriculum development. They embody the essence of the curriculum's purpose. Ongoing reference to the goals as the curriculum is developed supports the relevance and unity of the curriculum.

In contrast, the evidentiary basis of curriculum outcomes is not as extensive as that of curriculum goals. Accordingly, it cannot be assured that the outcomes are strongly related to the complete context, although they are related to the nursing context. The absence of core concepts and philosophical approaches in the outcome statements may lessen the visual unity of the curriculum. Therefore, outcomes statements do not necessarily reflect the foundations of an evidence-informed, context-relevant, unified curriculum.

CORE PROCESSES OF CURRICULUM WORK

Faculty Development

Faculty development can focus on how to write goal or outcome and competency statements. For some faculty, this will mean support to move away from the idea that content should determine the endpoint, to the idea that the abilities that nurses require is the starting point for determining and describing the educational destination and subsequent level expectations. Attention should be given to the components of either the goal or outcome statements. For some, an introduction to the taxonomies of learning would be helpful. A standard format for the outcome or goal statement and opportunities for practice and feedback could be provided.

Ongoing Appraisal

As curriculum developers proceed with defining the educational destination of the nursing curriculum, they appraise their work in an ongoing fashion. Questions they might ask of themselves and others include the following:

- Do the statements reflect our intent?
- Does each statement conform to the format we are using?
- In total, do the curriculum goal or outcome statements express what we believe is necessary for graduates to begin nursing practice?
- Are we missing something important?
- Are the curriculum expectations reasonable and achievable?
- Is the number of outcomes or goals reasonable?
- Are the expectations consistent with nursing education standards?
- Are the level expectations logical and sequenced with increasing complexity? Are they complete and achievable?
- Do the level expectations "add up" to the curriculum expectations?

Scholarship

Scholarship related to the development and confirmation of curriculum goals or outcomes in schools of nursing is limited. Therefore, manuscripts describing the processes undertaken and their inherent challenges would be a valuable contribution to the literature. A shift from generic instructions about how to write outcomes or goals to a concrete example of the process could be illuminating for other schools of nursing.

It would be worthwhile to conduct a Delphi survey of practicing nurses in staff positions and nurse leaders to determine their views about what the curriculum goals or outcomes should be. This could be completed early in curriculum development and at the time of curriculum revision. Such a project would provide evidence for the curriculum goals or outcomes and become the basis of a research manuscript.

Follow-up studies of graduates, to determine if the practice behaviors specified in the outcomes or goals are being enacted, would provide insight into the reasonableness of the goals and other aspects of the curriculum. The question that might be asked is: To what extent are the expected curriculum outcomes evident in practice?

CHAPTER SUMMARY

In this chapter, the formulation of curriculum goals and outcomes is addressed. The term *goals* is used in the Model of Evidence-Informed, Context-Relevant, Unified Curriculum Development; the term *outcomes* is in widespread use in the United Kingdom and the United States. There are similarities and differences in the components of goal and outcome statements, although both describe the educational destination of a curriculum and both incorporate the taxonomies of learning. The purposes of goal or outcome statements in curriculum development and for several groups are included. Further, the process of formulating goals and outcomes is described. The relationship of curriculum goals and outcomes to an evidence-informed, context-relevant unified curriculum is explained. Possible associated faculty development, ongoing appraisal, and scholarship related to formulating goals or outcomes are described.

SYNTHESIS ACTIVITIES

The case of the Southern Horizons School of Nursing is presented to illustrate ideas about formulating curriculum outcomes. This is followed by questions for analysis. Then, as in other chapters, questions and activities are offered to assist readers to formulate outcome or goal statements in individual settings.

Southern Horizons School of Nursing

Southern Horizons College is planning to open a school of nursing. This will be the first professional program at the undergraduate college. As such, the School of Nursing represents a change in the college's mission from the provision of liberal arts education to the inclusion of human service programs. The change in mission and the decision to initiate a nursing program arose from a long tradition of community service and social activism by college professors, an emphasis on service learning within the college, and a demand by the community for professional programs to be offered locally.

The founding director of the nursing program and two faculty members have been hired to plan a curriculum in advance of student admissions. The director was recruited from another nursing program in the state; the others are from other states. This group has met with healthcare and nursing leaders in the community, the leaders of social service agencies, and state health officials to learn about their needs and priorities. They have been particularly interested in the health profile of agency clients and the nursing leaders' views about what nurses need to be like now and 10 years into the future.

Believing that they have learned what is necessary, the group agrees that it is time to "put pen to paper" and start writing curriculum outcomes. They did not have to decide about whether to use goals or outcomes, because outcomes are standard in the college and are written as characteristics of the graduates. They meet to review the information they have collected and the *Essentials of Baccalaureate Education for Professional Nursing Practice* (American Association of Colleges of Nursing, 2009). Following the review and discussion, they decide that the essential attributes of nursing program graduates should be:

- Culturally competent
- Providers of safe, evidence-informed care
- Reflective practitioners
- Open to change
- Effective collaborators
- Responsive to clients' physical and psychosocial needs
- Skilled in the use of information technologies
- Respectful of professional boundaries in interpersonal and online environments
- Critical readers and users of research literature
- Committed to shared decision making with clients and other care providers

Questions and Activities for Critical Analysis of the Southern Horizons Nursing Program Case

1. Assess the process the group used to arrive at the attributes of graduates. If other activities might have been completed, what are they? In what ways could those other activities be helpful?

2. Examine the list of attributes.
   a. Does the list seem complete? If not, what might be missing?
   b. Are any items redundant or unnecessary? If unnecessary, what is the rationale for saying this?
3. How could stakeholders be involved in determining the curriculum outcomes?
4. Write outcome statements that incorporate the attributes decided upon for the Southern Horizons School of Nursing (or as modified in response to Question 2), the integrative action that will be performed, and the context of the action.

Questions and Activities for Consideration When Developing Goal or Outcome Statements in Readers' Settings

1. Describe a feasible process for the development of the curriculum goal or outcome statements. Who should be involved?
2. If there is a choice about using goal or outcome statements, what criteria should be the basis of the decision?
3. Who needs to be involved in the decision about the format of the statements of educational destination?
4. If goal statements are used, which components should be included? If outcome statements are used, which components should be included?
5. How can adherence to a consistent format be achieved?
6. Describe the advantages of presenting curriculum and level expectations as a completed package before seeking approval. Describe the advantages of gaining approval for the curriculum goals or outcomes before developing level expectations. Which approach would be more effective and why?
7. What is a reasonable time period for completion of this work?
8. Propose faculty development activities related to the development of goal or outcome statements.
9. What are the questions that could be asked in the ongoing appraisal as the goal or outcome statements and level expectations are prepared?
10. Suggest scholarship activities that should be considered and undertaken.

REFERENCES

American Association of Colleges of Nursing. (2009). *Essentials of baccalaureate education for professional nursing practice*. Retrieved from http://www.aacn.nche.edu/faculty/faculty-development/faculty-toolkits/BacEssToolkit.pdf

Anderson, L. W., Krathwohl, D. R., Airasian, P. W., Cruikshank, K. A., Mayer, R. E., Pintrich, P. R., . . . Wittrock, M. C. (Eds.). (2001). *A taxonomy for learning, teaching, and assessing: A revision of Bloom's taxonomy of educational objectives*. New York: Longman.

Atkinson, S. P. (2012). *Updated: Taxonomy circles—visualizations of educational domains*. Retrieved from http://spatkinson.wordpress.com/2012/11/13/updated-taxonomy-circles-visualisations-of-educational-domains/

Bloom, B. S., Englehart, M. D., Furst, E. J., Hill, W. H., & Krathwohl, D. R. (1956). *Taxonomy of educational objectives. The classification of educational goals: Handbook 1: Cognitive domain*. New York: David McKay.

Boland, D. (2012). Developing curriculum: Frameworks, outcomes, and competencies. In D. M. Billings & J. A. Halstead (Eds.), *Teaching in nursing: A guide for faculty* (4th ed., pp. 138–159). St. Louis, MO: Elsevier.

Gander, S. L. (2006). Throw out learning objectives: In support of a new taxonomy. *Performance Improvement, 45*(3), 9–15.

Glennon, C. D. (2006). Reconceptualizing program goals. *Journal of Nursing Education, 45*(2), 55–58.

Kennedy, D., Hyland, A., & Ryan, N. (2007). *Writing and using learning outcomes: A practical guide*. Retrieved from http://sss.dcu.ie/afi/docs/bologna/writing_and_using_learning_outcomes.pdf

Krathwohl, D. R., Bloom, B. S., & Masia, B. B. (1964). *Taxonomy of educational objectives: Handbook II: Affective domain*. New York: David McKay.

Mager, R. F. (1997). *Preparing instructional objectives: A critical tool in the development of effective instruction* (3rd ed.). Atlanta, GA: Center for Effective Performance Press.

Marzano, R. J., & Kendall, J. S. (2007). *The new taxonomy of educational objectives* (2nd ed.). Thousand Oaks, CA: Corwin Press.

Marzano, R. J., & Kendall, J. S. (2008). *Designing and assessing educational objectives: Applying the new taxonomy*. Thousand Oaks, CA: Corwin Press.

Oermann, M. H., & Gaberson, K. B. (2014). *Evaluation and testing in nursing education* (4th ed.). New York: Springer.

Oliva, P. F. (2009). *Developing the curriculum* (7th ed.). Boston: Pearson/Allyn & Bacon.

Simpson, E. J. (1972). *The classification of educational objectives in the psychomotor domain*. Washington, DC: Gryphon House.

Tyler, R. W. (1949). *Basic principles of curriculum and instruction*. Chicago: University of Chicago Press.

Western-Fanshawe Collaborative BScN Program. (2013). *Western-Fanshawe Collaborative BScN Program Guide*. London: ON: Author.

Wittman-Price, R. A., & Fasolka, B. J. (2010). Objectives and outcomes: The fundamental difference. *Nursing Education Perspectives, 31*, 233–236.

CHAPTER 12

Designing an Evidence-Informed, Context-Relevant, Unified Curriculum

Chapter Overview

This chapter begins with a presentation of information about curriculum design. Included are terminology, program type, structure, delivery, and models. General and health professional education designs, organizing strategies for nursing curricula, and patterns for nursing course sequencing follow. Then, the process of designing an evidence-informed, context-relevant, unified curriculum is described. Although presented in a linear fashion, curriculum design does not occur through a prescribed sequence, but rather through iterative discussion, generation of design ideas, and critique. Attending to curriculum implementation and planning curriculum evaluation are briefly addressed. The relationship of curriculum design to an evidence-informed, context-relevant, unified curriculum is described. A discussion of the three core processes of curriculum work (faculty development, scholarship, and ongoing appraisal related to curriculum design) is followed by a chapter summary. The synthesis section includes a case for analysis and questions to consider when undertaking curriculum design.

Chapter Goals

- Understand the process of designing an evidence-informed, context-relevant, unified curriculum.
- Identify factors important in curriculum design decisions.
- Appreciate variations in curriculum design.
- Consider human and financial implications of curriculum design.
- Gain insight into the value of curriculum evaluation planning as the curriculum is being designed.
- Appreciate the relationship of curriculum design to an evidence-informed, context-relevant, unified curriculum.
- Reflect on the core processes of curriculum work related to designing the overall curriculum.

CURRICULUM DESIGN

The term *curriculum design* refers to the configuration of the program of studies. It includes the courses selected, their sequencing, the relationships between and among courses, and associated curriculum policies. The design encapsulates the curriculum foundations and ought to present a picture of conceptual unity.

The process of designing the curriculum, or the *curriculum design process*, refers to the discussions and decision making that lead to the configuration of the program of studies. This process can feel like the heart of curriculum development, and its outcome is the written curriculum plan. The completed design makes the future curriculum tangible. Curriculum developers experience a strong sense of accomplishment, ownership, and satisfaction when they are able to say, "This is our curriculum."

It may be helpful to clarify some of the terminology used when undertaking the design phase of curriculum development. Terms such as *design*, *structure*, and *model* are often used interchangeably in the nursing education literature. To add to the confusion, descriptors such as "block," "integrated," "2 + 2," "accelerated," and "collaborative" have been referred to as designs, programs, structures, models, or patterns. For conceptual clarity, the following interpretations are used in this text and are more fully described in subsequent sections.

A program can be described according to the following characteristics, each of which can affect the configuration of courses:

- *Type*: Educational level (i.e., doctoral, master's, baccalaureate, associate degree, diploma, or practical nurse)
- *Structure*: Arrangement as to program length and semester or quarter divisions
- *Delivery*: Means by which faculty offer the curriculum
- *Model*: Overall organization of the curriculum that typically describes the arrangement of nursing and non-nursing courses (e.g., articulated, generic, or upper division nursing program)

Program Type and Structure

The program type, or educational level, has a significant influence on the curriculum design, because the nature and number of courses will be linked to the expectations for graduating students. The program type is evident in the curriculum or goal outcome statements, which should be internalized by curriculum planners.

Program structure refers to the duration of the program and the arrangement of divisions within the academic year. The duration is usually a function of program type, although alternative program lengths can be considered. For example, a prelicensure baccalaureate curriculum is typically 4 years in length, whereas accelerated curricula can be 12 to 24 months (Brandt, Boellaard, & Zorn, 2013). Once established, the program length is a boundary within which the curriculum must be designed. The division of the academic year into quarters, trimesters, semesters, or terms is established by the educational institution. These divisions are the temporal units in which year (or level), semester, and course goals or competencies must be achievable.

Program Delivery

Program delivery, another design element, refers to the method by which the curriculum is offered to students. Traditionally, this has been through provision of courses at the educational institution that awards the academic credential. Now, however, programs are extended through flexible delivery and partnerships.

Traditional Delivery

The traditional approach for delivering nursing curricula is through face-to-face instruction, in which the teacher and students are physically present in the same classroom, lab, or professional practice learning environment, at the same time, for a designated time period. This continues to be a fundamental feature of most undergraduate nursing programs.

This time- and place-dependent approach has been evolving to include more flexible scheduling and delivery. For example, nursing classes can be scheduled on one day of the week, in the evenings, or on weekends to accommodate students' work and family schedules. Additionally, faculty may travel to distant locations to offer classes for those unable to attend the credential-granting educational institution. Availability of faculty and suitable locations, as well as costs associated with time and travel, are some issues related to flexible, traditional delivery.

Distance Delivery

Distance delivery is a means to provide an educational offering when students are physically separate from the instructor and/or educational institution. Although generally understood to be technology based, distance delivery also includes print-based correspondence courses. Because of the predominance of online courses as a form of distance education, several terms are often used interchangeably or in conjunction with *distance delivery* to describe the educational process. These terms include: *distance education, distance learning, online education, online learning, web-based instruction, Internet-based instruction, Internet-based learning, distributed learning,* and *e-learning.* Whatever the mode of delivery, distance education entails planned experiences designed to support student learning (Frith & Clark, 2013).

The word "distance" is somewhat misleading as it may imply interpersonal and intellectual detachment and physical remoteness among participants engaged in the educational endeavor. However, physical distance should not automatically evoke images of students and instructors who are unconnected. Although course participants may be located around the globe, contemporary technology makes it possible for them to feel psychologically linked while actively and collectively engaging in learning experiences.

Flexibility ought to be a core element of distance delivery and uptake of programs and courses. Many variations are possible in the execution of distance courses, although they normally include the use of technology to connect students with faculty and each other. Courses can be conceptualized and offered using a single technology, or several, to accommodate students' learning styles, life roles, and inability to enroll in traditional on-campus programs. Also, courses can be paced or not paced. A paced course, typical in undergraduate and degree completion programs, is completed in a specified time period. Alternatively, if the course is not paced, students have more flexibility in timing. Course materials can be print based or computer based and include video and audio recordings, audio-enhanced online content, or a combination of these and/or other technologies.

Hybrid (Blended) Delivery

Hybrid delivery combines traditional face-to-face delivery with distance delivery. Courses or curricula offered via hybrid delivery can "provide moderate-to-high degrees of access and flexibility while offering the potential for moderate-to-high dialogue and low-to-moderate structure" (Millison & Wilemon, as cited in Ball, Mosca, & Paul, 2013). In other words, the design of the educational offerings can vary. Similarly, the amount of organization, interaction, fluidity of processes, and student choice can differ depending on the course or curriculum goals or outcomes.

From a review of research literature, Smythe (2011) asserts that in higher education, the dimensions of blended learning include combinations of:

- Traditional learning with web-based online approaches
- Media and technologies
- Pedagogical approaches, irrespective of the learning technology being used
- Synchronous and asynchronous components

Blended delivery can occur at the course, curriculum, or institutional level (Rietschel & Buckley, 2014). At the course level, online experiences may be an adjunct to regular face-to-face sessions. Or, the course could be divided between online and traditional delivery.

At the curriculum level, some courses may be face to face, and some may be delivered by technology. Alternatively, all courses might employ a blended approach. An institution might use a blended approach overall, with some courses using traditional delivery only, some online delivery only, while others use blended delivery.

Delivery Through Partnerships

Partnerships are formal arrangements that exist between and among institutions. In the nursing education literature, the terms *partnership*, *collaboration*, *collaborative partnership*, and *consortia* are often used without sufficient definition or differentiation. They do, however, refer to formal or informal affiliations or alliances developed by educational institutions with service agencies for professional practice or service-learning experiences, or to arrangements that exist between and among educational institutions for the purpose of providing nursing education. Within the educational partnerships, course delivery can occur by traditional, distance, or blended methods.

Educational institution partnerships are formed when more than one institution offers all or part of the same curriculum. These agreements require a high level of trust and cooperation. In collaborative partnerships and consortia with a common curriculum, negotiations and a willingness to let go of treasured aspects of individual curricula are necessary to achieve the larger purpose of the partnership. Contractual arrangements typically specify the responsibilities of all parties in developing, approving, implementing, and evaluating the curriculum, as well as administrative arrangements, including financial provisions. Additionally, details about the curriculum design can be specified.

The nature of contractual arrangements can have a profound effect on curriculum design. Clauses about design (e.g., where, how, and which courses will be offered), resource sharing, and requirements about faculty credentials could be written to ensure curriculum quality. Details such as course sequencing, or the provision of particular courses at specified sites, are sometimes seen as desirable to guarantee the role of partners. Yet, the more specific the curriculum detail in the signed agreements becomes and the greater the number of institutions involved, the more difficult it can be to modify the curriculum as time passes. Curriculum revision or complete reconceptualization of the curriculum will always require agreement by all partners. However, if specific design details are included in the partnership contract, new contracts must be developed. Therefore, it is wise to minimize references to curriculum details when agreements are first developed.

Three principal forms of partnerships exist between and among educational institutions. These are fee-for-service, collaborative partnerships, and consortium arrangements. There are no precise conceptual, functional, or quantitative demarcations between partnerships and consortia, so each grouping of schools of nursing uses the terminology it deems appropriate.

Fee-for-Service Partnership   In this arrangement, one institution purchases the course(s) of another. This is the least complex of the partnership agreements. Elements of the contract could include the nature of the course(s), number of students, delivery mode(s), and the fee, which may be based on enrollment numbers. The provider is unlikely to participate in the purchaser's curriculum development.

Collaborative Partnership   A collaborative partnership denotes a high degree of involvement between (or among) educational institutions. The collaborating partners share in curriculum development, implementation, and evaluation. Additionally, each partnership determines matters related to the following:

- Curriculum
  - All aspects of curriculum philosophy, goals or outcomes, design
  - Extent of allowable flexibility in response to local contexts
  - Admissions policies and procedures
  - Progression and appeals policies
  - Curriculum evaluation
  - Delivery modes
  - Sharing of human and physical resources
  - Faculty credentials
  - Approval and accreditation
  - Faculty development related to curriculum work
- Scholarship
  - Partnership-wide scholarship
  - Faculty development related to scholarship
- Governance
  - Committee structure, reporting requirements, approval processes, and so forth
  - Conflict resolution mechanisms
  - Procedures for partnership dissolution

A simple partnership involves two partners that support the same goal. There can also be several partners, and the more partners, the more intricate the contractual agreements between and among them.

In response to the baccalaureate-entry-to-practice requirement in Canada, universities and community colleges (the latter having formerly offered diploma, not degree, nursing programs) are collaborating to provide baccalaureate nursing education, with universities conferring the degree. In the province of Ontario, for example, universities have one or more college partner(s), with each partnership having one common curriculum. The formal arrangements include:

- Enrollment in either the college or university for the first 2 years of the program, with all students enrolled at the university for the final 2 years
- Simultaneous enrollment in both the college and university, with all students taking courses at both sites throughout the 4 years
- Simultaneous delivery of the entire program at each of the university and college sites, with students being enrolled in only one site.

Consortium   A consortium is a cooperative association of many partners formed to achieve common goals. It is an extended collaborative partnership. A well-known example is the Oregon Consortium for Nursing Education, a statewide consortium of university and community college nursing programs created to respond to the nursing shortage and the need for the type of nurse required to care for Oregon's changing demographics:

> It is an effort to increase capacity in schools of nursing by making the best use of scarce faculty, classrooms, and clinical training resources in the delivery of a standard curriculum on 13 campuses, including 8 community colleges and the 5 campuses of the OHSU [Oregon Health and Science University] School of Nursing. (Tanner, Gubrud-Howe, & Shores, 2008, p. 203)

There are common admission standards, a shared application process, a common curriculum, and student transferability among schools. The curriculum culminates in a bachelor of science in nursing (BSN) degree, although community college students can exit after the third year with an associate of applied science in nursing degree and eligibility to write the licensure examination. They can return to complete the fourth year to obtain the baccalaureate degree if they wish (Gubrud-Howe et al., 2003).

Advantages of Collaborative Partnerships and Consortia   The advantages of collaborative partnerships and consortia lie in the optimal use of resources to develop and share curricula and resources across institutions (Molzahn & Purkis, 2004). In addition, faculty development about teaching and scholarship are possible across the partnership. With the involvement of faculty from all partner sites in scholarship projects, there is a potential for a large sample size in nursing education studies. Further, collaboration among schools of nursing can lead to cohesion among nursing educators, who collectively can influence government funding and policies, nursing care, and healthcare organizations.

Program Models

The program model is the overall organization of the curriculum. This organization can vary according to the arrangement and numbers of required nursing, required non-nursing, and elective courses, as well as program length. All models are designed to facilitate students' achievement of the intended program goals or outcomes. In essence, the model determines where particular courses (including professional practice courses) can be placed in the curriculum. The name given to the model may include a reference to the type of program and/or the program length. It is important not to confuse *program model* with conceptual model or paradigm.

An integrated baccalaureate program is one example of a program model. Concepts are integrated throughout the curriculum in a meaningful way. In a 4-year, generic or basic program, nursing and non-nursing courses are given throughout the entire program, whereas in an upper division program, nursing courses are offered after foundation courses in other disciplines. Some 4-year baccalaureate programs may have an exit option to take licensure examinations after 3 years. In this model, courses deemed essential for registered nurse practice must be included in the first 3 years. The fourth year includes courses necessary to meet requirements for the nursing degree.

Articulated programs have a planned progression from a lower to a higher level of learning, for example, licensed practical nurse to associate degree in nursing (ADN), ADN to BSN or master of science in nursing. External degree models, for ADN or BSN study, are not centered on traditional patterns of institutional-based study. Rather, the focus is on the concept of providing credit on the basis of what one knows, not on how one has achieved it.

Accelerated programs represent another model. These nursing programs are built on students' prior degrees and are comprised primarily or entirely of nursing theory and practice courses.

A more recent program model is the dual degree partnership in nursing, with a 1+2+1 sequence, developed in Syracuse, New York. Students complete 1 year of arts and science courses at Le Moyne College, 2 years enrolled in the associate degree in nursing program at St. Joseph's College of Nursing at St. Joseph's Hospital Health Center, and then meet the remaining requirements for the bachelor of science degree at Le Moyne College (Bastable & Markowitz, 2012). This model is similar to the "sandwich" baccalaureate nursing programs that existed in Canada in the 1940s and early 1950s, whereby students completed 1 year of university study, 3 years in a hospital diploma nursing program, and then 1 final year at university.

The program model is an important element of design. If a nursing program is being created in an institution where nursing did not formerly exist, then there may be considerable freedom to choose the program model. However, if there is a desire to change an existing model, negotiation will be required, because there can be scheduling, faculty, and budgetary implications for the school of nursing and other departments.

CURRICULUM DESIGNS FROM GENERAL EDUCATION EVIDENT IN NURSING CURRICULA

Curriculum design, as noted at the beginning of this chapter, refers to the configuration of the program of studies, including the courses selected, sequencing, the relationships between and among courses, and associated curriculum policies. Two typologies of curriculum design in general education are evident in nursing curricula.

Selection and Organization of Content

Curriculum designs based on the selection and organization of content have been described and can be recognized in nursing curricula. Most nursing curricula do not use only one design, but rather a combination of these approaches.

In an *academic subject design*, particular subjects are included in each or most years of the curriculum (Henson, 2010). In public schools, an example is mathematics. In nursing, aspects of this design pattern are represented by nursing courses, such as professional nursing, which is often included more than once in a curriculum with increasing complexity. More generally, science courses are considered essential in nursing curricula and particular science courses can appear throughout a nursing curriculum, such as a chemistry course followed by a biochemistry course.

A *core curriculum* design includes subjects or topics that are required of all students (Henson, 2010). This core is essential to all curricula, although it may be addressed in different ways and to different depths in various curricula. An example is communication skills, which are addressed in all programs leading to a credential in nursing. The depth and nature of the skills expected is different in BSN and PhD curricula, but communication is a core skill that is included in the curricula. Furthermore, because communication is core to all nursing, the topic is considered in different contexts throughout the undergraduate curriculum.

Subjects are combined to form new content areas in a *fusion design*. A health promotion course would be an example. Knowledge from nursing, sociology, psychology, and education is combined so that the originating disciplines are not readily identifiable.

A *special topic design* is flexible. Content is drawn from several subjects to address important issues, problems, or areas of interest. As issues emerge, new courses are developed. They can become permanent, or they can be discontinued if no longer timely. In nursing curricula, the topic of international nursing or global health, for example, was often introduced as a special topic course and then became a regular part of the curriculum once it was apparent that the topic was an enduring one.

In *student-centered designs*, courses are provided in response to student interests. In nursing, giving choice about professional practice placement sites is an example of student-centeredness, as is the provision of elective courses in the curriculum.

Ordering or Construction of Knowledge

Wiles and Bondi (2011) describe five patterns of constructing or ordering knowledge (in contrast to content) in a curriculum. All can be identified within nursing curricula. The five patterns are described as follows, beginning with the most structured and ending with the most flexible.

In a *building blocks design*, a clearly defined body of knowledge or skills is organized into a pyramid-like arrangement. The base is made up of foundational knowledge, and the middle portion of the pyramid is composed of increasingly specialized material. The pinnacle contains in-depth, specialized knowledge. The sequence is prescribed and deviation is not allowed.

A *branching design* is a variation of the building blocks design. The endpoints of learning are known in advance. The curriculum starts with foundational knowledge, and then there is some choice within prescribed areas beyond the common experiences.

In a *spiral design*, the same knowledge areas are repeatedly revisited at higher levels of complexity. There can be some flexibility, but this is likely limited as curriculum designers decide what knowledge needs to be reexamined and when.

With a specific *tasks or skills design*, specific knowledge and experiences are intended to assist students to achieve predetermined competencies. There can be flexibility in the content and the ordering of content.

In a *process design*, there is a fluid organization of knowledge. The emphasis is on the process to be learned, and content is the medium through which specified processes are addressed.

Nursing curricula typically employ all five means of organizing or constructing knowledge. A building blocks approach is evident in a curriculum where students first encounter clients experiencing limited psychological stress and physiological alterations, then those with moderate levels of psychological and/or psychological problems, and, finally, clients with complex health and social problems. Curricula with course choices (i.e., branching) would reflect a belief that there is more than one path to reach the goals or outcomes. Many programs have a final professional practice practicum, and this experience provides an example of both branching and spiraling. A variety of placements for a practicum represents a branching design. Students who repeat a placement they have previously experienced are in a spiral situation; they are returning to the same practice area with more knowledge and experience and should be able to deepen their understanding of the clients and situations they encounter. Plans for psychomotor skills learning in many curricula are reflective of a specific task or skills design.

INTERPROFESSIONAL EDUCATION

Traditionally, health professional courses have been unidisciplinary. Curricula were planned by members of one health professional discipline for students in that discipline. However, there is now recognition that if students are educated in isolation from one another, they likely will have difficulty communicating and collaborating in meaningful ways once they are practicing professionals. As a consequence of faulty communication among health professionals, patient safety has been compromised. Therefore, there is increasing impetus to develop shared learning experiences for students of all health professions, with the ultimate goal of improving interprofessional communication and collaboration, patient care and safety, and organizational functioning.

Multidisciplinary, Interdisciplinary, or Transdisciplinary Learning

Shared learning experiences can be multidisciplinary, interdisciplinary, or transdisciplinary. "Multidisciplinarity brings two or more disciplines to bear on a problem without integrating disciplinary components, whereas interdisciplinarity is marked by a synthesis of disciplinary knowledge and methods that provides a more holistic understanding" (Knight, Lattuca, Kimball, & Reason, 2013, p. 144). Transdisciplinity is one step beyond interdisciplinary in that "it goes beyond drawing concepts from the disciplines to create new frameworks that break down (transgress) the traditional boundaries of the disciplines" (Mitchell, as cited in Park & Son, 2010). Some professional boundary blurring occurs as situations are considered within the new frameworks, while mutual trust and respect for discipline-specific expertise are developed.

In interdisciplinary learning, participant collaboration is the interaction mode and students learn to be knowledge collaborators. In transdisciplinary learning, students learn to be knowledge producers, and the knowledge production occurs through interdisciplinary collaborative learning (Park & Son, 2010). Transdisciplinary learning is the goal of interprofessional education (IPE).

Transdisciplinary Interprofessional Education

IPE is the provision of "occasions when members (or students) of two or more professions associated with health or social care engage in learning with, from, and about each other"

(Freeth et al., as cited in Reeves, Goldman, & Oandasan, 2007, p. 231). The goal is to facilitate students' development of attitudes, knowledge, skills, and behaviors that are expected to lead to successful collaboration. The expectation is that the preparation of a collaborative-practice-ready health workforce will result in collaborative professional practice, and that this will result in optimal health services (WHO Study Group on Interprofessional Education and Collaborative Practice, 2010). The core competencies for interprofessional practice delineated by organizations such as the Canadian Interprofessional Health Collaborative (2010) or the (U.S.) Interprofessional Education Collaborative Expert Panel (2011) provide frameworks for use in IPE.

Effective strategies include students from two or more disciplines engaging in problem-based learning, patient-focused case studies, or acquisition of clinical skills (Barnsteiner, Disch, Hall, Mayer, & Moore, 2007), either in practice or through simulation. Additionally, reflection on interactions and learning is an essential element of IPE. The metacognitive reflection is intended to assist students to extend their thinking beyond the healthcare situation and to illuminate the processes of learning, collaboration, and interprofessional collaborative functioning. Shared reflection extends interprofessional learning to transdisciplinary or transprofessional learning.

Whether courses or learning experiences shared by students in more than one health profession are multidisciplinary, interdisciplinary, or transdisciplinary depends on the extent to which faculty members from two or more health professions:

- Are committed to a shared vision that includes fostering collaborative interprofessional relationships
- Believe that healthcare knowledge is not the domain of only one discipline
- Recognize and value the contributions of members from other health professions to health care
- Are involved in shared course development, delivery, and evaluation
- Have an understanding of the goals, designs, and methods of transdisciplinary education in the health professions

Barnsteiner and colleagues (2007) propose the following five additional criteria for full engagement of IPE in an organization:

- Explicit and widely known organizational philosophy of IPE
- Embedding of IPE as a required part of curricula
- Inclusion of integrated and experiential opportunities to learn teamwork and collaboration, and how these group skills relate to safe care delivery
- Requirement that all students demonstrate competence in a single set of interprofessional competencies
- Presence of organizational infrastructure that fosters IPE

The WHO Study Group on Interprofessional Education and Collaborative Practice (2010) considers several conditions to be necessary for developing and implementing IPE:

- Presence of a champion who is responsible for coordinating IPE and identifying barriers to progress
- Preparation of instructors
- Compulsory attendance by students
- Use of adult learning principles
- Use of methods that reflect students' real-life experiences
- Interaction among students

More ambitious than the ideas previously cited about IPE are those proposed by the Lancet Commission (2010). This commission advocates radical changes in the education of health professions and in educational institutions to produce critically inquiring leaders who will transform health care globally. The Lancet Commission advocates for transformative learning, interdependence (among educational institutions, health systems, and global networks) in education, and a shared vision of all health professionals in all countries who can mobilize knowledge, engage in critical reasoning and ethical conduct, and "are competent to participate in patient-centered and population-centered health systems as members of locally responsive and globally connected teams" (p. 53). To this end, IPE should focus not only on technical skills, but also on:

> cross-cutting generic competencies, such as analytic abilities (for effective use of both evidence and ethical deliberation in decision making), leadership and management capabilities (for efficient handling of scarce resources in conditions of uncertainty), and communication skills (for mobilization of all stakeholders, including patients and populations). (p. 54)

ORGANIZING STRATEGIES FOR NURSING CURRICULUM DESIGN

A curriculum organizing strategy is the structure or scaffolding upon which courses are built. It gives direction to the nature and sequence of courses and learning experiences, which together must form a unified, coherent, and logical curriculum.

Nursing has always used an organizing strategy for curriculum design, beginning with Nightingale's statements about the person–environment relationship. Since then, numerous organizing strategies have been developed. The one selected should:

- Correspond with the curriculum philosophy
- Respond to the context of the program

- Ensure opportunities for students to achieve curriculum goals or outcomes
- Be logical and justifiable
- Provide optimal usefulness and consistency

Traditional Organizing Strategies

Medical Model

In the medical model of organizing nursing curricula, popular for more than half of the 1900s, content was organized according to the following components: disease (teaching by body system), knowledge (learning by parts and adding on), terms or vocabulary (precise definitions), concept of nurse (whose function is incidental and who "does things" to the patient and environment), and concept of patient (as a repository of disease and recipient of nursing care). In this organizing strategy, courses are ordered in specific sequences. The content to be learned and how it is to be learned are identified. Nursing courses and nursing skills are delineated first. Then, the required non-nursing courses, critical learning experiences, and evaluation methods to assess what students have learned are determined.

The traditional hospital clinical areas (maternity, medicine, pediatrics, psychiatry, surgery) are the focus of learning, with the addition of a community experience. Advantages of this organizing strategy include the wide availability of nursing textbooks written according to the medical model, a good fit with hospital organization and faculty members' areas of expertise, and a match with popular perceptions of nursing. However, a risk is that nursing knowledge may not be given prominence in the curriculum.

Use of the medical model has declined since the 1980s. However, remnants of this organizing framework are evident in course titles such as *Nursing Care of Psychiatric Patients*. Although classes might not follow the pattern of describing nursing care in relation to disease processes, the overall structure of the curriculum is organized in whole or in part according to the traditional medical specialties.

Simple-to-Complex

In a simple-to-complex organizing strategy, another traditional approach, knowledge is organized so that learning occurs sequentially. Students learn progressively more about a specific concept or process over time. For example, the curriculum might first address nursing care of individuals, then families, then aggregate groups. The advantage rests with the innate logic of incremental learning; students are expected to be responsive first to one person, then to a small group, and then to a community. However, this organization does not reflect the reality of nursing practice, because nurses typically respond to families along with individuals, to individuals within families and groups, and to individuals and small groups within aggregates.

Stages of Illness

Health and its meaning are considered first when employing stages of illness as the organizing strategy. Content addressing acute care nursing is followed by content about rehabilitative, and then chronic care nursing. Normal life processes such as pregnancy and aging do not fit easily into this approach, nor does health promotion of families and groups. Nonetheless, this strategy can encompass institutional and community-based practice.

Contemporary Organizing Strategies

Nursing Conceptual Framework, Model, or Theory

The curriculum can be organized according to one nursing conceptual framework, model, or theory, for example Orem's (1990) General Theory of Nursing or Watson's (2012) Human Caring Science. These can be employed individually. Each conceptual framework, model, or theory offers a somewhat different perspective of nursing with its own accompanying vocabulary. With this organizing strategy, the concepts and components of the selected theory or practice framework are predominant in all courses and experiences. The nursing focus is foremost in the curriculum and directs students to view theory and practice with a specific perspective. However, a single nursing conceptual framework, model, or theory may not reflect the views of all faculty and students, and may not easily fit all nursing practice contexts. Also, the language and critical concepts may be too abstract for some students. Finally, few textbooks and other references are likely to be organized according to the chosen perspective.

Multiple or eclectic nursing conceptual (or theoretical) frameworks can also be adopted. Curriculum designers select concepts and definitions that best fit their values and beliefs about nursing. Several conceptual frameworks, models, or theories within the curriculum (pluralism), might be used, with different ones being given prominence in different courses. Combining parts of two or more theories (eclecticism) is also possible. This would combine what is best understood from several nursing frameworks, models, or theories. Adaptation of elements from multiple perspectives could generate creative curriculum designs. Pluralism or eclecticism might be less constraining than reliance on only one framework. Nevertheless, a multiple-framework approach could jeopardize the body of knowledge from one model, or take away from that which is uniquely nursing. Distortion of original concepts, definitions, characteristics, and attributes of one or more of the original models or theories might result.

Use of nursing frameworks and theories continues in nursing education, albeit often only in selected courses or as a component of a philosophy, and not as a basis for an entire curriculum. Their decreasing prominence as organizing strategies for curricula is related to the fact that they have not been sufficient for all aspects of the nursing curriculum and there has been little uptake of the frameworks in nursing practice. The language of the theories and frameworks has, at times, been a barrier to understanding between students and practicing nurses.

Outcomes

An outcomes approach is another organizing strategy. When curriculum developers focus on outcomes, design proceeds from this point. In this way, curriculum designers would initially identify the outcomes students will be required to demonstrate, and accordingly shape the concepts embedded in the outcomes and competencies. For example, if health promotion, critical thinking, collaborative skills, and shared decision making are necessary outcomes, these concepts or competencies will form components of the curriculum. Curriculum developers would first identify essential qualities of graduates, then identify competencies or competency statements for each year or level of the program necessary to attain the outcomes (which also become the evaluation criteria). Curriculum developers would then determine the antecedents or factors necessary for achieving the competencies, the learning experiences, teaching methods, learning resources, and assessment strategies (Boland, 2012).

Dalley, Candela, and Benzel-Lindley (2008) have proposed developing curriculum outcomes as the starting point of curriculum design. They then suggest that faculty list all the possible content, concepts, and abilities pertinent to their teaching area, and then organize items from that list into the following categories:

- Foundational content, concepts, and abilities that should be mastered in early nursing courses and be evident in all subsequent courses
- Specialty concepts and abilities associated with specialized areas of nursing practice
- Content that students can discover for themselves

Once this is completed, faculty make decisions about leveling and placement of content based on the outcomes.

Other Theories, Concepts, and Philosophies

Theories, concepts, and philosophies, which influence the development of the curriculum philosophical approaches, could also be the basis of the curriculum design. For example, views related to theories of knowledge development, domains of practice, feminism, or existentialism, singly or in combination, can be used to organize the curriculum or parts of the curriculum.

In the Model of Evidence-Informed, Context-Relevant, Unified Curriculum Development, concepts, abilities, and educational and philosophical approaches are the foundations of the curriculum and all courses and classes. The evidence-informed concepts and abilities are derived from an analysis of the context in which the curriculum is offered and in which graduates will practice nursing. With reference to concepts only, Giddens and Brady (2007) advocate their use to organize the nursing curriculum and to be the foci of courses. In their approach, a benchmarking of curriculum concepts exercise was undertaken by schools and consortia using concept-based curricula. Three broad categories of concepts emerged: attribute concepts, health and illness concepts, and professional nursing concepts (Giddens, Wright, & Gray, 2012).

Many ideas have been proposed for concepts to include in a curriculum, either throughout the curriculum or as the foundation of a single course. Some of these ideas are:

- Incorporating *caring* throughout the curriculum (Brown, 2011)
- Including *culture* (Sairanen et al., 2013) or *multiculturalism* (Bagnardi, Bryant, & Colin, 2009) in the curriculum
- Integrating concepts of *evidence-based practice* and *best practices* throughout the curriculum (Finotto, Carpanoni, Turroni, Camellini, & Mecugni, 2013)

The abundance of concepts to include in a curriculum, or ideas about concepts to use in particular courses, highlight that one conceptual framework is probably not suitable for all situations and that nurse educators accept pluralism as a sound basis for curriculum development. Moreover, it is evident that curricula are evolving as new ideas are proposed within nursing and other disciplines, and in response to contextual realities. If pluralism is the basis of curriculum design, the frameworks must be consistent with the philosophical approaches and with each other.

Course-Sequencing Patterns

Within the organizing strategy used to design the curriculum, courses can be sequenced in block, concurrent, mixed, or immersion-residency patterns. A block pattern specifies theory and professional practice courses in sequence, each separate from the other and becoming the foundation for those that follow. In a concurrent pattern, theory and professional practice courses are scheduled simultaneously throughout the curriculum.

A mixed pattern is also possible, with different parts of the curriculum having different patterns. A program with concurrent theory and practice, followed by a concentrated professional practice practicum without formal classes, is an example of a mixed pattern for course sequencing.

A newer pattern is the immersion-residency pattern, developed by the University of Delaware School of Nursing. Students have nursing theory courses and lab-based experiences in the first 3 years of the curriculum, with professional practice experiences reserved for a full-year immersion residency in the final year of the program (Diefenbeck, Plowfield, & Herman, 2006; Paulson, 2011).

DESIGNING AN EVIDENCE-INFORMED, CONTEXT-RELEVANT, UNIFIED NURSING CURRICULUM

Creating an evidence-informed, context-relevant, unified nursing curriculum design involves many processes. These include confirming the goal of the design process; organizing, defining, and refining curriculum concepts; defining curriculum parameters; deliberating about delivery approaches, program models, organizing strategies, and course sequencing; identifying courses; mapping the curriculum; planning curriculum evaluation; and attending to program policies and resources. Iterative discussions lead to the generation of design proposals, critique, and decision making. Although the processes of designing a curriculum are described in the following sections as separate components, much occurs concurrently and iteratively.

There is no formula for curriculum design, so that a particular program model and organizing strategy result in a predetermined design. Each design team establishes its own procedures and through use of creative and logical thinking produces a design relevant for its own context. Invariably, the design group's work will be characterized by ongoing deliberation and negotiation.

Confirming the Goal of the Curriculum Design Process

Nurse educators strive to develop evidence-informed, context-relevant, unified nursing curricula that will build students' professional knowledge and skills so that graduates will practice nursing competently in a changing healthcare environment, thereby contributing to the health and quality of life of those they serve. It is valuable to clarify the goal of the curriculum design process, because members of the development team may have varying expectations. The goal is to design a curriculum that:

- Is evidence informed, context relevant, and unified
- Adheres to the chosen philosophical and educational approaches
- Will be feasible within the context in which the curriculum will be offered
- Has the support of faculty members and the educational institution
- Allows for the continuous and evident presence of the curriculum foundations, that is, core curriculum concepts, key professional abilities, and philosophical and educational approaches
- Provides opportunities for students to achieve the curriculum outcomes or goals
- Meets requirements for approval and accreditation

Defining Curriculum Parameters

Attention to curriculum design (i.e., the configuration of the program of studies) cannot occur in isolation from the context in which the curriculum will be offered. The context and previous curriculum decisions determine the curriculum parameters, that is, the limits within which the curriculum must be designed and operationalized.

Many curriculum parameters will have been identified during collection and analysis of the contextual data, although they might not have been labeled in this way. A review of contextual data can highlight relevant information that curriculum designers should keep in mind. Internal contextual data include information about faculty numbers, infrastructure, institutional policies, partnerships, and the ability of other departments to mount new courses. Critical data from the external context to keep in mind include the types of health services available in the community and standards for state or provincial approval and national accreditation.

In addition to contextual influences, the design is affected by all curriculum decisions made to date. These decisions give direction to the design, while also requiring curriculum developers to limit themselves to ideas that are congruent with the philosophical and educational approaches, core curriculum concepts, and key professional abilities. These prior decisions make some designs possible, while ruling out others. It is important for curriculum designers to be clear about the parameters that affect the design so that a realistic, feasible, and logical curriculum can be created.

Facilitating the Design Process

Designing the curriculum, which requires time and considerable intellectual effort, can be facilitated by reviewing current literature, visiting other schools, consulting with colleagues regionally and nationally, and attending nursing education conferences. Surveys of catalogues of highly rated schools (particularly those using similar philosophical approaches), with attention to program designs, could prove beneficial and move the process forward.

To solicit input, the design team might develop a template and ask stakeholders to respond to the designated elements. Following formulation of statements about the philosophical approaches, core curriculum concepts, key professional abilities, and curriculum goals or outcomes, the template could include space for year goals or outcomes, semester outcomes, possible courses, credit allocations, sequencing, professional practice experiences, and other items deemed relevant. The collation of this information can provide a basis for curriculum design.

Another way to depict the developing curriculum visually is in a matrix format with relevant horizontal and vertical headings. The matrix indicates the plan for continuity of concepts. It is a recording of prominent ideas for each nursing course and the basis for detailed course and evaluation planning. Once finalized, the matrix (along with the concept map described later in this chapter) becomes a blueprint against which the operationalized curriculum can be compared and assessed. However, the matrix cannot be finalized in isolation of other aspects of the design process. A draft matrix can serve as a focus for discussion and then be confirmed after all other aspects of design are discussed. See **Figure 12-1** for a template of a curriculum matrix.

Deliberating About Curriculum Design

It can be worthwhile to review the curriculum work done to date to rekindle agreed-upon perspectives. As in all aspects of curriculum development, similarities should be capitalized upon, previous decisions recalled, and differences negotiated. A review of the analysis of the contextual data will refresh members about previously proposed design ideas.

Deliberations about curriculum design encompass integrative discussion about all aspects of design and focused discussion about the specific components of design.

Figure 12-1   Template for curriculum matrix.
© C. L. Iwasiw.

	Year 1			Year 2			Year 3			Year 4		
	Year Goals/ Competencies 1. 2. etc.			Year Goals/ Competencies 1. 2. etc.			Year Goals/ Competencies 1. 2. etc.			Curriculum Goals/ Competencies 1. 2. etc.		
Nursing Course Titles												
Course Goals or Competencies												
Major Concepts												
Knowledge and/or Professional Practice Focus												
Interprofessional Courses or Experiences												
Non-nursing Courses												

If diagrammed, discussion would resemble many overlapping and repeated zigzags among the design components, not a segmented, linear progression of ideas. The dialogue could address the following questions:

- How might the philosophical approaches be operationalized?
- How should the core curriculum concepts be addressed throughout the curriculum?
- How can the curriculum be designed so students will have opportunities to achieve the curriculum goals or outcomes?
- What design ideas stem from the chosen educational approaches?
- Which ideas from the analysis of the contextual data warrant further discussion?
- If there is a choice about the program model, which is preferred? Why?
- What could be the overall organizing strategy for the design?
- Which pattern for sequencing learning experiences matches the agreed-upon ideas about learning?
- What are the learning experiences (theory and professional practice) that students require to achieve curriculum goals or outcomes?
- What are the necessary nursing and non-nursing courses?
- Is shared education for health professional students a possibility? Are multidisciplinary, interdisciplinary, or transdisciplinary experiences preferred? How could IPE be initiated, advanced, and/or supported?
- Which courses could be optional for students?
- What configurations of courses are possible to maximize learning?
- What is the rationale for the delivery approach, model, organizing strategy, and configuration chosen?
- How feasible are the ideas?
- What academic policies require consideration as part of the design?

In the following paragraphs, some design components are addressed in detail. Notably, these include selecting delivery approaches, a program model, an organizing strategy, and a course-sequencing pattern.

Selecting a Delivery Approach

Decisions about delivery (traditional, distance, or hybrid) form an important part of the overall discussion, if this has not already been defined as a design parameter. When referring to contextual data about faculty, institutional support for distance delivery, and available infrastructure, designers might ask questions such as:

- Is the use of only one delivery approach congruent with the philosophical approaches and curriculum outcomes, or could a combination be used?

- Which modalities best suit the nature of the curriculum?
- What resources would faculty require?
- What resources will students require for distance or blended delivery?
- How might delivery approaches affect the configuration of courses?

Selecting a Program Model

When curriculum designers have the option of creating a new program model, their deliberations are strongly guided by beliefs about learning and nursing education. They might discuss the following matters:

- The arrangement of nursing and non-nursing courses that best match the curriculum foundations (philosophical and educational approaches, curriculum outcomes or goals, core curriculum concepts, and key professional abilities)
- Arrangements that can be ruled out
- The most suitable model that will likely be feasible and acceptable to students, faculty, and the educational institution

Selecting an Organizing Strategy and a Course-Sequencing Pattern

The choice of an organizing strategy will depend on the philosophical approaches previously determined for the curriculum and the core curriculum concepts identified from the analysis of the contextual data. Curriculum designers might ask themselves questions such as the following:

- What are appropriate criteria for choosing an organizing strategy and sequencing pattern?
- Which organizing strategies can be ruled out?
- Which organizing strategies might best fit with the philosophical and educational approaches?
- Is there a natural fit with core curriculum concepts and one of the organizing strategies?
- Can some of the organizing strategies be combined in a meaningful way?
- Could a model unique to our school be developed?
- Should a block, concurrent, mixed, or immersion-residency pattern of course sequencing be used?

These, and other points of discussion, will occur in a recursive fashion, leading to a conclusion about an organizing strategy and sequencing pattern. Like other aspects of curriculum development, ideas are proposed, and, following exploration, debate, and review of previous decisions, modifications are made and new ideas are added.

Organizing and Defining Curriculum Concepts

The concepts derived from the contextual analysis, and additional concepts present in the statement of philosophical approaches, must be organized in a meaningful way to form a framework for further curriculum design. This first requires synthetic thinking to combine and (re)name similar concepts. Then, they can be grouped into three to five categories that are consistent with curriculum ideas that have been developed so far.

Consensus is essential about the concept list and categorization of concepts. Then, the concepts must be carefully defined. Additionally, agreement is needed about how the concepts will be used in the curriculum (Giddens et al., 2012). A common understanding of the concepts by curriculum developers and all faculty implementing the curriculum is crucial. This will ensure that use of the concepts in the curriculum is consistent and unambiguous to students. This consistency contributes to curriculum unity.

Identifying Courses

Discussion about courses to include in the curriculum requires attention to many ideas concurrently. The depth of concepts (i.e., what is to be learned), the knowledge context in which the concepts will be addressed, the sequence (order of the units), and continuity (logical relationship or progression from one unit to another) are significant concerns for curriculum designers. The balance between process and content can be a source of much deliberation, possibly reflecting differing values in the group.

Identifying appropriate courses begins with an examination of the curriculum goals or outcomes, followed by discussion about prerequisite knowledge and experiences (Boland, 2012; Doll, 1996; Friesner, 1978; Gagné, Briggs, & Wager, 1992). Recognition of courses that are not suitable occurs as part of the discussion and helps to define which ideas are relevant. The integration of concepts and substantive knowledge and prerequisite knowledge and experiences form the basis of nursing and non-nursing courses.

Typically, the curriculum goals or outcomes are those for the graduating year or final semester of the program. Working backward from these, level (year) or semester competencies are identified and then analyzed to derive goals or competencies for the nursing courses. In this way, the link between individual units of learning (courses) and the curriculum outcomes is evident. Further refinement is required for individual courses.

The curriculum goals or outcomes encompass the key professional abilities and the core curriculum concepts that have been derived from the analysis of contextual data. Therefore, during the delineation of prerequisite professional abilities and subconcepts, the interrelationships among the professional abilities, and among the concepts, are revealed. Ultimately, this process results in a logical progression from the learning expectations and experiences in the first courses to those in subsequent courses, and to the expected curriculum goals or outcomes.

Nursing Courses

Nursing courses are typically defined first. The interface between level and semester competencies or goals and the organization of identified concepts gives rise to decisions about the nature, number, and configuration of nursing courses. These decisions rest upon the program model, structure, organizing strategy, course-sequencing pattern, and all previous decisions about the curriculum.

As ideas for courses are being proposed, it is helpful to examine all the curriculum possibilities that were proposed when contextual data were analyzed. Among the possibilities may be ideas for courses, or several possibilities might be combined to form a course. The value of the time spent in analyzing the contextual data and brainstorming about curriculum possibilities becomes readily apparent when nursing courses are being defined.

When thinking about nursing courses, curriculum designers consider whether courses in other disciplines or within other health science disciplines would be suitable instead of developing their own courses. The following questions could shape the discussion:

- Which of the curriculum possibilities that were proposed during the analysis of the contextual data fit best with philosophical approaches and program goals or outcomes?
- Are there curriculum possibilities that logically combine to form meaningful courses?
- Which ideas about curriculum possibilities warrant further development?
- How can core curriculum concepts be integrated with increasing depth throughout the curriculum?
- How could concepts be grouped into courses?
- How many nursing courses are possible within the program structure?
- Which nursing courses could be included?
- How will the overall focus of each course contribute to curriculum outcomes?
- What could be the competencies or goals for the proposed courses?
- What is a reasonable sequence for these courses?

In defining the general substance of each course, curriculum designers may struggle with the tension between substantive knowledge for nursing practice and adherence to a conceptual approach. Although course details will be defined later, at this time it is important to be clear about the predominant concepts and general focus of each course. Brief course descriptions and course competencies or goals should be drafted. These will give members of the curriculum development team an understanding of the intent of all nursing courses.

Titles of nursing courses are important. Generic titles, such as *Nursing Care of Adults* or *Clinical Practicum*, do not provide sufficient information about the concepts or professional abilities that will be addressed. As much as possible, nursing course titles can be created to match the organization of the major curriculum concepts. The use of nomenclature aligned with the major curriculum concepts conveys the intellectual dimension of nursing and gives conceptual and visual unity to the curriculum.

Each course title should convey the main conceptual, process, and/or contextual focus of the course in accordance with the overall curriculum design. For example, the course title, *Health Promotion and Caring: Families and Communities*, includes the concepts and processes of health promotion and caring, and specifies families and communities as the context. Similarly, the title, *Professional Practice: Families and Communities*, makes evident the process of the course (professional practice) and the context in which students will engage in the process. Collectively, course titles ought to present a picture of a unified curriculum. **Table 12-1** lists selected nursing course titles for a curriculum whose metaconcepts are *Health Promotion* and *Caring*, and which has adopted the terminology of *professional practice* for all lab and client-based learning experiences.

Table 12-1	Selected Nursing Course Titles to Reflect Curriculum Concepts*
Year 1:	Foundations of Professional Practice
	Health Promotion and Caring for Self, Colleagues, and Clients
	Holistic Health Assessment
Year 2:	Health Promotion and Caring: Families and Communities
	Professional Practice: Families and Communities
	Ways of Knowing: Research
Year 3:	Health Promotion and Caring in Rural Contexts
	Professional Practice in a Global Context
	Ways of Knowing: Data Analysis
Year 4:	Reflecting on Professional Practice and Context
	Transitions to Professional Nursing Practice

*Metaconcepts: caring, health promotion. Other curriculum concepts: holism, health, ways of knowing, culture, context, transitions, professional practice

© Western-Fanshawe Collaborative BScN Program (2010). Used with permission.

Non-nursing Courses

Consideration should be given to non-nursing courses that contribute to students' knowledge and understanding of nursing. These courses do not merely support the curriculum; they are an integral and significant part of it.

Substantive knowledge from liberal arts and psychosocial and health sciences is essential to the development of open-minded, educated, and informed practitioners. Students' interaction with an array of concepts, processes, and worldviews expands the depth and scope of their learning and helps them think critically from a broader, more comprehensive knowledge base. Therefore, consideration should be given to which required non-nursing courses to include, prerequisites, and the number of electives. Modification of existing non-nursing courses, or development of new ones, could be discussed. In all probability, these ideas will require negotiation with the departments offering the courses. Conclusions about non-nursing courses are reached through discussion about their nature, contribution to students' achievement of curriculum outcomes or goals, and fit in the curriculum.

Interprofessional Courses

Courses shared across health science disciplines can form part of the curriculum as elective or required classroom or professional practice courses. Because it is important for nursing students to respect the goals and perspectives of other disciplines, and to learn to work collaboratively with members of many health disciplines, they require opportunities to learn and interact in multidisciplinary teams and practice settings. Faculty committed to interdisciplinary education, IPE, and practice need to design and schedule courses in concert with faculty from other disciplines, bearing in mind each discipline's curriculum outcomes, philosophies, and roles. It is important that intellectual cross-pollination among students be a constant feature of courses through discussion, shared projects, and shared professional practice learning.

A decision to include interprofessional experiences in the curriculum requires attention to operational and logistical matters. These include:

- Identifying faculty from other disciplines committed to IPE, or at least willing to learn about and test such courses
- Developing a shared vision and philosophy (Barnsteiner et al., 2007)
- Reaching agreement about when IPE best belongs in the curricula of all disciplines: before or after students' socialization to their own professions
- Achieving consensus about the nature, goals, and processes of the courses
- Interpreting shared professional practice experiences to agencies
- Developing expert facilitators

- Scheduling
- Building enthusiasm for the endeavor in the organization and among students and clinicians

Elective Courses

Elective or optional courses, within and outside of nursing, can be a valuable component of the curriculum design. The purpose of elective courses is to provide students the freedom to explore interests in nursing and other disciplines. The design team may require electives at a specific academic level or from particular disciplines. Conversely, faculty may believe that students should choose elective courses freely, without constraint. These decisions will hinge on the institutional mission, and the philosophical approaches and intended outcomes of the nursing curriculum.

Developing Curriculum Maps

Curriculum maps are the plan for curriculum implementation. They are a visual representation of the intended curriculum (prospective maps). As curriculum implementation proceeds, they can be modified to depict what actually happened (retrospective maps). A comparison of the prospective and retrospective maps allows curriculum developers to assess the consistency between the design and the implementation, one aspect of curriculum evaluation. Any differences become a basis for further planning, either at the course or curriculum level.

Curriculum Concepts

Once agreement is reached about the overall course design, concepts are then mapped across the curriculum. This requires locating the courses in which the concepts will be addressed, the depth to which the concept will be considered, and expectations of what students will do with the concept. According to Iwasiw (2012), the following are descriptions of the depth of concepts and expectations of students:

- *Introduction*: The concept is introduced. Students are expected to explain the concept and its importance to nursing practice in a basic way.
- *Beginning*: More depth is added to the meaning of the concept. Students are expected to propose how it is applied in nursing practice. They should identify and use the concept in nursing practice, possibly with guidance.
- *Developing*: Complexity is added to the meaning of the concept. This complexity can arise from expanded theoretical explanations and/or contextual applications. Students are expected to apply the concept readily in assignments and nursing practice.

- *Advanced*: Sophisticated interpretations or applications of the concept are evident. Students are expected to analyze the concept and its use in nursing practice.
- *Integrated*: The concept forms part of the "gestalt" of class discussions, students' nursing practice, and assignments. Students are expected to use the concept and recognize its presence easily and accurately. (p. 1)

Adoption of this typology allows for mapping of the concepts across the curriculum with a two-way matrix. On one axis, nursing courses are listed and on the other axis are the curriculum concepts. Then the level of the concept in each course is identified. In this way, the increasing depth of the concepts becomes readily evident. There is no expectation that all concepts will be considered in all nursing courses. However, in final practicum or capstone courses, students should be working with the concepts at an *integrated* level.

Other Aspects of the Curriculum

Other curriculum maps can be developed. For example, educational strategies, written assignments (Hale, 2008), and/or exemplars used to illustrate concepts might be mapped. Such planning would ensure that educational approaches are consistent, assignments are reflective of course goals or outcomes, the timing of assignments is reasonable for students, and suitable exemplars are used to illuminate the concepts. In addition, sufficient variety could be planned across the curriculum. Also, in a content-focused curriculum, content can be mapped (Landry et al., 2011), and in an outcomes-focused curriculum, competencies can be mapped (Perlin, 2011).

Attending to Implementation Matters

As design ideas are presented and discussed, thoughts naturally turn to how the ideas can be implemented. Curriculum developers ask themselves if the design proposals are feasible within the school and community contexts. Additionally, they consider the logistical arrangements that are required for the design to be implemented. Consideration of the feasibility and practicalities of ideas is an important element of creating a realistic curriculum. No matter how elegant a curriculum design is, it has no value if it cannot be realized. Therefore, matters related to curriculum implementation form an important part of the deliberations about design.

Determining Policies and Guidelines

Developing new policies, or modifying existing ones, is part of the curriculum design process. A policy is a firm course of action that must be adhered to in every situation (e.g., appeals policy). The function of policies is to support and guide the achievement of the program and institutional mission and outcomes (Applegate, 1998). When devising policies, curriculum designers need to differentiate between policies and less formal guidelines for action. Guidelines, or guiding principles, present an appropriate course of action for a specific situation, although there may be some context-dependent flexibility (e.g., dress code for professional practice).

Some policies will be in place within the educational institution and apply to all academic constituencies, while others will be discipline specific. The latter must be consistent with those of the larger institution, and with the philosophical approaches of the curriculum. Policies ought to be readily available to all members of the academic community so that the "rules" are known. The number and nature of policies will vary among nursing programs. Nevertheless, there are some fundamental matters about which policies will be evident in all programs. The following are examples:

- *Admissions and progressions*: Admissions policies state the criteria used to determine whether an applicant meets admission standards. Progressions policies address advancement in the curriculum specifically the requirements to progress to subsequent semesters or levels. These normally include statements about passing grades for classroom and professional practice courses, required grade point average, and whether failing courses can be repeated.
- *Academic rights and responsibilities*: Academic rights and responsibilities include, among others, an appeals policy and a code of student conduct. An appeal is a formal request by a student to have an academic decision about a grade or adherence to a policy reviewed and changed. Normally, the institution will have a formal process for students and faculty to follow. A code of student conduct outlines what is viewed as acceptable behavior in the institution and may be an example of a policy with more flexibility than an admission policy.

Other policies and guidelines can be formulated specifically for the nursing program, such as attendance at professional practice experiences, laboratories, and/or class, definition and consequences of unsafe professional practice, immunization requirements, language proficiency standards, and dress code. Additional institutional policies can include those related to transfer from other institutions (Purcell, 2006), student involvement in institutional governance, scholastic discipline, student support, enrollment status, graduation requirements, nondiscrimination, and human rights.

Considering Human and Financial Implications

Each curriculum has human and financial implications; therefore, it is essential that the school leader be kept informed of the emerging design. A successful design depends on the availability of adequate resources for implementation, and the school leader is in the best position to know if those resources will be present.

If, for example, the new curriculum includes more nursing courses than previously, more professional practice time, or new opportunities for international placements, there will be increased teaching costs. If financial resources in the school cannot support the proposed design, then the school leader knows how and with whom to negotiate for additional funding. Modifications to the design will be necessary if adequate financial resources are not forthcoming.

Alternately, a curriculum redesign may mean that some faculty will no longer be required. A change from supervised professional practice to more independent practice, for example, could result in reduced numbers of faculty. The school leader may need to inform long-standing, part-time faculty that their employment will be decreased in amount or cease entirely. Concomitant with decreased faculty costs could be a decreased budget for the school. If so, strategic planning will be necessary to at least retain the school's budget.

A reconceptualized curriculum design might mean significantly changed teaching assignments for some faculty. Again, the school leader needs to be fully apprised of the emerging design so that teaching assignments and faculty development can be planned.

It is essential that possible financial implications for students be taken into account when designing a curriculum. An increased reliance on flexible delivery could make it possible for geographically dispersed students to enroll in the nursing program. Yet, if those students must then travel a considerable distance for dispersed professional practice experience, the associated costs could preclude their enrollment. Similarly, on-campus students may find travel to new practice sites difficult. It is important that the anticipated costs to students are considered and that accurate information will be provided to prospective applicants.

Deciding on the Design

When deciding on a curriculum design, developers can construct several designs, with different configurations of courses, and judge the advantages and disadvantages of each. Ultimately, one design will be proposed that is optimally useful, responsive to current and future social contexts, flexible enough to allow for ongoing refinement, and congruent with the curriculum goals or outcomes and philosophical and educational approaches.

Like other aspects of curriculum development, it is important that the design subcommittee's work be reviewed and approved by the total faculty group. The subcommittee presents the level or semester goals or competencies, configuration of courses, draft course goals or competencies, and brief course descriptions to the total faculty group, as well as the matrix of concepts. The matrices can facilitate the group's understanding. It is important that the faculty group is satisfied that the design represents an evidence-informed, context-relevant, unified curriculum.

Creating Course Templates

Creating templates for course syllabi and guidelines for student learning activities facilitates subsequent course development. These models provide a cognitive scaffold as curriculum work proceeds. Templates can also be created to map the details of courses (Hagler, White, & Morris, 2011). Use of the same templates in all courses adds to the unified nature of the curriculum.

Summary of Design Processes

There is no formula for developing an overall curriculum design. Curriculum developers will create processes that are useful to them. However, in all cases, the processes are iterative, because firm decisions can be made only when an overall design is created. Activities such as defining and mapping concepts, proposing course titles, and sequencing occur in a concurrent and recursive fashion, reflective of logical and creative thinking. The core curriculum concepts, key professional abilities, philosophical and educational approaches, and curriculum goals or outcomes are the touchstones for assessing a proposed design. With persistent attention to these, and to implementation matters, curriculum developers can be confident that they are creating a feasible, evidence-informed, context-relevant, unified curriculum.

PLANNING CURRICULUM EVALUATION

Concurrent with the curriculum design process is creation of a plan for curriculum evaluation. It is recommended that curriculum evaluation be planned along with the curriculum design process, because curriculum foundations are uppermost in faculty members' minds at this time. Therefore, it is relatively easy to think about curriculum evaluation processes that would be consistent with them. The philosophical approaches lead to ideas about *how* to evaluate, that is, methods that are congruent. Additionally, faculty members' focus on the foundations and the curriculum design leads to ideas about the content of the evaluation, that is, *what* to evaluate.

Planning curriculum evaluation is often overlooked because of urgency to complete the design. Yet, if curriculum evaluation is considered, faculty can be sure that it will indeed be possible to evaluate the curriculum components. Attention to curriculum evaluation is one form of ongoing appraisal of the design. For example, faculty members can ask themselves how they might determine students' achievement of the curriculum goals or outcomes, or how they could assess the relationships among curriculum components.

If the responses are robust, they can feel confident about the design; if not, then some revisions may be necessary so that sound evaluation data can be obtained in the future.

Complete planning of curriculum evaluation will likely not occur until after implementation begins. However, it is worthwhile to consider and record ideas about evaluation as the curriculum is designed.

RELATIONSHIP OF CURRICULUM DESIGN TO AN EVIDENCE-INFORMED, CONTEXT-RELEVANT, UNIFIED CURRICULUM

The curriculum foundations, that is, core curriculum concepts, key professional abilities, and the philosophical and educational approaches, are developed from data about the context in which the curriculum will be offered and graduates will practice. From these, the curriculum goals or outcomes are formulated. Thus, the evidence-informed, context-relevant nature of the curriculum foundations and goals is evident.

The unified nature of the design is expressed in the expectations of students throughout the curriculum. First, the curriculum goals or outcomes are developed and from these, the level goals or competencies are derived. Then, course expectations are derived from level expectations. Thus, there is a logical and visible progression and alignment in what students are expected to achieve. Additionally, the nature and sequence of courses that will allow students to achieve the curriculum expectations reflect unity between curriculum outcomes or goals and courses. Moreover, the designation of concepts for courses throughout the curriculum, with increasing depth, indicates that courses are not separate from one another, but rather connected by the increasing level of student expectations in relation to their understanding and use of the concepts. Course titles that consistently reflect the curriculum's conceptual bases are important in the visual unity of the curriculum. Further, the creation of course templates for use during course development assists in the development of course materials that are unified in appearance and conceptual orientation. Finally, attention to the processes and content of curriculum evaluation heightens the unity between the design and the future evaluation.

CORE PROCESSES OF CURRICULUM WORK

Faculty Development

The overall goal of faculty development in relation to curriculum design is to expand members' knowledge and appreciation of curriculum design. As with all aspects of faculty development, the precise activities will be dependent on faculty needs.

Faculty development can include a brief review of the goals of the curriculum design process and the parameters that constrain it. Then, attention can be given to the processes of designing an evidence-informed, context-relevant, unified curriculum. This might include reviewing the curriculum work completed to date and an explanation of the connections between that work and designing the curriculum.

In a workshop setting, a draft curriculum matrix might be introduced for small groups to consider and modify. In this way, the faculty development activity would contribute directly to the design process. Additionally, a matrix of courses and concepts could be introduced and faculty asked to complete the cells, delineating the level at which concepts should be addressed in each course. This would help them appreciate how concepts are built across the curriculum and addressed in courses.

Ongoing Appraisal

While designing the curriculum, curriculum developers repeatedly ask themselves questions such as:

- Is the organization of the concepts reasonable?
- Are we satisfied with the definitions of the concepts? Are they understandable? Is there a reasonable progression in the depth of concepts?
- Does the design represent a context-relevant curriculum?
- Is the design congruent with the philosophical and educational approaches?
- Will the design allow for the continuous and evident presence of the core curriculum concepts and key professional abilities? Is the unity visible?
- Are there opportunities for students to achieve the intended curriculum outcomes or goals?
- Does the design seem logical?
- Are the draft course descriptions convincing?
- Is the design feasible within our school of nursing and the external context?
- Have the logistics of implementation been adequately considered?
- Does the design support the institutional mission?
- Is anything missing?
- Can faculty and other stakeholders commit to this curriculum?
- Is this curriculum design of the quality that we expect of ourselves?
- Is this design of the quality that will likely be acceptable to external reviewers?
- How can curriculum evaluation be planned to be consistent with the curriculum tenets?

Scholarship

Faculty undertaking curriculum design might consider scholarship about the processes they are experiencing, analyzing reasons for the challenges faced, and describing how those challenges were resolved. Publications about student and stakeholder involvement in curriculum design would be a valuable addition to the literature. A comparison of design processes in several schools of nursing could be instructive to schools undertaking curriculum development. Furthermore, increased sharing of curriculum designs would be a benefit to faculty everywhere who are struggling with designing curricula in the face of expanding and intensifying expectations by external organizations associated with higher education and health care. Research about curriculum design might include studies of the processes used in several health professional programs with the intent of identifying common processes that could be relevant to the development of IPE.

CHAPTER SUMMARY

The curriculum design is the configuration of the program of studies. The design must be congruent with the institution and school's mission and purpose, and with the faculty's values and beliefs. It should be directed and oriented to student learning, and reflect the curriculum concepts, outcomes or goals, and context of nursing. Curriculum developers need to have a clear sense of purpose and commitment to completing the task of design in a timely fashion. Because of human resource and financial implications, it is necessary that the school leader be apprised of the emerging design.

The chapter includes descriptions of elements important in curriculum design such as the program type, structure, and delivery approaches. Information is provided about educational designs, strategies to organize knowledge, and IPE. The process of designing an evidence-informed, context-relevant, unified curriculum is detailed, beginning with confirming the goal of the design process and identifying curriculum parameters. Attention is given to identifying courses and mapping the curriculum. Policy development is addressed, as are human and financial implications of curriculum design. Consideration of curriculum evaluation is included. The relationship of curriculum design to an evidence-informed, context-relevant, unified curriculum is explained. Finally, the core processes of faculty work in relation to designing the curriculum are described.

SYNTHESIS ACTIVITIES

Stonecastle University College of Nursing is undertaking curriculum design, and information about this process is presented for review, analysis, and discussion. Questions are suggested to stimulate critique. Following the case, questions and activities are offered about designing curricula in readers' settings.

Stonecastle University College of Nursing

Stonecastle University is a public university that began when a large stone house (locally called *The Castle*) was bequeathed to a mining town to become the location of a technical college to support the mining industry. Over time, the college became a degree-granting institution with graduate programs in disciplines such as engineering, chemistry, and physics. Programs for health and social service professionals were introduced, beginning with nursing. From the outset, nursing faculty members have been committed to progressive education, and they continue to be educational leaders in the health sciences.

There has been some shared teaching in a course that is elective in both the nursing and medical colleges: *International Health Care*. This course was developed through the mutual interests of Dr. Gallia Rostova from nursing and Dr. David McLeod from medicine.

The College of Nursing is undergoing curriculum redesign under the leadership of the undergraduate program chair, Dr. Keisha Jefferson. The revised baccalaureate degree curriculum will emphasize humanism and phenomenology, educational approaches consistent with brain-based learning, and institutional and community-based nursing. Major concepts include evidence-informed care, community as client, physiological concepts, and health promotion. The outcomes address collaboration with professionals and clients in the provision of evidence-informed, client-centered care, effective communication, ethical and cultural competence, and advocacy to enhance social justice.

During the data-gathering phase of curriculum development, faculty members took note of students' enthusiasm for both the processes and content of *International Health Care*. They agreed that they would strive to include mandatory interprofessional experiences in the curriculum to ensure that students would have opportunities to achieve the curriculum outcome related to collaboration. Dr. Rostova was asked to investigate whether there was interest in medicine for more interprofessional opportunities, and if faculty members in physical therapy and occupational therapy might be interested.

Representatives of the other professional programs met and agreed that IPE would be a valuable addition to their curricula. However, there was considerable discussion about how it could be integrated into the overcrowded curricula of the four programs, each with different class and professional practice schedules. Moreover, there was some skepticism about including undergraduate nursing students in shared learning experiences with graduate students in physical therapy and occupational therapy. Concern was expressed that the nursing students would lack the knowledge and maturity to contribute meaningfully. Dr. McLeod assured them that the nursing students had valuable perspectives to offer and had been equal participants in the *International Health Care* course. The group agreed to convene a meeting of faculty members interested in learning more about IPE, with the expectation that possible course foci could emerge.

Drs. Rostova and Jefferson reported back to the nursing faculty that they should not plan on expanded IPE in the near future. However, the group reaffirmed their commitment to providing experiences that would help students to become skilled in interprofessional collaboration.

Questions and Activities for Critical Analysis of the Stonecastle University College of Nursing Case

1. How will the curriculum concepts, outcomes, and philosophical approaches influence the curriculum design?
2. Consider whether it is reasonable to include a curriculum outcome related to collaboration when IPE is not immediately possible.
3. In the absence of formalized IPE, how can nursing faculty plan experiences that will allow students to achieve the curriculum outcome? How could these experiences be mapped?
4. How should the curriculum committee proceed with the curriculum design?
5. What would be the advantages of inviting faculty members from the other health professions to participate in some aspects of curriculum development?
6. Design the interprofessional component of a nursing curriculum that would directly address the outcome of collaboration with professionals and clients in the provision of evidence-informed, client-centered care.

Questions and Activities for Consideration When Designing an Evidence-Informed, Context-Relevant, Unified Curriculum in Readers' Settings

1. Which program structure is most appropriate for the type of program being developed? Why?
2. Select the program model that best reflects faculty beliefs about learning. Explain why this is the *best*. If this is not the program model currently in use, what should be done?

3. Should a partnership be considered to extend access to the program? Why or why not? If yes, who could the partners be?

4. Identify delivery method(s) supported by the educational institution and by faculty. How will the supported delivery method(s) affect the curriculum design?

5. Determine the organizing strategy that best assures students' logical progression to, and achievement of, curriculum outcomes or goals.

6. Develop a curriculum map to reflect the developing ideas about curriculum design.

7. Create a process for defining curriculum concepts expeditiously. How can consensus about the definitions be achieved?

8. Recommend nursing, non-nursing, and elective courses that will best facilitate achievement of the curriculum outcomes or goals. Should there be interdisciplinary, multidisciplinary, and/or transdisciplinary courses? Describe the process for developing interprofessional courses or experiences.

9. Develop two or more possible configurations of courses that should be considered.

10. How can courses be titled to ensure conceptual and visual unity?

11. Assess the influence of existing institutional policies on the curriculum design.

12. What negotiations should take place with other academic units to operationalize the envisioned curriculum?

13. Consider whether curriculum policies need to be developed or modified.

14. Make recommendations about the resources required to support the curriculum design process.

15. Identify the resource implications of the curriculum design.

16. Draft a tentative plan for curriculum evaluation.

17. Plan faculty development activities related to curriculum design.

18. Suggest questions for ongoing appraisal of the emerging curriculum design.

19. Propose scholarship activities that could be undertaken.

REFERENCES

Applegate, M. A. (1998). Educational program evaluation. In D. M. Billings & J. A. Halstead (Eds.), *Teaching in nursing: A guide for faculty* (pp. 423–457). Philadelphia: Saunders.

Bagnardi, M., Bryant, L., & Colin, J. (2009). Banks multicultural model: A framework for integrating multiculturalism into nursing curricula. *Journal of Professional Nursing, 25*, 234–239.

Ball, D. R., Mosca, J. B., & Paul, D. P. (2013). Evaluating the effectiveness of audio in hybrid courses. *American Journal of Business Education Online, 6*(1), 73–84.

Barnsteiner, J. H., Disch, J. M., Hall, L., Mayer, D., & Moore, S. M. (2007). Promoting interprofessional education. *Nursing Outlook, 55,* 144–150.

Bastable, S. B., & Markowitz, M. (2012). Dual degree partnership in nursing: An innovative undergraduate educational model. *Journal of Nursing Education, 51,* 549–555.

Boland, D. L. (2012). Developing curriculum: Frameworks, outcomes, and competencies. In D. M. Billings & J. A. Halstead (Eds.), *Teaching in nursing: A guide for faculty* (4th ed., pp. 138–159). St. Louis, MO: Elsevier Saunders.

Brandt, C. L., Boellaard, M. R., & Zorn, C. R. (2013). Experiences and emotions of faculty teaching in accelerated second baccalaureate degree nursing programs. *Journal of Nursing Education, 52,* 377–382.

Brown, L. P. (2011). Revisiting our roots: Caring in nursing curriculum design. *Nurse Education in Practice, 11,* 360–364.

Canadian Interprofessional Health Collaborative. (2010). *A national interprofessional competency framework.* Retrieved from http://www.cihc.ca/files/CIHC_IPCompetencies_Feb1210.pdf

Dalley, K., Candela, L., & Benzel-Lindley, J. (2008). Learning to let go: The challenge of de-crowding the curriculum. *Nursing Education Today, 28,* 62–69.

Diefenbeck, C. A., Plowfield, L. A., & Herman, J. W. (2006). Clinical immersion: A residency model for nursing education. *Nursing Education Perspectives, 27,* 72–79.

Doll, R. C. (1996). *Curriculum improvement* (9th ed.). Boston: Allyn & Bacon.

Finotto, S., Carpanoni, M., Turroni, E. C., Camellini, R., & Mecugni, D. (2013). Teaching evidence-based practice: Developing a curriculum model to foster evidence-based practice in undergraduate student nurses. *Nurse Education in Practice, 13,* 459–465.

Friesner, A. (1978). Curriculum process for developing or revising a baccalaureate nursing program. In National League for Nursing, *Curriculum process for developing or revising a baccalaureate nursing program* (pp. 13–22). New York: Author.

Frith, K. H., & Clark, D. J. (2013). *Distance education in nursing* (3rd ed.). New York: Springer.

Gagné, R. M., Briggs, L. J., & Wager, W. W. (1992). *Principles of instructional design* (4th ed.). Fort Worth, TX: Harcourt Brace Jovanovich.

Giddens, J. F., & Brady, D. P. (2007). Rescuing nursing education from content saturation: The case for a concept-based curriculum. *Journal of Nursing Education, 46,* 65–69.

Giddens, J. F., Wright, M., & Gray, I. (2012). Selecting concepts for a concept-based curriculum: Application of a benchmark approach. *Journal of Nursing Education, 51,* 511–515.

Gubrud-Howe, P., Shaver, K., Tanner, C. A., Bennett-Stillmaker, J., Davidson, S., Flaherty-Robb, M., . . . Wheeler, P. (2003). A challenge to meet the future: Nursing education in Oregon, 2010. *Journal of Nursing Education, 42,* 163–167.

Hagler, D., White, B., & Morris, B. (2011). Cognitive tools as a scaffold for faculty during curriculum redesign. *Journal of Nursing Education, 50,* 417–422.

Hale, J. A. (2008). *A guide to curriculum mapping.* Thousand Oaks, CA: Corwin Press, A Sage Company.

Henson, K. T. (2010). *Curriculum planning: Integrating multiculturalism, constructivism, and education reform* (4th ed.). Long Grove, IL: Waveland Press.

Interprofessional Education Collaborative Expert Panel. (2011). *Core competencies for interprofessional collaborative practice: Report of an expert panel.* Washington, DC: Interprofessional Education Collaborative. Retrieved from http://cabarizona2011.org/sites/cabarizona2011.org/files/u9/IPECReport.pdf

Iwasiw, C. L. (2012). *Definitions of concept levels*. Unpublished paper. Arthur Labatt Family School of Nursing, Western University.

Knight, D. B., Lattuca, L. R., Kimball, E. W., & Reason, R. D. (2013). Understanding interdisciplinarity: Curricular features of undergraduate interdisciplinary programs. *Innovations in Higher Education, 38,* 143–158.

Lancet Commission. (2010). *Education of health professionals for the 21st century: A global independent commission*. Retrieved from http://www.healthprofessionals21.org/docs/HealthProfNewCent.pdf

Landry, L. G., Alameida, M. D., Orsolini-Hain, L., Boyle, A. R., Privé, A., Chien, A., . . . Leong, A. (2011). Responding to demands to change nursing education: Use of curriculum mapping to assess curricular content. *Journal of Nursing Education, 50,* 587–590.

Molzahn, A. E., & Purkis, M. E. (2004). Collaborative nursing education programs: Challenges and issues. *Nursing Leadership (CJNL), 17*(4), 41–53.

Orem, D. E. (1990). A nursing practice theory in three parts, 1956-1989. In M. E. Parker (Ed.), *Nursing theories in practice* (pp. 47–60). New York: National League for Nursing.

Park, J. Y., & Son, J. B. (2010). Transitioning toward transdisciplinary learning in a multidisciplinary environment. *Journal of Pedagogies and Learning, 6,* 82–93.

Paulson, C. (2011). The experiences of faculty teaching in an innovative clinical immersion nursing curriculum. *Nursing Education Perspectives, 32,* 395–399.

Perlin, M. (2011). Curriculum mapping for program evaluation and CAHME accreditation. *The Journal of Health Administration Education, 28(1),* 27–47.

Purcell, F. B. (2006). Smooth transfer: A once mundane administrative issue re-emerges as a key tool for equity. *Connection: New England's Journal of Higher Education, 21*(1), 20–21.

Reeves, S., Goldman, J., & Oandasan, I. (2007). Key factors in planning and implementing interprofessional education in health care settings. *Journal of Allied Health, 36,* 231–235.

Rietschel, M. J., & Buckley, K. M. (2014). Blended learning. In C. A. O'Neil, C. A. Fisher, & M. J. Rietschel (Eds.), *Developing online learning environments in nursing education* (3rd ed., pp. 85–99). New York: Springer.

Sairanen, R., Richardson, E., Kelly, H., Bergknut, E., Koskinen, L., Lundberg, P., . . . De Vlieger, L. (2013). Putting culture into curriculum: A European project. *Nurse Education in Practice, 13,* 118–124.

Smythe, M. (2011). Blended learning: A transformational process. Retrieved from http://akoaotearoa.ac.nz/community/national-teaching-and-learning-conference-2010/resources/files/smythe-blended-learning-transformative-process

Tanner, C. A., Gubrud-Howe, P., & Shores, L. (2008). The Oregon Consortium for Nursing Education: A response to the nursing shortage. *Policy, Politics, & Nursing Practice, 9,* 203–209.

Watson, J. (2012). *Human caring science* (2nd ed.). Burlington, MA: Jones & Bartlett Learning.

WHO Study Group on Interprofessional Education and Collaborative Practice. (2010). *Framework for action on interprofessional education and collaborative practice*. Retrieved from http://whqlibdoc.who.int/hq/2010/WHO_HRH_HPN_10.3_eng.pdf

Wiles, J. W., & Bondi, J. C. (2011). *Curriculum development: A guide to practice* (8th ed.). Boston: Pearson Education.

CHAPTER 13

Creating Courses for an Evidence-Informed, Context-Relevant, Unified Curriculum

Chapter Overview

Following completion of the curriculum design, attention turns to the creation of individual courses. In this chapter, descriptions of course components are offered, including a synopsis of strategies to ignite learning. Information about design parameters and approaches to course design are presented. The process of creating evidence-informed, context-relevant, unified courses is detailed. Ideas about creating individual concept-based classes are offered. Matters about course implementation and evaluation are addressed. The relationship between creating courses and an evidence-informed, context-relevant, unified curriculum is explained. Ideas about faculty development, ongoing appraisal, and scholarship associated with creating courses are proposed. The chapter concludes with a summary and synthesis activities.

Chapter Goals

- Identify course components.
- Consider parameters influencing course design.
- Examine approaches to course design.
- Understand the process of creating conceptually based courses.
- Gain insight into the value of planning course evaluation concurrently with designing courses.
- Appreciate the relationship between creating courses and an evidence-informed, context-relevant, unified curriculum.
- Reflect on the core processes of curriculum work related to creating courses.

COURSE DESIGN

An academic course is a recognized unit of learning within an overall curriculum. It is created with components that outline the purpose of the course, what students are to accomplish, and what they are to do. The intent of creating courses is to achieve unity and coherence within each course and among courses. Course design begins as soon as a curriculum design has been approved and truly never ends, because courses are refined throughout the life of the curriculum. It is a cyclical process: after implementation, courses are evaluated and modified.

The term *course design* refers to the configuration of a course. The design encompasses all components (title, purpose, and description; goals or competencies; strategies to ignite learning; concepts and substantive content; classes; opportunities for students to demonstrate learning; and faculty evaluation of student achievement), and the relationships between and among them. The process of designing courses, or the *course design* process, refers to the discussions and decision making that lead to the configuration of a course. The course design process personalizes the impending curriculum by giving faculty members a sense of ownership about the courses they create and will teach.

The course design begins once the curriculum design is approved. The starting points of the design of each course are the decisions (level, year, or semester competencies or goals) and the draft documents (brief course descriptions, course competencies or goals, and the concepts mapped for each course) prepared during curriculum design. In total, the courses should lead to the curriculum outcomes or goals. The agreed-upon philosophical and educational approaches are enacted within courses.

The terminology used to describe course components varies among nursing programs. Nonetheless, they are present in all academic courses, whether they are theory, professional practice, or laboratory, and whether offered through traditional, distance, or hybrid delivery. Designing courses is an iterative process, with ideas about each component influencing ideas about all others. Therefore, although they are described separately, decisions about each component will lead to reexamination and possible modification of other components.

Course Title, Purpose, and Description

The course title should convey the main conceptual, process, and/or contextual focus of the course in accordance with the overall curriculum design. The title will immediately create expectations in the faculty, students, and professional practice stakeholders about the intent of the course, and this intent is described in the purpose statement.

A statement of purpose makes evident why the course is part of the curriculum and how it contributes to students' achievement of curriculum outcomes or goals.

Although the purpose may be readily apparent to curriculum designers, the reason for the existence of the course in the curriculum might not be obvious to students. Therefore, explicit statements about the course purpose and how it contributes to students' development as professional nurses make evident the value of the course in their progress toward career goals.

Each course requires a brief description that is published in the institutional catalogue, or calendar. Class or professional practice hours, course credits, and pre-, co-, or anti-requisites are generally stated. This would have been drafted during the overall curriculum design and is the basis of an extended course description.

The brief description is expanded in a course syllabus to provide more detail for students. The expanded explanation provides information about the scope of the course, preparation required for classes, the nature of class meetings, expected participation and interactions, and other information that faculty consider important to explain the intent and character of the course. This can be written in the second person to personalize the ideas so they will have more impact for each student.

Course Competencies or Goals

Competency or goal statements are another component of courses. They describe the abilities expected of students at the end of the course and are written in the same format as the curriculum and level goals or outcomes.

Learning, a process that leads to the acquisition or development of new knowledge, understandings, and abilities, is the ultimate purpose for which courses are designed. The nature of the desired learning achievement is expressed in the course competency or goal statements. Preliminary course competencies or goals, derived from curriculum and level expectations, are formulated when courses are identified and configured as part of curriculum design. It is important that these be refined so they are specific and feasible for each course.

Course competency or goal statements delineate the achievements expected of students. Important concepts should be evident in the statements. The number of competencies or goals may exceed the number written for each level because the course expectations are more specific. Expectations for all courses in the same level need to collectively "add up" to the semester outcomes or goals, although each course may not address every semester outcome or goal.

Course Concepts and Content

The course concepts and their depth are delineated in the concept mapping activities of curriculum design. Additionally, each course has a substantive focus. This content focus is typically of most immediate interest to students. Within all courses, the concepts and scope of content are conveyed in the form of titles or topics for each session, along with required readings. Although students may initially focus on the substantive content, it is through the course concepts that this content is addressed.

The substantive knowledge (facts, concepts, hypotheses, methods, etc.) is selected to illuminate the concepts and provide an avenue for students to develop the thinking processes of nursing practice. Because all content cannot be addressed, the course topics must be judiciously selected. Students require content as one of the building blocks of their thinking; therefore, substantive content remains an important aspect of concept-based courses.

In a concept-based theory course, professional practice exemplars are selected to illuminate the concepts and to direct students to essential substantive content. Therefore, when determining course content, it behooves faculty to consider two layers of knowledge: the concepts to be addressed and the required substantive facts or theories. Additionally, they must decide the best fit between the two layers as they develop the schedule of class topics. In this planning, attention is given to exemplars for which there is evidence about nursing practice so that students will learn about evidence-informed nursing practice in a way that is seamless, and not as a separate "add-on" to other ideas.

Content in professional practice courses is comprised of the following:

- Concepts, knowledge, and professional abilities
- Thinking processes
- Attitudes and professional comportment
- Client situations
- Interactions with clients and other professionals
- Insights and understandings developed during the experience

Being in the situation, applying previously held and new knowledge and abilities, seeking learning opportunities, and formulating new understandings are the intent of professional practice courses. Therefore, a weekly topical schedule is not applicable. However, faculty can identify particular concepts or professional abilities as the focus of experiences.

Faculty members' intentional focus on concepts in professional practice courses is important to assist students to:

- Understand the relevance and importance of the concepts for practice
- Apply the concepts in practice
- Identify the concepts in the situations they encounter
- Analyze factors influencing the expression of the concepts
- Plan interventions that will affect clients' experience of the concepts

A focus on concepts in professional practice courses will contribute to bridging the theory-practice gap and make evident the unity of the curriculum.

Strategies to Ignite Learning

"The mind is not a vessel to be filled, but a fire to be ignited" (Plutarch, n.d.). This quotation encapsulates the intent of student-centered teaching, that is, teaching that has student learning and not teacher activities as the central focus. The teaching responsibilities in such situations are to:

- Plan classes and professional practice experiences that will appeal to students, be meaningful to them, and propel them to "devote physical and psychological energy" (Astin, as cited in Popkess & McDaniel, 2011) to a learning endeavor
- Facilitate learning activities that will require students to "work with" knowledge and not merely absorb or recall it
- Encourage students' development of their own understandings, insights, and connections to previous knowledge and experiences, and to anticipated experiences

Teaching-learning strategies are specific actions planned by a faculty member to ignite students' learning. These are termed *teaching-learning strategies*, rather than merely *teaching strategies,* to emphasize that learning is the purpose of the activities. Moreover, through planning for students' learning and through interaction with them, faculty members expand their own understanding and insights, and thus are learners themselves.

Contemporary teaching-learning strategies promote active learner engagement and motivation. Students take an active role in learning in a variety of ways. These can include the following:

- Simulated professional practice
- Virtual reality experiences
- Cooperative and collaborative projects, possibly using cloud computing spaces, social media, or online forums
- Database searching
- Creation and synthesis of knowledge in the classroom

Other active learning strategies might involve the use of games, visual art, literature, film, music, narrative dialogue, problem-/context-based techniques, and purposeful reflection (Crookes, Crookes, & Walsh, 2013). In general, these strategies have cognitive constructivism as the underlying theory of learning.

Strategies to ignite learning for professional practice courses are influenced by the size and level of the student group and the learning opportunities available in the setting. Direct client care and interaction, pre- and postconferences, on-the-spot consultations, and questioning are commonly employed, as are observational experiences, peer teaching, preceptoring, interprofessional rounds, and reflective journaling.

Currently, there is a paradigm shift in higher education from teacher-centered to student-centered teaching (Stanley & Dougherty, 2010). As a consequence, the literature is replete with strategies to engage students in active learning. However, it is beyond the scope of this text to examine them all. **Table 13-1** provides a summary of selected newer strategies to ignite learning.

Outlined in **Table 13-2** are characteristics of many strategies to ignite learning that a novice nurse educator might find helpful. In this table, *group size* indicates the student numbers for which the strategy is suitable. *Learner engagement* is the extent to which students participate actively in the learning process. *Learning curve* is a term that refers to the rate at which learning about the strategy is necessary for students to feel comfortable

Table 13-1 Summary of Selected Strategies to Ignite Learning	
Strategies	**Key Features**
Consensus boards (charts)	Working in groups of four, each student takes one quadrant of a chart to write his or her understanding of the main ideas of a topic. The students then reach consensus on the top three ideas and write these in the center of the chart (Hsu & Malkin, 2011).
Flipped (inverted) classroom	Instead of taking classroom time to introduce concepts, the instructor prepares a vodcast, video lecture, or screencast that students view in advance of the class. Traditional classroom activities have "homework" status, and class time is spent in interactive learning activities (Milman, 2012; Missildine, Fountain, Summers, & Gosselin, 2013).
Graffiti boards	Several students write their response to an instructor's prompt on the chalkboard. The class then discusses similarities, differences, and further ideas (O'Connor, 2013). Alternatively, all students write their responses on flip charts for everyone to see (Hsu & Malkin, 2011).
Inquiry-based critical self-reflection	Semi-structured and guided exercises that pose challenges and are somewhat ambiguous are used to help students develop self-regulated learning behaviours and learn content. Questioning, interpretation, investigation, and guidance help students to "systematically criticize, justify, solve and appraise the right answers" (Rusche & Jason, 2011, p. 341). Students prepare written reflection questions in response to readings and pose questions about the readings. These questions form part of class discussion.
Mobile devices in the classroom (M-learning)	Mobile devices are acknowledged as a legitimate means to access current information. Their use is incorporated into classroom activities in a planned way so students seek and evaluate information and hone search skills (Smith, 2012).

Table 13-1 Summary of Selected Strategies to Ignite Learning (*continued*)

Strategies	Key Features
Peer teaching, reciprocal learning	Students assume responsibility for teaching other students. They can be at the same or different levels in the program. Students work in pairs to instruct or guide a peer for a specified purpose (Goldenberg & Iwasiw, 1992; Iwasiw & Goldenberg, 1993). This can be used with lab, professional practice, and theory courses.
Social media	Social media are a means to engage others electronically, supported by Internet sites or software. Through the use of Twitter, Facebook, Google+, or similar applications, students can exchange information related to nursing courses. Groups can be formed within some applications for collaborative student work. The creation of blogs and e-portfolios could form part of course work through access to publicly available software (Schmitt, Sims-Giddens, & Booth, 2012).
Student-created dramas	Students interview individuals having a particular experience and write a reflective paper. Then, student teams prepare a script based on the interviews and present their dramas to peers (SmithBattle, 2012).
Team-based learning	Students form learning teams for the length of a course, which is divided into modules. There are specified pre-class activities, individual and team testing in each class with immediate feedback, and activities to apply content during the remainder of the class (Mennenga, 2013).
Unfolding case studies	An unfolding case study (simulated or paper-based) presents a client situation in a way that promotes the development of students' clinical reasoning. Students respond to a practice situation in the absence of full information, as occurs in nursing practice. Further information is progressively revealed, prior decisions reviewed, and further problem solving undertaken (Day, 2011; Reese, 2011).
Quick writes	Students are asked to respond in writing to a class concept, film, narrative, etc. They immediately reflect on their thoughts, feelings, and understandings (Hsu & Malkin, 2011).
Virtual worlds	A virtual world is "a synchronous, persistent network of people, represented by avatars, facilitated by computers" (Bell, as cited in De Gagne, Oh, Kang, Vorderstrasse, & Johnson, 2013, p. 392). Students enter the virtual world through their computers and interact with the characters, or respond to actions in the simulated world. The virtual world "combines the collaborative properties of [a] virtual community" (De Gagne et al., 2013, p. 392) with the graphics of an online game.

Table 13-2   Characteristics of Strategies to Ignite Learning

Strategies	Group Size	Student Engagement	Learning Curve	Appropriate Cognitive Processes[1]
Algorithms	All	Active	Minimal	Analyze, evaluate
Audio-conferencing	Small	Passive	Minimal	Understand, apply, analyze, evaluate
Buzz groups	All	Active	Minimal	Apply, analyze, evaluate
Case studies, unfolding case studies	All	Active	Steep	Apply, analyze, evaluate, create
Clinical observation	Small	Active	Moderate	Understand, analyze, evaluate
Computer-assisted instruction	Large	Active	Moderate	Understand, apply, analyze
Consensus boards	All	Active	Minimal	Analyze, evaluate, create
Concept mapping	Small	Active	Moderate	Analyze, create
Debate	All	Active	Minimal	Analyze, evaluate
Direct client care	Small	Active	Steep	Apply, analyze, evaluate, create
Discussion	All	Active	Minimal	All processes
High-fidelity simulations	Small	Active	Steep	Apply, analyze, evaluate, create
Film/video	All	Passive	Minimal	Understand, analyze, evaluate
Flipped classroom	All	Active	Moderate	Apply, analyze, evaluate, create
Gaming	All	Active	Minimal	Apply, analyze, evaluate,
Graffiti	All	Active	Minimal	Understand, apply, analyze, evaluate, create
Inquiry-based critical self-reflection	All	Active	Moderate	All processes
Laboratory practice	Small	Active	Moderate	Apply, analyze, evaluate
Lecture	Large	Passive	Minimal	Remember, understand
Live patient simulations	Small	Active	Moderate	Apply, analyze, evaluate, create
M-learning (mobile devices)	All	Active	Moderate	Understand, apply, analyze, evaluate
Metaphor	All	Active	Moderate	Analyze, evaluate, create

Table 13-2 Characteristics of Strategies to Ignite Learning (*continued*)

Strategies	Group Size	Student Engagement	Learning Curve	Appropriate Cognitive Processes[1]
Narrative dialogue	Small	Active	Minimal	Analyze, evaluate, create
Online forums	Small	Active	Steep	Understand, apply, analyze, evaluate, create
Oral examinations	Small	Active	Steep	All processes
Peer teaching	Small	Active	Steep	Understand, apply
Podcast, vodcasts	Large	Passive	Minimal	Understand
Preceptorships	Small	Active	Minimal	All processes
Pre-/postconferences	Small	Active	Minimal	All processes
Problem-/context-based learning	Small	Active	Steep	Understand, apply, analyze, evaluate, create
Questioning	All	Active	Minimal	All processes
Quick write/1-minute paper	All	Active	Minimal	All processes
Reflective journaling	Small	Active	Steep	All processes
Response systems (e.g., clickers)	Large	Active	Minimal	Remember, understand, apply, analyze, evaluate
Role-play	Small	Active	Moderate	Analyze, evaluate
Social media	Large	Active	Moderate	Analyze, evaluate, create
Student-created dramas	All	Active	Steep	Understand, apply, analyze, create
Student presentations	All	Active	Steep	Create
Team-based learning	All	Active	Moderate	Apply, analyze, evaluate, create
Think-pair-share	Large	Active	Minimal	Apply, evaluate
Video-conferencing	Small	Active	Steep	All processes
Virtual worlds	All	Active	Steep	Apply, analyze, evaluate, create
Written assignments	All	Active	Moderate	All processes

[1]As described by Anderson, L. W., Krathwohl, D. R., Airasian, P. W., Cruikshank, K. A., Mayer, R. E., Pintrich, P. R., . . . Wittrock, M. C. (Eds.). (2001). *A taxonomy for learning, teaching, and assessing: A revision of Bloom's taxonomy of educational objectives*. New York: Longman.

about participating in, and learning from, the strategy. The column *Appropriate Cognitive Processes* refers to the levels of the cognitive taxonomy for which the strategies are most appropriate.

Although some strategies, such as high-fidelity simulation, can require students to use a wide array of cognitive and psychomotor processes, the complexity of the strategies makes them impractical if learning goals or outcomes are directed toward the lower levels of the cognitive or psychomotor taxonomies. Therefore, judicious selection of strategies is important. Additionally, a variety of strategies throughout a course reflects attention to brain-based learning guidelines and respect for diversity in students' learning styles.

Use of evidence-informed strategies in classrooms and practice settings adds to the academic rigor of the curriculum. For example, the outcomes and efficacy of strategies such as problem-based learning, simulation, or service-learning have been documented. Anecdotal and research reports about a host of strategies are available in nursing education and higher education literature, and these can provide ideas to course developers.

Individual Classes

Each course has a specified number and duration of formal sessions when faculty and students interact. These sessions can be conducted in classrooms, professional practice settings, labs, or through cyberspace. In classroom courses, a topic is typically identified for each session. Although the structure of courses offered through distance delivery methods may vary, the courses generally retain the idea of a "class" in which a conceptually meaningful unit of content is addressed weekly. For professional practice or laboratory courses, the "class" is each practice session.

Guidelines for student learning activities can be planned for each class, and, if created, they become part of the course syllabus. These describe the preparatory, in-class, and follow-up activities that students are expected to complete. The preparatory activities can include reading, interviews with clients, visits to community agencies, writing a vignette from a professional practice experience, and so forth. The intent is that students arrive at class ready to engage with the content (both conceptual and substantive) and not merely to receive it. The in-class activities typically include opportunities to process information and experiences, and work toward achievement of course goals or competencies through interaction with course content, faculty, peers, clinicians, and/or clients.

The amount of detail that is given in the guideline varies. Some faculty prefer to describe this in a general way (e.g., discussion, review), so that there is room for more specific planning as the class approaches. Others provide more precise details (e.g., view a video entitled *Evidence for Nursing Practice*). The follow-up activities provide suggestions for reflection, application, and development of deeper understandings.

The <u>key feature</u> of the guidelines is that the <u>learning activities require active engage</u>-ment of students. Thus, they reflect a belief that <u>learning is optimized when students are</u> <u>responsible for acquiring basic knowledge</u>, and <u>participating in the development of under</u>-<u>standings, analysis, and synthesis of that knowledge</u>. In **Figure 13-1** is an example of class guidelines for a first-year bachelor of science in nursing course entitled *Foundations of Professional Nursing*.

Figure 13-1   Example of a guideline for student learning activities for *Foundations of Professional Nursing*.
Developed by Karen Ferguson, RN,MHSc(N). © Western-Fanshawe Collaborative BScN Program (2013). Used with permission.

Developing a Personal Philosophy of Nursing

Overview

This year you have been introduced to the metaparadigm concepts: person, environment, health, and nursing. Together, these concepts capture the key features of what is the broad and complex practice of nursing (Fawcett, 1984). To develop a personal philosophy of nursing, you need to reflect on the learning journey of becoming a nurse, and consider how your values and judgements regarding who the client is (person), the context of care (environment), your beliefs about health, and what constitutes nursing, have evolved.

Fawcett, J. (1984). The metaparadigm of nursing: Present status and future refinements. *Image, 16*(3), 84-87.

Goals

Learners will have the opportunity to:
- Explore how the metaparadigm concepts contribute to a personal philosophy of nursing.
- Understand how personal values and judgments of person, environment, health, and nursing change over time.
- Consider the importance of a personal philosophy of nursing.

In Preparation

Read:

Barnett, P. (2012). What does it mean to be a professional nurse? *New Jersey Nurse & Institute for Nursing Newsletter*. April, p. 3.

Lee, R.C., & Fawcett, J. (2013). The influence of the metaparadigm of nursing on professional identity development among RN-BSN students. *Nursing Science Quarterly, 26*(1), 96-98. doi: 10.1177/0894318412466734

In Class

Exploration of the class concept(s) may be guided by the following:
Review of how values and beliefs affect nursing practice
Examination of how the metaparadigm concepts are the building blocks of all philosophies of nursing
Attention to the steps in writing a personal philosophy of nursing

In Reflection

Consider the implications if no one in nursing had a philosophy.

Opportunities for Students to Demonstrate Learning and Faculty Evaluation of Student Achievement

Students are required to demonstrate achievement of course competencies or goals so faculty can be assured that they are ready to progress in the curriculum and ultimately, to graduate. Therefore, opportunities for students to demonstrate learning and faculty evaluation of student achievement are viewed as a single course component. This view is taken because the student activity of demonstrating learning and the faculty activity of evaluating the products of learning are inextricably linked.

The phrase *opportunity to demonstrate learning* is used in this text for what are typically called assignments, course requirements, or simply evaluation of student work. The terminology connotes a more positive, student-oriented perspective and conveys the idea that students have a responsibility to provide evidence that they are achieving course expectations.

The opportunities for students to demonstrate learning can include a host of activities. In theory courses, the activities might be undertaken by individuals or groups of students in face-to-face or online environments. The opportunities might be:

- True-false, multiple-choice, multiple-response, short-answer, and essay tests and examinations; term papers and other written assignments (Oermann & Gaberson, 2014)
- Class presentations and other oral reports
- Oral examinations

In laboratory or professional practice courses, students generally demonstrate their achievement of course goals or outcomes individually. Their performance might be observed and evaluated as they participate in:

- Objective structured clinical examinations
- Direct client care (which is observed by a faculty member or preceptor)
- Simulated care scenarios

In addition to performing in real or simulated professional settings, students could complete process recordings, care plans, case studies, teaching plans, portfolios, and/or self-evaluation to demonstrate their achievement (Oermann & Gaberson, 2014).

Once students fulfill their responsibility and present their evidence of learning, the faculty member's reciprocal obligation is to evaluate the completed work fairly. This means that the processes, standards, and timeframes need to be clear and known to students and faculty members. In theory courses, faculty members can develop and use rubrics for assessment of written work, and these can be shared with students. The rubrics state the criteria against which the work is being assessed, and the allocation of marks for different aspects of the project. This contributes to consistency in the assessment of student work. In evaluation of professional practice, students are generally required to complete a self-evaluation, using the same form as faculty members. Student self-evaluations and descriptions of acceptable performance contribute to the perceived fairness of evaluation procedures.

Another element of fairness is authentic assessment. *Authentic assessment* has been described as "an assessment requiring students to use the same competencies, or combination of knowledge, skills, and attitudes that they need to apply in the criterion situation in professional life" (Gulikers, Bastiaens, & Kirschner, 2004, p. 69). Because the combination of knowledge, skills, and attitudes forms part of the course goals or competencies, the assessment contributes to the unity of the course. Elements of authentic assessment include but are not limited to:

- Alignment of learning goals or competencies, classroom instruction, and assessment techniques
- Fidelity of the task or problem to professional practice, including complexity, physical and social context, and necessity for students to use integrative thinking
- Requirement for a product or performance that is reflective of real-life demands and that could be presented to others
- Meaningfulness of the task and product to students
- Clear criteria that are known to students, or created with them
- Provision of feedback about performance, including self, peer, and faculty assessment (Gulikers et al., 2004)

Evaluation of students' performance in real or simulated professional practice situations is authentic assessment. Authentic assessment in theory classes is also possible (e.g., analysis of client cases, preparation of health teaching materials). Some traditional assessment strategies may also have aspects of authenticity. For example, although the task of completing a multiple-choice examination might not reflect professional practice, the thinking necessary in professional practice can be tested if high-level questions are constructed. Moreover, students often consider multiple-choice examinations to be important and meaningful practice for licensure or registration examinations.

In addition to certifying learning (summative evaluation) and providing feedback (formative evaluation) about course learning through assessment, faculty can plan procedures that provide a foundation for lifelong learning (Boud & Falchikov, 2006). Specifically, the aforementioned authors propose that the assessment task ought to prepare students for "the tasks of making complex judgements about their own work and that of others and for making decisions in the uncertain and unpredictable circumstances in which they will find themselves in the future" (p. 402). This means that students should be involved in establishing criteria for evaluating success, in assessing their performance and that of others, and in working in groups on a task, similar to what they will experience after graduation. An approach such as this would require consistency through several courses to achieve the goal of helping students to become accurate self-assessors able to identify their own learning needs in complex situations.

Decisions about opportunities for students to demonstrate learning and faculty evaluation of student achievement will be influenced by many factors, including: philosophical and educational approaches, course competencies or goals, purpose of the evaluation (formative/summative), content, course level, learning domain, class size, educational delivery medium, reliability, validity, utility, evaluation frequency, and availability of resources. The opportunities that are developed for students to demonstrate their learning ought to be carefully aligned with the educational and philosophical approaches of the curriculum and the course goals or competencies. Students' completion of the activities inherently involves learning, and hence a dual purpose is served: students learn and they demonstrate their achievement.

This course component requires thoughtful attention because the consequences are significant. Faulty evaluation can result in the loss of a competent student from the profession or graduation of an incompetent nurse.

In **Figure 13-2** are portions of a course syllabus that includes the course components described earlier. Although there is no heading entitled *Strategies to Ignite Learning* or *Teaching-Learning Strategies*, these can be discerned in the expanded course description and in the section entitled, *How We Will Work Together.*

APPROACHES TO COURSE DESIGN

The approach to course design is strongly influenced by faculty members' abilities, interests, and comfort level, as well as the background knowledge, life experiences, and capabilities of students. Often, faculty use a familiar approach without giving careful thought to what is consistent with the curriculum foundations. If it seems that some courses are not being designed in accordance with the agreed-upon philosophical and educational approaches, then broader faculty discussion may be needed about the amount of flexibility that is acceptable in each course.

Irrespective of the approach to course design, attention should be given to student diversity. Accordingly, course designers strive to ensure the following:

- Written course materials and oral expression are clear, unambiguous, and complete.
- Important ideas receive prominence in course materials.
- Course websites are readily understandable and intuitive.

Figure 13-2   Edited course syllabus.
Developed by Marilyn Evans, RN, PhD; Beverly Leipert, RN, PhD; Yvette Laforet Fliesser RN, MScN; Karen O'Brien, RN, MScN; Katie Studnicka, RN, MScN. © Western-Fanshawe Collaborative BScN Program, 2013. Used with permission.

HEALTH PROMOTION & CARING: FAMILIES and COMMUNITIES

Calendar Description:

This course provides students with the opportunity to deepen their understanding of health, empowering health promotion, and caring in the context of family, community, and populations across the lifespan. Normal growth and development, family health, and community health are addressed.

Expanded Description:

The process of promoting the health of individuals, families, groups, and communities is an integral component of professional nursing practice. This course provides a philosophical and theoretical foundation for understanding family and community health issues and implementing nursing interventions guided by practice standards to promote family and community health.

In this course you will have the opportunity to develop a basic understanding of community health nursing through exploring sociological, psychological, philosophical, and nursing concepts and theories that support family and community health promotion practice across the lifespan. Focus will be on nursing practice with family and community as "partner". Primary health care, health education, health promotion, and social determinants of health are critically examined as they relate to family and community health nursing practice. This course enhances your critical thinking skills through course readings and lectures, in class discussions, and various learning activities.

Course Goals:

1. To develop an understanding of the foundational pillars of community health nursing in Canada.
2. To outline and analyze the implications of societal trends and social determinants of health on the health of individuals, families, groups, and communities.
3. To demonstrate an appreciation of the diversity, trends, and evolving nature of families, groups, and communities.

Etc.

Major Concepts in the Course:

- Client-centered care/individual, family, groups and community
- Health/Wellness
- Health promotion
- Disease/injury prevention
- Etc

How this Course Will Contribute to Your Development as a Professional Nurse:

The professional nurse needs to establish, build, and nurture professional relationships that promote maximum participation and self-determination of individuals, families, groups, and communities (Community Health Nurses of Canada, 2011). Using a variety of creative activities, this course will assist you to develop knowledge, appreciation, and abilities to collaboratively and effectively work with diverse clients to address determinants of health.

How We Will Work Together:

In this course teaching and learning are considered a **shared** responsibility. The professor's role is to guide, facilitate and support your learning; your responsibility is to use the resources, and to actively engage in dialogue and reflective, critical thought on the topics being covered. The course is designed to foster discussion, debate, and critical examination of concepts relevant to the promotion of family and community health. To facilitate an interactive classroom environment, the professor will seek individual and collective student input.

(continues)

Figure 13-2   Edited course syllabus. (*continued*)

The various learning activities, readings, and lectures will help you to develop insights, see patterns, and critically reflect on real-life experiences as you learn about the nurse's role in working with communities. Your commitment and active participation in these activities are critical to your own learning as well as to the learning of your colleagues. Attendance at class and participation in learning activities is therefore expected and will promote your success not only in this course but also in nursing practice in the community. Suggestions to help you be successful in this course include: 1) Ask questions of the professor, teaching assistant, and your classmates; 2) Allow time every week (2-3 hours) for readings, preparation for lectures, assignment preparation, and online postings; 3) Read the syllabus and make note of assignment requirements; and 4) Participate in class on an ongoing basis.

Weekly Schedule (partial)

Week	Topic	Concepts	Course Goals
1	Introduction to Health Promotion and Caring of Family and Community Health	Clients (individuals, family, groups, community) Health promotion/disease prevention; primary health care; health/wellness; caring; time/transition	1,2,3
3	Nurses' Ways of Knowing: Use of Health Assessment Tools	Social determinants of health; ways of knowing; clients; diversity; relational practice	2,3,8
6	Caring and Social Justice with Clients in Diverse Contexts	Social justice; diversity; context/ culture; advocacy; caring; ethical practice	2,3,4,5,7
8	Health Promotion and Caring: Empowerment and Capacity-building with Families and Communities	Health promotion; social justice; primary health care; ways of knowing; ICP; growth and development	4,7,8

Opportunities to Demonstrate Learning

1. Scholarly paper: Community health and its impact on family

The purposes of this assignment are for you to:
- Identify a current nursing-related issue within the community. Explain the impact this issue is having on the community and on the families living in the community from a strengths-based perspective.
- Critique scholarly sources of information.
- Discuss solutions and implications for nursing practice with families and communities.

Part A – Purpose statement - Due Week 6 - (5%)

Assignment process:
1. Choose a current nursing-related issue from the community.
2. Review nursing literature related to the issue.
3. Develop a purpose statement for your paper and initial reference list including 5 current references excluding the course texts and assigned readings.

Figure 13-2   Edited course syllabus. (*continued*)

Criteria for evaluation:

- Use APA (6th ed.) formatting and referencing
- Include title page, 12 point Times New Roman font, 2.5cm (1") margins
- Grade: 5%

Scholarly paper - Part B — Due: Week 10 – (25%)

Assignment process:

1. Choose a current nursing-related issue from the community.
2. Explain why it is an issue and why it is important to the community.
3. Discuss the impact the issue is having on the community and families within the community from a strengths-based approach.
4. Research the nursing literature related to the community issue. Utilize a minimum of 5 current scholarly nursing sources (within last 5 years) excluding course texts and assigned readings.
5. Discuss potential realistic solutions to the issue.
6. Discuss the implications for nursing practice.

Criteria for evaluation:

- Scholarly writing and use APA (6th ed.) formatting and referencing.
- Maximum of **2500** words (not including title page and references). Include word count on title page.
- Use 12 point Times New Roman font, double spaced, 2.5cm (1") margins.
- Plain white paper, stapled, no cover or binder.
- Minimum of 5 current nursing sources not related to course content.
- Due date:
- Grade: 25% - See the marking template for this assignment for further guidance.

2. **Mid term exam: Week 7 (30%)**
3. **Scholarly paper: Week 10 (25%)**
4. **Final exam: (40%)**

Summary of Opportunities to Demonstrate Learning

OPPORTUNITIES TO DEMONSTRATE LEARNING	COURSE GOAL(S) ADDRESSED	VALUE	DUE DATE
1. Scholarly paper: Purpose statement	2, 3, 6	5%	Week 6
2. Mid-term exam	1, 2, 3, 4, 5	30%	Week 7
3. Scholarly paper	1, 2, 3, 4, 5, 7	25%	Week 10
4. Final exam	All	40%	Exam period

- Class norms (e.g., preparation for class, attendance) are specified or negotiated.
- Class and evaluation activities are varied to account for differences in learning styles (Bowe, 2000; Higbee, 2009).

Extending from the idea of making courses intellectually and physically accessible is the belief that courses should be culturally comfortable for students of differing sociocultural backgrounds. Therefore, deliberate effort is made to ensure that language, texts, readings, and learning experiences avoid ethnocentric, gender-limited, and class-limited perspectives. Additionally, authors with varied backgrounds and viewpoints should be represented in course readings (Saunders & Kardia, n.d.). The intent is to make the course as inclusive as possible so all students feel welcome and accepted in an environment conducive to learning.

Traditional Approaches

In traditional approaches to course design, planning proceeds in a logical, step-wise fashion, starting with objectives. The intent is to design a course and lessons that will lead students to achieve specific objectives and learn specific content in a readily identified and prescribed way. The traditional, behaviorist course design is structured, supports knowledge as being absolute, and is teacher-centered. Faculty have responsibility for identifying the nature, purpose, and objectives of the course, as well as content, teaching-learning strategies, and evaluation methods. Students are the recipients of knowledge and decisions.

With this approach, a course description is written first. Then, course objectives are formulated according to taxonomies that address cognitive, psychomotor, and affective learning domains. The course objectives state what students will be able to do, think, or feel. They are drawn from program and level objectives, the course description, and content necessary for desired behaviors to occur. In addition, unit or module objectives are specified, with the units being defined by content groupings. "Courses are constructed around the content deemed necessary to produce the desired target behaviors" (Bevis, 1982, p. 195). Teaching strategies, media, and evaluation methods are then selected.

Gagné, Briggs, and Wager (1992) propose a more detailed approach, whereby following the specification of curriculum outcomes, an instructional analysis is completed to identify the skills involved in reaching those outcomes. This entails a task analysis to delineate the steps or skills in the behavior and an information-processing analysis to identify the mental processes required to enact each outcome. From these, objectives are prepared. Next, criterion-referenced evaluation procedures are created and instructional strategies and media are selected.

Lesson planning is an important element of traditional approaches. For each lesson, objectives are delineated and appropriate instructional events are defined. Written lesson plans specify activities that the teacher will carry out. See **Table 13-3** for an example of a traditional lesson plan.

Table 13-3   Traditional Lesson Plan for a 2-Hour Class

Teaching Purpose: Ensure students acquire necessary information for health promotion with families

Learning objectives	Content	Teaching-Learning Strategies	Time	Resources	Evaluation Methods
Identify 3 goals of health promotion	Health promotion goals	Lecture/discussion	10 min	Smartboard PowerPoint slides	Question and answer (pretesting)
Describe how the Health Belief Model can be used to influence behavior	Health Belief Model	Lecture/discussion	25 min	PowerPoint slides	Question and answer
Assess health promotion needs of families	Assessment of family health and learning readiness	Case study analysis in small groups and large-group discussion	35 min	Case and case questions on course website Flip charts	Question and answer
Recall guidelines for health promotion	Provincial guidelines for health promotion	Brainstorming Large-group discussion	20 min	Student access to Internet	Question and answer
Propose pertinent health promotion measures		Small-group discussion	30 min	Student laptops	Group e-submission of health promotion plan at end of class

The following criteria for judging the quality of a lesson plan have been suggested:

- Coherence is evident in the link between what students should know, understand, and be able to do.
- Activities in the lesson are motivating and designed to suit students with a variety of learning styles.
- The lesson supports the intent of the curriculum and is worthy of the time given to it (Erickson, 2007).

These criteria are applicable for all classes, whether or not traditional lesson plans are used.

Contemporary Approaches

With a more contemporary or conceptual approach to course design, courses are planned so the focus of learning is on inquiry and the active pursuit of experiences that contribute to learning. These learning-centered course designs incorporate recognition and acceptance of the values, beliefs, knowledge, and experience that students bring. Courses are designed in accordance with the premises that learning and contextual knowledge:

- Evolve from processes such as discussion, dialogue, debate, and other heuristics that promote active engagement and sharing of knowledge
- Occur in an environment that advances trust and critique among all participants

This approach to course design is based on adherence to values of human freedom and self-reflection, and an epistemology of transactional constructivism. Therefore, course procedures are designed to emphasize students' information processing and construction of understandings and meanings through transactions with others (Sutinen, 2008). Process-oriented courses promote integrative learning, de-emphasize specific content, and reduce reliance on the lecture method. Attention is given to how students, faculty, and clients, together, bring life experiences to knowledge and learning. Understanding develops through thoughtful deliberation and critical analysis of information, dialogue about its meaning, and reflection on its fit with personal beliefs and values.

Faculty and students share course design, jointly creating the climate and cultural reality in which collaboration flourishes. Together, they determine course competencies or goals, establish appropriate methods for students to achieve them, and agree on the evaluation procedures. Students become active constructors of knowledge and meaning (Seaton-Sykes, 2003), and shape their learning through participation in course design and activities. They gain a sense of ownership for the course and become autonomous learners, consistent with adult learning principles (Conklin, 2013). The faculty member is an expert learner, metastrategist, and facilitator (Bevis, 2000), who empowers, fosters creativity, stimulates intellectual inquiry, and maintains rigor. Importantly, the faculty member retains authority while trusting that students, individually and collectively, will make wise decisions about course matters (Conklin, 2013).

Central to contemporary course design is conceptualizing learning activities for classes, and then the associated guidelines for students. As stated previously, guidelines enable students to process information and work toward achievement of course competencies or goals through interaction with course content, peers, and faculty. They specify activities that students undertake, with the intent that learning occurs, and they can be developed as a part of course design. Development of the guidelines (which can occur collaboratively with students) and students' subsequent completion of the learning activities for each session reflect the idea of a flipped or inverted classroom: Preparation is necessary to work with the content in class in contrast to merely receiving it. The collaborative development of the guidelines for the classes increases students' investment in the course.

The success of this approach to course design is highly dependent on the interpersonal dynamics between and among faculty and students. Student maturity is necessary, because many decisions are required at the beginning of a course and the decisions need to align with academic standards. For students to engage in the process of designing a course together, or some aspects of it, faculty ought to be welcoming, convey respect for all class members, be relaxed about self, encourage students as they offer ideas and perspectives (Higbee, 2009), and convey belief in students' potential (Read, Vessey, Amar, & Cullinan, 2013). Moreover, authentic communication among all participants is essential.

Combined Approaches

In a combined approach, there is a mixture of contemporary and traditional approaches. In small classes, a contemporary approach may be possible because faculty and student collaboration could occur in all aspects of course design. In large undergraduate courses, however, some predetermined structure is required because of class size, agreements with healthcare agencies, and policies of educational institutions. Faculty who support constructivism and adult learning principles might rely upon an approach to course design that combines traditional and contemporary perspectives.

For the most part, faculty members design the course structure (i.e., define the description, competencies or goals, concepts and general scope of content, and opportunities to demonstrate learning) in a way that appears to mirror traditional approaches. Nonetheless, there can be opportunities for student choice within specified limits (Iwasiw, 1987). For example, students may choose from a number of broadly defined opportunities to demonstrate learning, determine the weighting of assignments, collectively decide due dates, and/or negotiate ground rules for class and professional practice sessions.

While courses are designed with a predetermined structure, their intent is to support process learning. A contemporary approach becomes apparent in the strategies to ignite learning. For example, the use of peer teaching (Iwasiw & Goldenberg, 1993), learning teams, unfolding case studies, games, narrative pedagogy, and problem-based learning, among others, requires students to be active participants in learning and knowledge construction. With these strategies, students are in charge of their learning.

Additionally, faculty can develop guidelines that emphasize process learning in course sessions and make these available to students. The guidelines are learning-centered, specify class preparation activities, make evident the information-processing skills expected, and allow fluidity in the conduct of classes. Thus, there is a predetermined structure, including plans for each session, in a combined approach to course design. However, within that structure the following are provided:

- Opportunities for students' participation in course decisions
- Expectations of students' active involvement in learning activities
- Fluidity in class processes

PROCESSES TO CREATE EVIDENCE-INFORMED, CONTEXT-RELEVANT, UNIFIED COURSES

Like all aspects of curriculum development, creating a course is an iterative process with decisions about each course component affecting deliberations about other components. The process involves writing, modifying, critiquing, and revising before plans are finalized. The intent is to devise a course that adheres to curriculum philosophical and educational approaches, facilitates students' achievement of course expectations, and is effective within the school's context. There should be unity within the course, so that the relationships among the course components are apparent.

Course titles, brief descriptions, placement in the program, draft competencies, major curriculum concepts, philosophical and educational approaches, and so forth are determined as part of the curriculum design process. These, along with ideas about curriculum possibilities (content and learning experiences) generated during the analysis of contextual data, and the level goals or outcomes, are reviewed as intensive course design begins.

Typically, courses are designed in the order in which they are to be implemented. During the design process, courses should be compared to the curriculum matrix or maps to maintain adherence to the original curriculum intent. Reasons for deviations should be explained and agreement reached about their acceptability. Variations from the curriculum plan might necessitate changes in subsequent courses (Heinrich, Karner, Gaglione, & Lambert, 2002).

Course design is not an activity undertaken in isolation. Ongoing consultation is required among course designers to ensure the following:

- The curriculum intent and integrity are maintained.
- Concurrent courses are complementary.
- Sequenced courses build in depth and complexity without redundancy.
- Curriculum outcomes or goals can be achieved.
- Student and faculty workloads are reasonable.

The process begins with a review of parameters that influence the design and selection of a course design approach. Then, creation of the course components begins. Use of curriculum templates can be helpful as discussion proceeds. Although attention is given to the components individually, ideas arise about all of them simultaneously. This concurrent thinking leads to a unified course. The iterative process concludes when course developers are satisfied with their ongoing appraisal of the course design. The final step is preparation of information for students.

Reviewing Course Parameters

Course parameters are boundaries within which courses can be created. The parameters limit the range faculty have in creating courses, yet compel them to exercise creativity and ingenuity in designing courses that are motivating and promote positive learning experiences. Reviewing these parameters and how they will affect the course design is a necessary beginning.

Curriculum Foundations and Goals or Outcomes

The overriding parameters for all courses are the curriculum foundations: philosophical and educational approaches, core curriculum concepts, and key professional abilities. These are evident in curriculum goals and partially present in outcomes. From curriculum goals or outcomes, level goals or competencies are derived, and from these, course expectations are defined. If the curriculum is being organized according to specific theories, concepts, or frameworks, these must be evident in course components. Importantly, the philosophical approaches influence all aspects of course design and define the desired learning climate.

Course Level, Structure, and Delivery

The course level, that is, the semester and year in the curriculum, gives course designers information about students' prior learning, which determines the depth and scope possible in the course to be designed. Course structure (i.e., course length; number, frequency, and duration of class sessions) also has a direct bearing on the competencies to be achieved, the extent of the subject matter, and evaluation. Course delivery approaches establish how students access and engage in the course.

Student Characteristics

Student numbers, and their attitudes toward learning, technology, participation, and evaluation, are important to know. These characteristics, plus students' cultural and generational diversity, maturity, motivation, interests, and other commitments, have a bearing on course design.

Physical Environment

Desk arrangements, temperature, windows, ventilation, and lighting affect attention, fatigue, and interactions. Availability of Internet access in classrooms and access to an online course site can also influence course design. The details about a classroom cannot always be known in advance of creating a course, and indeed, the finalized design will influence the classroom space that is required. Moreover, for professional practice courses, the physical setting and the presence of other healthcare students can affect learning opportunities.

Human and Material Resources

The numbers of faculty and graduate teaching assistants, and their experience, have a bearing on the decisions made about individual courses. Importantly, clients and personnel in healthcare and community agencies influence professional practice courses. Library and computer resources and technical equipment in classrooms, among other material resources, require consideration.

Policies and Contractual Agreements

Finally, educational institutions have policies or regulations that must be respected in course design. For example, there may be requirements about the timing of evaluation and examinations. For professional practice courses, contractual arrangements with healthcare or community agencies regulate learning experiences.

Limitations and Administrative Issues

It is prudent to review the limitations and administrative issues identified during analysis of contextual data. These may provide insights relevant for course design. To reinforce the parameters in the minds of those designing courses, they might ask:

- What are the institutional requirements related to course design?
- Which core curriculum concepts and major professional abilities will be addressed in this course?
- What are the implications of the philosophical approaches for course design?
- What are the educational approaches of the curriculum?
- What is the learning climate we wish to achieve in the course?
- Which delivery method(s) will be employed? Could multiple methods be used? Is the infrastructure sufficient to support the preferred method(s)?
- What resources to support teaching and learning will be available for the course?
- What knowledge and experiences do students bring to this course?

- How many students are likely to be enrolled? What are their characteristics?
- Will the students be:
  - Directly from secondary institutions?
  - Those with previous diplomas, degrees, or some postsecondary education?
  - Adults with strong values about lifelong learning and continuing their education?
  - Individuals who, in addition to academic responsibilities, manage multiple life roles?
  - Students with special needs for whom certain accommodations need to be made?
  - Diverse or homogenous?

Choosing an Approach for Course Design

The choice of an approach for course design could be guided by the alignment between a traditional, contemporary, or combined approach with:

- Philosophical and educational approaches of the curriculum
- Faculty and student preferences
- Feasibility
- Institutional requirements

Confirming the Course Title, Purpose, and Description

Confirming or modifying the draft course title and description established by the curriculum design team may seem as though it should be the first step in course design. However, the final confirmation of these components is not possible until all other aspects of course design start to become firm. Nonetheless, the course title and description are the starting point for discussion. Course designers need to be clear about the:

- Conceptual, process, and substantive focus of the course
- Reason the course is in the curriculum

Faculty can determine whether the draft title adequately reflects the course intent or whether it needs to be modified, remembering that course titles are important in visually conveying the conceptual bases and the unity of the curriculum.

Once a title is tentatively decided upon, a preliminary course description is written, based on the draft prepared during curriculum design. The description undergoes many revisions during course design. The initial description represents the ideas that faculty first discuss as possibilities for the course. The course description is not finalized until all other design components are completed. In general, the following questions are raised as the description is discussed and written:

- What is the purpose of the course in the curriculum?
- Which curriculum possibilities, identified during the analysis of the contextual data, should be considered? What other learning experiences could be suitable?
- What would be the nature of interactions in these learning experiences?
- How can the course concepts be addressed? What could be the scope of the exemplars and substantive content, or the nature of practice experiences?
- How should students participate in this course?
- If there is choice about delivery modes, which one(s) would be most fitting?
- If face-to-face delivery, what is suitable scheduling?

In addition, the course purpose needs to be drafted and finalized. A clear narrative about how the course will contribute to students' development as professional nurses influences the value that students will attach to the course.

Formulating Course Goals or Competencies

The level goals or outcomes, derived from the evidence-informed, context-relevant curriculum goals or outcomes, are the basis on which course goals or competencies are developed. The level expectations are examined to identify those pertinent to the course. Then, course expectations are written to include concepts, processes, and contexts particular to each course. Formulation of course expectations centers on the following queries:

- Which of the level outcomes or goals should be addressed in this course?
- Which curriculum concepts and professional abilities should be most evident in the course competencies or goals?
- What is the context in which achievement of the competencies or goals will be evident?
- How can the level competencies or goals be modified to be particular to the course, ensuring that the language of the curriculum is retained?

Determining Exemplars to Match Concepts

Matching exemplars to course concepts requires logical and imaginative thinking. First, discussion occurs about the concepts designated to be emphasized according to the curriculum matrix, and how they are evident in professional practice situations particular to the practice context of the course. Subsequent to this, faculty members consider the professional practice situations that are most relevant for students to understand in order to meet the course expectations. Then, they deliberate about which concepts are best illuminated through which practice situations and the scope of substantive content that could be addressed in these situations. As they determine the exemplars to match concepts, faculty members might pose the following questions:

- Which curriculum concepts are to be included in this course?
- What practice situations are relevant for the course?
- Which practice situations would best illuminate particular concepts?
- Are the possible exemplars suitable for students to practice the thinking processes expressed in the course goals or competencies?
- What is a reasonable depth and scope of content at this stage of the nursing curriculum?
- What is the available evidence for the concepts and substantive content that should become part of the content?
- Which curriculum possibilities, identified during analysis of the contextual data, would be suitable in this course?
- How can the course topics be sequenced to emphasize philosophical approaches and facilitate students' achievement of the course goals or competencies?

Deciding on Classes

Classes are created through the placement of the conceptual and substantive content into meaningful and logically sequenced units. This involves determining the best match between concepts and exemplars. Course designers consider:

- Concepts and professional abilities that should be emphasized through the content
- Possible organization and sequence of concepts and content to match the number of class sessions
- Possible class titles to ensure that they:
  - Reflect the curriculum foundations
  - Convey unity within the course and curriculum

Selecting Strategies to Ignite Learning

Selection of strategies to ignite learning is of vital concern to course designers because these define, in part, what faculty will do. Faculty could begin with a review of curriculum possibilities identified during analysis of the contextual data. These may be directly suitable for the course, or suitable with modification. As faculty members ponder the wide range of strategies and techniques available to them, they give thought to strategies that:

- Are consistent with the agreed-upon philosophical and educational approaches
- Will best facilitate students' achievement of course expectations
- Are feasible within the course parameters
- Are suitable for the delivery method(s)

- Best suit students' learning needs and styles
- Would be most useful for the course
- Have sufficient research or anecdotal evidence to support their use

Finally, when decisions have been made, faculty give thought to how they can become prepared to use strategies that are new to them.

Creating Guidelines for Student Learning Activities

Formulating student learning activities for each class calls upon the creativity of course designers. Decisions about strategies to ignite learning will be foundational to the creation of the guidelines that will help students maximize their learning in each class. Some questions faculty might ask as they create the guidelines include:

- What types of student engagement with content will promote achievement of course goals or competencies?
- Which curriculum possibilities, identified during analysis of the contextual data, would be suitable in this course?
- What is a reasonable amount of work to expect of students in preparation for classes?
- Which preparatory, in-class, and post-class activities can facilitate students' achievement of course competencies or goals?
- What readings and other resources will enhance student learning?
- What types of practice experiences will enable students to achieve course expectations?
- How well do our proposed learning activities match the educational and philosophical approaches?
- What is the likelihood that the proposed learning activities will allow students to achieve the expectations at the desired depth?

Planning Opportunities for Students to Demonstrate Learning and Faculty Evaluation of Student Achievement

When considering how students might demonstrate learning in the course, faculty simultaneously give thought to how they will evaluate the evidence of learning. They are cognizant that both the evidence they are asking for, and the way they evaluate it, must be consistent with the curriculum foundations. Decisions about the nature and frequency of evaluation, student choice, and whether to provide grading criteria to students, are among the decisions that faculty make when designing courses. Questions faculty should consider include:

- In what ways could students demonstrate achievement of course competencies?
- Which evaluation methods are consistent with the philosophical and educational approaches, and course competencies or goals?

- What are the advantages and disadvantages for students and faculty with respect to
  ~~the ideas proposed?~~

~~present authentic~~

develop specific criteria or marking ~~rubrics. If so,~~
  along with other course material information?
- What will be reasonable due dates for students to submit their work? Could the dates
  be negotiated with the class?

Attending to Implementation Matters

As course design ideas are presented, discussion includes ideas of implementation: *How can we do that? How would that work?* Course designers ask themselves what is possible and feasible within the course, and what is reasonable within the context of all other courses within the curriculum level. Furthermore, they consider the logistical arrangements that are required for the course design to be implemented. The latter requires ongoing consultation with faculty members who are designing other courses within the curriculum level. Consideration is also given to the preparation that faculty members might require to implement the courses as designed.

Preparing the Course Syllabus

Once decisions about course design have been finalized, a syllabus is prepared, according to a template previously determined for the curriculum. Generally, this is posted on a course website. Although the terminology and precise nature of syllabi can vary, they typically include an expanded course description; course competencies or goals; class topics and schedule; information about opportunities for students to demonstrate their learning; due dates of work to be submitted; required texts; and possibly, guidelines for individual classes. Other information may be added, such as participation guidelines for the course, the need for Internet access, policies about plagiarism, and so forth. The structure of the syllabus can reinforce the unified nature of the course. For example, in **Figure 13-2**, course concepts and goals are identified in the weekly schedule, and the goals which the projects address are made explicit in the *Summary of Opportunities to Demonstrate Learning*. In addition, a consistent template for guidelines for student learning activities contributes to visual unity.

CREATION OF INDIVIDUAL CLASSES

The overall course design provides the framework for individual classes. Each class must contribute to the course purpose, with student learning activities particularized. When planning classes, faculty might ask the following questions:

- How can we title this class so that its relationship to the course and the curriculum foundations is evident?
- How can the class be designed to clearly relate to course competencies or goals?
- What should students achieve in this class?
- What learning activities can be planned so that the desired balance of concepts and substantive content is achieved? How can the two be integrated?
- What is the evidence pertinent to the substantive content?
- What are useful learning activities? How can the faculty member facilitate learning in the activities?
- What is a reasonable sequence and time allotment for the activities?

If a traditional approach to course design is employed, lesson plans can be developed to organize each class. If a blended approach is used, class guidelines for students can be beneficial. With either approach, class planning generally involves determining the following:

- Purpose students should achieve
- Scope of concepts and substantive content
- Appropriate exemplars
- Strategies to ignite learning
- Sequence and timing of class activities

Many teachers strive to obtain feedback about each class. Therefore, they plan a few minutes at the conclusion of each session to ask questions such as:

- What did you like about this class?
- What worked well for you?
- What might we have done differently, and how?

This information allows for refinement of the class if it is going to be offered again. Additionally, if a pattern of responses emerges in reaction to the predominant strategies to ignite learning, it is possible to take this into account for later classes.

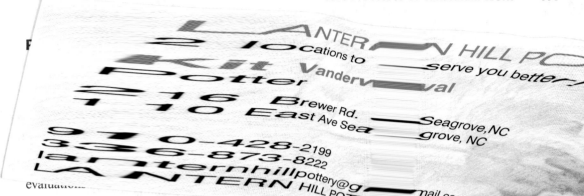

RELATIONSHIP OF COURSE CREATION TO AN EVIDENCE-INFORMED, CONTEXT-RELEVANT, UNIFIED CURRICULUM

Nursing courses and individual classes are the culmination of the development of an evidence-informed, context-relevant, unified curriculum. Concepts that were identified from analysis of contextual data are the focus of the courses. Core concepts and key professional abilities, deduced from contextual data, along with philosophical approaches, are expressed in the curriculum goals or outcomes. Level goals or competencies are then derived from these, and course expectations from the level goals or competencies. Therefore, the conceptual foci and course goals or competencies are evidence-informed and context-relevant. Moreover, because all competencies or goals within a curriculum level are directed toward achievement of these level expectations, there is unity among the courses. This unified nature of the curriculum is also evident in the course titles, use of common templates for course syllabi and guidelines for learning, and adherence to the curriculum's educational and philosophical approaches.

The evidence-informed nature of courses is strengthened by plans to use evidence-informed strategies to ignite learning, and the inclusion of evidence for nursing practice as content. The logical consistency between the goals or competencies and the ways in which students demonstrate their learning also contributes to the unified nature of each course. Finally, when individual classes are titled in accordance with the course concepts, and are planned to align with course expectations and curricular educational and philosophical approaches, there is unity within each course.

CORE PROCESSES OF CURRICULUM WORK

Faculty Development

Faculty development is directed toward facilitating members' knowledge and expertise in designing courses and classes. Depending on faculty needs, and following an initial review session on the parameters involved, faculty development activities can include discussion about some or all of the course components.

Discussion about the approach to course design is appropriate. This would help team members appreciate whether a traditional, contemporary, or combined approach is most relevant to the curriculum foundations. Mentorship for those less familiar with course and class design could be beneficial. Likely, some attention will have to be given to drafting course and class designs. Attention to the creation of concept-based classes would be wise. Sharing, critiquing, and discussing can be facilitated by experienced faculty members. Faculty might also gain from peer learning about strategies to ignite learning, and from microteaching sessions to practice any new strategies proposed for courses. This could be followed by member feedback.

Ongoing Appraisal

As course design proceeds, faculty members engage in ongoing appraisal. Before finalizing the course design, they critique it in an holistic fashion, asking themselves questions such as:

- Does this course seem to fulfill its purpose in the curriculum?
- Is this course feasible within the design parameters?
- Is the course consistent with the curriculum foundations?
- How strongly are the course expectations deduced from, and aligned with, the level outcomes or goals?
- Is there an appropriate balance between concepts important for nursing practice and substantive content?
- Will course processes and content lead students to achieve course competencies or goals?
- Are the preparatory activities of sufficient depth and interest?
- Does the syllabus reflect our intent in a way that will be meaningful to others? Is the language consistent with curriculum tenets?
- Will the teaching-learning strategies ignite learning?
- Do the course components fit together in a unified and logical fashion?
- Are this course and its individual classes of the quality that we expect of ourselves?
- Have we taken student diversity into account?
- Are the opportunities for students to demonstrate learning aligned with the course goals or outcomes? Are they reasonable? Are they consistent with authentic assessment?
- Will the workload for students be feasible when considered in conjunction with other courses in the semester?

- Does this course result in a reasonable workload for faculty?
- Have we attended to the necessary implementation matters?
- Has our consideration of course evaluation been sufficient? Are there other ideas to consider?
- Is this curriculum work of the quality that is satisfactory to us and that will likely be acceptable to external reviewers?

Scholarship

Because the process of designing concept-based courses is relatively new in nursing education, expository articles about the experiences of faculty groups, and the provision of examples of courses, would be important additions to the nursing education literature. Faculty undertaking course design might consider scholarship about the processes they are experiencing, analyzing reasons for the challenges faced and describing how those challenges were resolved. A study that examines the development of concept-based courses by faculty and stakeholders in more than one institution would be illuminating, particularly if it resulted in recommendations about how others could proceed smoothly. Another idea might be to prepare a manuscript about the development and conduct of a concept-based class. Specific information such as this could serve as a model for faculty members beginning this initiative.

Another possible scholarship project is the creation of a textbook. Some nursing textbooks continue to be based on a medical model and do not match conceptually based courses. Therefore, faculty who create, implement, and evaluate innovative courses could undertake the writing of a text suitable for their courses.

CHAPTER SUMMARY

In this chapter, course components (title, purpose, and description; competencies or goals, strategies to ignite learning, concepts and content; classes; opportunities for students to demonstrate learning and faculty evaluation of student achievement) are described and course design parameters are detailed. Several approaches to creating courses are included. Attention is given to the process of course design, and ideas are presented for the creation of individual concept-based classes. The intent is that courses incorporate the curriculum foundations in a consistent manner. Course implementation and evaluation are briefly described. The relationship between creating courses and an evidence-informed, context-relevant, unified curriculum is explained. Ideas about the core processes of faculty development, ongoing appraisal, and scholarship related to creating courses are proposed. The chapter concludes with a summary and synthesis activities.

SYNTHESIS ACTIVITIES

The Blue Seas College School of Nursing case includes information about three faculty members who are creating a course entitled *Supporting Health Through Life's Milestones*. Questions follow that provide a basis for analysis of the situation. Subsequently, questions and activities are suggested that might assist readers when creating courses in their own settings.

Blue Seas College School of Nursing

Blue Seas College is an undergraduate college offering degrees in liberal arts and sciences, as well as education and nursing. As can be expected from its name, the college is located in a medium-sized city overlooking the Pacific Ocean. The college began as a normal school in 1872 to train high school graduates to become school teachers. Over time, the normal school became a college and expanded the program offerings, with the School of Nursing program beginning 40 years ago. With education as the foundation of the college, the quality of teaching has always been a priority in all disciplines.

The School of Nursing is comprised of 16 full-time faculty and 22 part-time faculty who engage mainly in professional practice teaching. All full-time faculty are expected to maintain some professional practice in addition to their teaching and research requirements. Faculty members and supportive stakeholders have just redesigned the nursing curriculum. The nursing program model is 4 years and integrated. The curriculum philosophical approaches include elements of humanism, feminism, and phenomenology. There is agreement to adhere to ideas about cognitive constructivism and brain-based learning in the educational approaches.

Professors McInnes and Suarez are assigned the task of developing a course to be offered in the second semester of the curriculum, *Supporting Health Through Life Transitions*. Among the concepts determined for this introductory theory course are *growth and development, death and dying, health, health promotion, nursing, support,* and *transitions*. In subsequent courses, life transitions, such as pregnancy and birth, major illness events, and death and dying, will be addressed in more detail and depth.

The draft description prepared by the curriculum design team is: *An introduction to significant life transitions from birth to death and supportive nursing for individuals and families during periods of change.* The course competencies have not been prepared in detail. Instead, the curriculum designers have proposed that the competencies relate to an understanding and application of the concepts in individual and family situations, and understanding and application of supportive nursing strategies during normal life transitions.

Within the current curriculum, Professor McInnes is teaching theory and professional practice courses focused on maternal-infant-child health. Her practice area is labor and delivery. Professor Suarez's theory and professional practice teaching is in the areas of acute and chronic illness, and her practice is with adults undergoing surgery.

Questions and Activities for Critical Analysis of the Blue Seas College of Nursing Case

1. Consider the brief course description and course competencies provided by the curriculum design team. Describe the ideas that immediately come to mind about the nature of this course.
2. Review the information about the course competencies provided by the curriculum design team. What are your thoughts about this information as a starting point for developing course competencies? If there is more information that you would like to have, what would it be?
3. Analyze how the teaching and practice experiences of Professors McInnes and Suarez might influence the creation of the course.
4. What might be the scope of content that would be reasonable to include in this introductory course?
5. How could the concepts and content be matched?
6. Develop a draft of this course, including an expanded description, competencies, class titles, strategies to develop learning, and opportunities to demonstrate learning.
7. Create the guidelines for student learning activities for one class.

Questions and Activities for Consideration When Creating Courses in Readers' Settings

1. Identify the parameters of course design. How will these influence decisions about course creation?
2. Which approach(es) to course design would be appropriate and why?
3. Consider the merits of creating course templates to facilitate discussion and decision making.

4. What should be the purpose, description, and outcomes of the courses?
5. How can the scope of content for the courses be determined?
6. How can course concepts and content be matched?
7. Describe strategies to ignite learning that would match the educational and philosophical approaches of the curriculum.
8. Design opportunities for students to demonstrate learning that are aligned with course competencies.
9. Propose a strategy to follow if a final course design does not match the previously determined curriculum map(s).
10. Plan faculty development activities related to creating courses.
11. Suggest questions that could be asked in the ongoing appraisal of courses as they are being created.
12. Propose scholarship activities that could be undertaken.

REFERENCES

Anderson, L. W., Krathwohl, D. R., Airasian, P. W., Cruikshank, K. A., Mayer, R. E., Pintrich, P. R., . . . Wittrock, M. C. (Eds.). (2001). *A taxonomy for learning, teaching, and assessing: A revision of Bloom's taxonomy of educational objectives.* New York: Longman.

Bevis, E. O. (1982). *Curriculum building in nursing: A process* (3rd ed.). St. Louis, MO: Mosby.

Bevis, E. O. (2000). Teaching and learning: The key to education and professionalism. In E. O. Bevis & J. Watson (Eds.), *Toward a caring curriculum: A new pedagogy for nursing* (pp. 153–188). Sudbury, MA: Jones and Bartlett.

Boud, D., & Falchikov, N. (2006). Aligning assessment with long-term learning. *Assessment & Evaluation in Higher Education, 31,* 399–413.

Bowe, F. G. (2000). *Universal design in education: Teaching nontraditional students.* Westport, CT: Bergin & Garvey.

Community Health Nurses of Canada. (2011). *Canadian community health nursing: Professional practice model and standards of practice.* Toronto, ON: Author.

Conklin, T. A. (2013). Making it personal: The importance of student experience in creating autonomy-supportive classrooms for millennial learners. *Journal of Management Education, 37,* 499–538.

Crookes, K., Crookes, P., & Walsh, K. (2013). Meaningful and engaging teaching techniques for student nurses: A literature review. *Nurse Education in Practice, 13,* 239–243.

Day, L. (2011). Using unfolding case studies in a subject-centered classroom. *Journal of Nursing Education, 50,* 447–452.

De Gagne, J. C., Oh, J., Kang, J., Vorderstrasse, A. A., & Johnson, C. M. (2013). Virtual worlds in nursing education: A synthesis of the literature. *Journal of Nursing Education, 52,* 391–396.

Erickson, H. L. (2007). *Concept-based curriculum and instruction for the thinking classroom.* Thousand Oaks, CA: Corwin Press.

Gagné, R. M., Briggs, L. J., & Wager, W. W. (1992). *Principles of instructional design* (4th ed.). Fort Worth, PA: Harcourt Brace Jovanovich.

Goldenberg, D., & Iwasiw, C. L. (1992). Reciprocal learning among students in the clinical area. *Nurse Educator, 17*(5), 27–29.

Gulikers, J. T. M., Bastiaens, T., & Kirschner, P. A. (2004). A five-dimensional framework for authentic assessment. *Educational Technology, Research and Development, 52*(3), 67–85.

Heinrich, C. R., Karner, K. J., Gaglione, B. H., & Lambert, L. S. (2002). Order out of chaos: The use of a matrix to validate curriculum integrity. *Nurse Educator, 27*(3), 136–140.

Higbee, J. L. (2009). Implementing universal instructional design in postsecondary courses and curricula. *Journal of College Teaching and Learning, 6*(8), 65–77.

Hsu, A., & Malkin, F. (2011). Shifting the focus from teaching to learning: Rethinking the role of the teacher educator. *Contemporary Issues in Education Research, 4*(12), 43–49.

Iwasiw, C. L. (1987). The role of teacher in self-directed learning. *Nurse Education Today, 7,* 222–227.

Iwasiw, C. L., & Goldenberg, D. (1993). Peer teaching among students in the clinical area: Effects on student learning. *Journal of Advanced Nursing, 18,* 659–668.

Mennenga, H. A. (2013). Student engagement and examination performance in a team-based learning course. *Journal of Nursing Education, 52,* 475–479.

Milman, N. B. (2012). The flipped classroom strategy: What is it and how can it best be used? *Distance Learning, 9*(3), 85–87.

Missildine, K., Fountain, R., Summers, L., & Gosselin, K. (2013). Flipping the classroom to improve student performance and satisfaction. *Journal of Nursing Education, 52,* 597–599.

O'Connor, K. J. (2013). Class participation: Promoting in-class student engagement. *Education, 133,* 340–344.

Oermann, M. H., & Gaberson, K. B. (2014). *Evaluation and testing in nursing education* (4th ed.). New York: Springer.

Plutarch. (n.d.). *The mind is not a vessel to be filled, but a fire to be ignited.* Retrieved from http://edgalaxy .com/education-quotes/

Popkess, A. M., & McDaniel, A. (2011). Are nursing students engaged in learning? A secondary analysis of data from the National Survey of Student Engagement. *Nursing Education Perspectives, 32,* 89–94.

Read, C. Y., Vessey, J. A., Amar, A. F., & Cullinan, D. M. (2013). The challenges of inclusivity in baccalaureate nursing programs. *Journal of Nursing Education, 52,* 185–190.

Reese, C. E. (2011). Unfolding case studies. *Journal of Continuing Education in Nursing, 42,* 344–345.

Rusche, S. N., & Jason, K. (2011). "You have to absorb yourself in it": Using inquiry and reflection to promote student learning and self-knowledge. *Teaching Sociology, 39,* 338–353.

Saunders, S., & Kardia, D. (n.d.). Creating inclusive college classrooms. Center for Research on Learning and Teaching, University of Michigan. Retrieved from http://www.crlt.umich.edu/gsis/p3_1

Schmitt, T., Sims-Giddens, S., & Booth, R. (2012). Social media use in nursing education. *The Online Journal of Issues in Nursing, 17*(3), 2.

Seaton-Sykes, P. (2003). *Teaching and learning in Internet environment in Australian nursing education* (Unpublished doctoral dissertation). Griffith University, Queensland, Australia.

Smith, C. M. (2012). Harnessing mobile devices in the classroom. *Journal of Continuing Education in Nursing, 43,* 539–540.

SmithBattle, L. (2012). Learning to see the other through student-created dramas. *Journal of Nursing Education, 51*, 591–594.

Stanley, M. J. C., & Dougherty, J. P. (2010). A paradigm shift in nursing education: A new model. *Nursing Education Perspectives, 31*, 378–380.

Sutinen, A. (2008). Constructivism and education: Education as an interpretative transformational process. *Studies in Philosophy and Education, 27*(1), 1–14.

PART V

Implementation and Evaluation of an Evidence-Informed, Context-Relevant, Unified Curriculum

Ensuring Readiness for Curriculum Implementation

Chapter Overview

Implementing an evidence-informed, context-relevant, unified curriculum requires planning and effort throughout the curriculum development process so that the curriculum will be actualized as conceived. Ensuring that the curriculum is ready to be introduced, and that there will be fidelity of implementation, requires engaging stakeholders, logistical planning, and preparation of faculty and students, matters that are discussed in this chapter. The relationship of readiness and fidelity of implementation to an evidence-informed, context-relevant, unified curriculum is described. The core components of curriculum work (i.e., faculty development, ongoing appraisal, and scholarship) are presented. A case is included for analysis, and questions are posed for readers to consider as they prepare to introduce a redesigned curriculum in their own settings.

Chapter Goals

- Consider the meaning of *readiness* in relation to curriculum implementation.
- Integrate ideas of *fidelity of implementation* into understandings of curriculum work.
- Examine the roles of stakeholders, faculty, and students in contributing to readiness for, and fidelity of, implementation.
- Consider the logistical aspects of preparing for curriculum implementation.
- Appreciate the relationship of readiness and fidelity of implementation to an evidence-informed, context-relevant, unified curriculum.
- Reflect on the core processes of curriculum development as they relate to readiness for, and fidelity of, curriculum implementation.

READINESS FOR CURRICULUM IMPLEMENTATION

Readiness for curriculum implementation connotes being in a state of preparedness to introduce the curriculum and fully enact its tenets. Readiness encompasses:

- Willingness of faculty, stakeholders, and students to engage in the processes inherent in the redesigned curriculum
- Sufficient intellectual and behavioral preparation and support to enact the willingness
- Adequacy of external conditions and resources to make enactment of the curriculum possible

Readiness builds as the curriculum is being developed and attention is given to engagement of stakeholders, logistics, and preparation of faculty and students.

FIDELITY OF CURRICULUM IMPLEMENTATION

The term *fidelity of implementation* refers to the extent to which a program is implemented as conceived by the developers, or "how well an intervention is implemented in comparison to the original program design" (O'Donnell, 2008, p. 33). Criteria for assessing intervention fidelity that are relevant for curriculum implementation planning are related to structure and process.

The structure criteria relevant to educational programs are: (1) *adherence*, whether the components are being delivered as designed; and (2) *duration*, or the number, length, and frequency of sessions implemented. The process criterion is *quality of delivery*, that is, the style in which the program is delivered through use of the approved techniques and processes (Harn, Parisi, & Stoolmiller, 2013; O'Donnell, 2008). *Participant involvement*, how participants respond to or are engaged by an intervention, is another criterion that has aspects of both the structure and process dimensions (Ruiz-Primo, as cited in O'Donnell, 2008). Achievement of these criteria is related, in part, to the readiness for curriculum implementation.

To ensure readiness and attain fidelity of implementation, faculty members forecast the conditions that must be in place for the curriculum to be operationalized as conceived, and then make the arrangements for these conditions to be realized. Therefore, implementation planning is a simultaneous and constant feature of curriculum development. Among the matters that curriculum developers consider when planning for implementation are engagement of stakeholders, logistics, and preparation of faculty and students.

ENGAGING STAKEHOLDERS TO ENHANCE READINESS FOR, AND FIDELITY OF, IMPLEMENTATION

Implementation of a redesigned curriculum should not be a surprise to the community because relevant stakeholders (such as members of community and healthcare agencies) have been included in the data gathering that leads to an evidence-informed, context-relevant, unified curriculum. They have participated in curriculum development and served on advisory committees. All who have been involved in, and will be affected by, the curriculum redesign ought to be thoroughly prepared for its implementation. Informing others of evolving plans, and involving them in implementation planning, best occurs simultaneously with curriculum development. In this way:

- Curriculum plans are feasible.
- Stakeholders are ready for a redesigned curriculum.
- Practical steps are taken to ensure structural and process aspects of implementation fidelity.
- It is possible to implement the curriculum as conceived.

Informing Stakeholders

Stakeholder involvement in the creation of an evidence-informed, context-relevant, unified curriculum results in a sense of curriculum ownership and a desire to ensure its successful implementation. To this end, stakeholders can become regular and effective messengers, keeping others apprised of forthcoming changes and their rationale. The stakeholders help shape the path for a smooth transition from one curriculum to another.

Students

Current students ought to be informed about ongoing curriculum development because they are naturally interested in the planned curriculum changes and what the changes will mean for them. This information sharing can be accomplished by faculty and students who are involved in the curriculum development process. Students can be very helpful in explaining and promoting the developing curriculum to their peers. Therefore, it is prudent for faculty members to be diligent in keeping students informed.

The Educational Institution

As curriculum development proceeds, consultation with senior administrators and chairpersons of relevant institution-wide committees is ongoing. Keeping these people apprised of the developing curriculum will expedite approval. In addition, negotiations about non-nursing courses and their scheduling have to be concluded before the curriculum is finalized.

Similarly, arrangements for financial resources, student services, library resources, technological support, and so forth are necessary before curriculum approval is requested. Assurance about these matters is gained by engaging administrators and directors of relevant services in discussion early in the curriculum development process. In this way, they can alert the leader of the school of nursing, or the curriculum leader, about any anticipated problems, and attend to financial and personnel implications within their units.

Healthcare and Community Agencies

Involvement and support of stakeholders outside the educational institution are foundational to a curriculum with a practice component. Steering committee members serve as ambassadors for the new curriculum to nursing professional practice and community agencies. However, support from these and other nursing leaders, while essential, may not be sufficient to ensure successful implementation in placement sites.

Personnel with whom students will be working in professional practice placements require information about the curriculum redesign. Information sharing can be accomplished, in part, through formal presentations and the provision of written materials. More detailed, small-group meetings are also necessary to orient nursing and other staff to new learning goals or outcomes, activities students will pursue, scheduling, and any plans related to the placement of students in the new curriculum who are completing a different program level from those currently there. Faculty members, whose work intersects with nursing personnel, have a critical role in this latter activity. Answering questions and allaying any apprehensions that might surface about the curriculum will be helpful in reducing misconceptions and subsequent misaligned expectations.

If placements are planned in agencies or units where students have not had previous professional practice experiences, curriculum orientation will be particularly important. Discussion can focus on expectations of students, the nature of student interactions with clients and staff, the desired nature of staff-faculty-student interactions, and logistical details. Interpreting the role of nursing education and explaining how nursing students will contribute to the agency mission and client well-being are particularly important.

Attending to Contractual Arrangements with Healthcare and Community Agencies

Nursing programs are usually required to have formal agreements with agencies in which students have professional practice experiences. Educational administrators negotiate these affiliation or contractual agreements. Signed copies of the agreements are retained in the school of nursing and the agencies providing learning experiences.

If new placements are desirable for a redesigned curriculum, it is important to develop productive working relationships with agency personnel. During early meetings, the nature and expected outcomes of the practice experience can be explored and clarified. Agency personnel can explain the requirements of the setting and their expectations for students and faculty. These first meetings provide the basis for establishing a letter of agreement or a formal contract, both of which are later negotiated by administrative and legal personnel from both settings.

Meetings between faculty and agency staff are also necessary to complete the arrangements and discuss details of the learning experiences, such as:

- Nature of the experience
- Intended goals or outcomes for students
- Numbers and levels of students
- Students' schedules and roles
- Faculty members' roles
- Staff expectations and roles
- Other details important to individual experiences

These discussions confirm the appropriateness of faculty members' prior decisions about agencies and units to be used for clinical placements. The choices are linked to intended learning outcomes or goals, nature of available learning experiences, clients, compatibility of school and agency philosophies, practice model in use, staff, and resources and support for students (Gaberson & Oermann, 2010; Goldenberg & Iwasiw, 1988; Peters, Halcomb, & McInnes, 2013; Rodger et al., 2008; Schofield, Keane, Fletcher, Shrestha, & Percival, 2009). Because professional practice placements require negotiation, it is wise to create a plan for placements that covers several years. A tentative plan that takes into account the phasing out of one curriculum and the introduction of a redesigned curriculum allows members of healthcare and community agencies to assess the impact on their services and staff, and thus, the plan's feasibility within agencies. It is likely that modifications to the proposed plan will be necessary, and these can be determined within the context of readiness and fidelity of implementation.

Legal Areas of Concern

Nurse educators are concerned about issues related to student-educational-institutional relationships and their own professional liability if students make errors in their care activities. The calendar (bulletin) and other school documents, such as the student handbook, represent an agreement between students and the educational institution, and typically include a policy about safe professional practice. In professional practice settings, these documents have legal implications as they guide student and faculty behavior.

The responsibility and accountability of the educational institution, healthcare or community agency, faculty, students, and agency staff should be clarified. All matters related to the legal aspects of clinical education are addressed when contracts are negotiated and arrangements are made for student practice.

Insurance

Contracts with community and healthcare agencies generally stipulate that the educational institution must have insurance for student practice. The insurance policies should be made known to faculty and students and address matters such as harm to clients, faculty and student liability, student injuries, and equipment loss or breakage. Additionally, the educational institution might require that students and faculty have their own professional liability insurance (Rodger et al., 2008).

Additional Considerations

Other matters may be addressed in discussions, formal contracts, or letters of agreement between the school of nursing and the healthcare or community agency. These might include considerations, such as:

- Whether full names of all students and instructors be specified prior to the experience (O'Connor, 2001)
- The maximum student-to-faculty ratio (O'Connor, 2001)
- An orientation of faculty and students to agency policies and procedures
- Health requirements
- Cardiopulmonary resuscitation and first-aid certification of faculty and students
- Effect of faculty absence on student experience
- Patients' or clients' rights with respect to care by students
- Responsibilities of staff in relation to student learning

Completion of contractual arrangements with healthcare and community agencies fulfills the requirement that satisfactory arrangements are in place for the professional practice aspects of the curriculum to be enacted. These arrangements are pertinent for the criteria of *adherence* and *duration*. Moreover, discussions about the details of learning experiences contribute to the *adherence* and *participant involvement* criteria of fidelity of implementation.

Maintaining Ongoing Communication with Stakeholders

During curriculum development, regular meetings with students, nurses, and others interested in knowing about the curriculum will serve to maintain open dialogue and facilitate a feeling of inclusion. Similarly, an electronic newsletter or a regularly updated website outlining progress and responses to frequently asked questions makes the process transparent and keeps interested parties informed about curriculum development progress and implementation plans.

Once implementation of the redesigned curriculum begins, follow-up meetings at placement sites to review and discuss student experiences will promote ongoing successful implementation. These meetings can address:

- What is working well
- Concerns expressed by staff and/or students
- Appropriate actions to resolve concerns and capitalize on successes

Further to facilitating learning experiences for students, these meetings provide opportunities to:

- Demonstrate the educational institution's interest in the views of practitioners
- Express appreciation for practitioners' involvement in student learning
- Bring to light learning experiences not previously considered
- Build commitment to student learning

Regular meetings of this nature contribute to healthy relationships with healthcare and community agencies. Importantly, they provide opportunities to reinforce ideas about the curriculum with agency personnel, thereby contributing to the readiness of agency personnel to support the curriculum and to achievement of the *adherence*, *quality of delivery*, and *participation* criteria of fidelity of implementation.

LOGISTICAL PLANNING FOR STRUCTURAL ASPECTS OF FIDELITY OF IMPLEMENTATION

Planning for fidelity of implementation for the nursing curriculum necessitates attention to structural features, that is, the conditions that will allow the curriculum to proceed as envisioned. Success requires a commitment by all curriculum participants to the institutional mission, purposes of education in general and nursing education in particular, the curriculum philosophical and educational approaches, and goals or outcomes. Additionally, sufficient finances and human resources are mandatory to mount and implement the curriculum, matters that require attention while the curriculum is being developed.

Attention to scheduling, requests for classrooms, laboratories, and professional practice placements is important as the existing curriculum is phased out and the redesigned curriculum introduced. All these matters affect the criterion of *adherence*, which subsequently affects the *quality of delivery* criterion of fidelity of implementation.

Ensuring Necessary Personnel

Faculty

Having sufficient numbers of qualified faculty to teach the courses is of paramount importance. Nursing school leaders will need to plan whom to retain, recruit, and appoint. Characteristics of suitable faculty include expertise, teaching skills, practice competence, effective interpersonal relationships, attributes of effective teachers, and willingness to accept and operationalize the tenets of the curriculum.

Some faculty will probably be required to teach in the existing and redesigned curricula simultaneously, and they may feel overstretched as they strive for excellence in both. It would be wise for the school leader to consider suitable teaching assignments carefully to ensure that not too much is expected of some individuals. Conversely, some faculty may be faced with the prospect of a lightened teaching assignment, or even with no obvious teaching responsibilities for a semester or an academic year, as the redesigned curriculum is being introduced. The school leader is responsible for maintaining teaching loads that are consistent with workload agreements so that there is a perception of fairness, and so that faculty and students are well served in the process.

In the event that additional faculty will be required, hiring becomes necessary and adjunct faculty could be engaged for some of the teaching. Inevitably, this would necessitate planning and organizing faculty orientation and development sessions that would require experienced and willing faculty to conduct these activities.

It is also possible that fewer faculty, or faculty with different expertise from those currently employed, will be required. This could result in the loss of valued members who do not hold permanent appointments. It is incumbent upon the school leader to minimize the pain to these individuals and their teaching colleagues.

Support Staff

Administrative, secretarial, and clerical services are necessary to implement the curriculum successfully. Personnel such as administrative assistants, secretaries, staff to manage student practice placements, and information technology support staff are to be aligned with the redesigned curriculum.

Scheduling Courses and Requesting Classrooms, Laboratories, and Professional Practice Placements

A student timetable that includes nursing and non-nursing courses, and laboratory and professional practice time, needs to be developed for each semester. Some aspects of the plan will likely have to be negotiated with other departments in the institution. Schedules and space requirements ought to be determined far enough in advance of the semester in which they are required so that institutional deadlines for classroom and laboratory requests can be met.

Similarly, healthcare and community agencies have deadlines for placement requests and the school of nursing is obliged to adhere to these. Scheduling for student placements likely requires joint planning with personnel from other programs and educational institutions. Students in other nursing programs, medicine, physical therapy, occupational therapy, psychology, and social work also need practice experiences. Therefore, it is vital that placement schedules for all these groups be coordinated within each healthcare and community agency where learning experiences occur.

If satisfactory timetables and other arrangements are achieved, then the organizing structures are in place to meet the criterion of *duration,* one aspect of fidelity of implementation. In addition, the assurance of some external conditions necessary to offer the curriculum is an aspect of readiness for implementation.

Phasing Out the Existing Curriculum and Introducing the Redesigned Curriculum

The process of phasing out the existing curriculum and introducing the redesigned one requires careful attention. It is common for experiences in a changed curriculum to be sequenced differently from how they had been in the previous one. Accordingly, students in both curricula may require similar classroom courses and access to the same practice sites at the same time. This curriculum overlap must be taken into account so neither group feels disadvantaged and practice sites are not overwhelmed by student numbers.

Attending thoughtfully to the sensitivities of students in the existing and in the redesigned curriculum is important. References by faculty to the "old" and "new" curriculum can engender negative feelings. Students in the existing curriculum might feel that their program is outdated and that faculty interest lies with the altered curriculum. Special attention ought to be given to this group so they do not harbor resentment. In contrast, the first students admitted to the redesigned curriculum often feel that they are "guinea pigs," an experimental group on which new educational approaches are being tested. This perception may be reinforced by the fact that some curricular refinements will likely occur for the next class that is admitted. Faculty need to consistently demonstrate confidence in both curricula and convey their belief that all students are receiving an education that will lead to competent nursing practice.

Further, faculty would be wise to think about how much overlap from the redesigned curriculum into the existing one is permissible. Understandably, as faculty members become immersed in altered philosophical and educational approaches, and emphasize different concepts, they might introduce these into the current curriculum. They may be influenced by changed curriculum goals or outcomes and can unintentionally modify their expectations of students in the curriculum that is being phased out. It is worthwhile to discuss this overlap and come to agreement about alterations (if any) that will occur so that a suitable balance is achieved between introducing students to new perspectives and maintaining the integrity of the existing curriculum.

Planning for Fidelity of Implementation with Nursing Faculty and Students

Nursing Faculty

Faculty development throughout the curriculum development process is preparation for implementation. As faculty learn about curriculum processes and develop the curriculum, they become imbued with the tenets of the redesigned curriculum. Scales (1985) commented, "Faculty [who have] developed the curriculum . . . will own, honor, and respect the curriculum and will aggressively and actively implement it" (p. 108). However, the ability to elevate curriculum plans to reality cannot be assumed.

Adherence and *quality of delivery*, two aspects of fidelity of implementation, hinge on faculty adoption (Woolley, Rose, Mercado, & Orthner, 2013). Therefore, active preparation of faculty and ongoing support as the redesigned curriculum is introduced are foundational to implementation that adheres to the original intent and is of the quality expected. Without such support, curriculum planning may be little more than an academic exercise (Wiles, 2005), with some faculty reverting to previous approaches.

It is wise to identify core teaching skills that are consistent with the philosophical and educational approaches chosen for the curriculum, and to provide opportunities for faculty to practice the skills. Small-group learning and practice with peer feedback can lessen the discomfort of "learning to teach." These microteaching sessions are best led by a trusted, nonjudgmental colleague who can demonstrate the desired skills and coach others. In a concept-based curriculum, faculty can find it helpful to witness how a concept-based class is conducted. A large-group session could be planned, with one faculty member leading the "class" of a small group of colleagues. Then, the observers, "students," and "teacher" might discuss the conduct of the class, sharing observations, questions, insights, doubts, and additional suggestions. If such a session is undertaken as course creation begins, faculty will have a solid basis for planning individual classes.

Additionally, faculty development could be directed at methods to evaluate student learning that are reflective of the curriculum foundations. Ideas could be presented and discussed, with attention given to how the ideas are aligned with the intent of the curriculum. It would be important to allow time for faculty members to consider how new ideas could be applied in their courses. If a particular method has been chosen for use throughout the curriculum, such as the use of reflective reports of professional practice, faculty members may need practice in responding to the reflections.

Ongoing faculty development is an essential component of curriculum implementation. Typically, faculty members experience doubts and questions when they actualize the plans, and these become the basis of faculty development sessions. As faculty become familiar with the curriculum tenets and methods, new questions will arise, and these will require attention in individual or small-group mentoring sessions, or larger group settings.

Informal faculty development sessions can be planned to discuss issues related to implementation. For example, biweekly or monthly "lunch and learn" meetings can be scheduled. During these sessions, peer discussion and problem solving could provide a basis for deeper understanding and adherence to curriculum tenets.

For faculty members who have not been involved in curriculum development, such as part-time professional practice instructors, planned faculty development is vital. If the curriculum is to have fidelity of implementation, it is essential that all members with a responsibility for facilitating and evaluating student learning be fully immersed in its tenets.

Fidelity and sustainability of curriculum implementation have been positively related to ongoing, meaningful professional development (Penuel, Fishman, Yamaguchi, & Gallagher, 2007), professional development customized for participants, contextualized coaching, and modifications to the teaching intervention to suit local contexts (Harn et al., 2013). Noteworthy is a study of fidelity of implementation of research-based instructional strategies in engineering science courses. Study findings were that the more complex the intervention (e.g., service-learning), the lower the fidelity, that is, the implementation of all components of the strategy (Borrego, Cutler, Prince, Henderson, & Froyd, 2013). These findings have relevance for nursing curriculum implementation. Specifically, ongoing faculty development is necessary for new educational approaches; some flexibility in implementation can be appropriate; and the more complex the educational approach, the more sustained support is necessary. In these ways, *adherence* and *quality of delivery* are addressed and fidelity of implementation is strengthened.

Students

Students can be prepared and supported to participate in the redesigned curriculum through:

- Provision of information to prospective students that includes some detail about the:
  - Educational approaches and how students are expected to participate
  - Evaluation approaches and standards
- Explanations of expected student participation at the start of each course and in all course syllabi
- Adherence to expectations for student participation in the curriculum, possibly by including an evaluation aspect
- Opportunities for academic, personal, and financial support to enhance participation and success

Student readiness for participation in the curriculum will contribute to meeting the criteria of *adherence*, *quality of delivery*, and *participant involvement*, all of which are aspects of fidelity of implementation.

RELATIONSHIP OF ENSURING READINESS FOR AND FIDELITY OF IMPLEMENTATION TO AN EVIDENCE-INFORMED, CONTEXT-RELEVANT, UNIFIED CURRICULUM

Whereas course creation constitutes the culmination of the *development* of an evidence-informed, context-relevant, unified curriculum, it is curriculum *implementation* that is the embodiment of the ideas agreed to during the development process. All matters that influence readiness for implementation, and thus, fidelity of implementation, affect the integrity of the curriculum. Planning for and creating circumstances that will support readiness and fidelity of implementation will lead to the enactment of the evidence-informed, context-relevant, unified curriculum as it was designed.

CORE PROCESSES OF CURRICULUM WORK

Faculty Development

Faculty development activities in relation to planning for fidelity of implementation are described in the section entitled, *Planning for Fidelity of Implementation with Nursing Faculty and Students*. These activities should not be delayed until implementation is imminent, because it can take time to learn to enact new philosophical and educational approaches and integrate them fully into individuals' repertoires of action.

Ongoing Appraisal

As attention is given to implementation simultaneously with curriculum development, and immediately prior to implementation, faculty appraise readiness to deliver the curriculum as conceived. Their questions might be:

- Have the necessary steps been taken to negotiate for the needed professional practice placements? If the desired placement sites cannot accommodate our plans, what are our alternatives?
- How clear are we and agency personnel about the nature of the desired learning experiences and the roles of students, faculty, and staff?
- Do the plans for ongoing communication with healthcare and community agencies seem reasonable and sufficient?
- Do we have or can we acquire the classroom and laboratory space we need?
- Are the necessary technological resources available?
- Do faculty members feel ready to implement the curriculum as conceived? If not, what are the matters that need further attention?
- Are plans sufficient to help students participate fully in the curriculum?
- To what extent do we believe our plans will support fidelity of implementation? How can our plans be improved?

Scholarship

Scholarship activities could include a qualitative study about faculty members' and stakeholders' sense of readiness to implement a redesigned curriculum. A similar study could be conducted with healthcare and community agency personnel. Matters that might be addressed are their level of knowledge about the educational and philosophical approaches, comfort with enacting the new approaches, and confidence in the curriculum plans. Factors contributing to readiness and ideas to enhance readiness could emerge.

As the curriculum is being implemented, it would be worthwhile to note the logistical arrangements that work well, do not work, or were inadvertently omitted. Information of this nature would contribute to curriculum evaluation and refinement, and could form the basis of an article that would add to the literature about curriculum development in nursing education.

CHAPTER SUMMARY

Readiness for curriculum implementation includes willingness by individuals to enact the curriculum and the existence of external conditions that make the enactment possible.

Fidelity of implementation is the extent to which the curriculum is implemented as planned. Ensuring readiness and planning for fidelity of implementation are essential to fulfill the intentions of curriculum designers who have created an evidence-informed, context-relevant, unified curriculum. This preparation requires focused attention concurrently with curriculum development. The relationship of readiness and fidelity of implementation to an evidence-informed, context-relevant, unified curriculum is described. Ideas related to the core components of curriculum work, faculty development, ongoing appraisal, and scholarship are presented.

SYNTHESIS ACTIVITIES

Planning for implementation of a revised nursing curriculum at Sunset Meadows School of Nursing is described and followed by questions and activities related to the case. Then, questions and activities are presented to stimulate thinking when readers are planning curriculum implementation in their settings.

Sunset Meadows School of Nursing

Sunset Meadows School of Nursing offers a 20-month accelerated bachelor of science in nursing degree program. Following an internal curriculum evaluation, faculty members agreed that curricular changes were necessary. There was consensus that a revision, and not a complete curriculum change, would be appropriate.

Accordingly, Dr. Suzanne La Forêt, the school leader, requested that the undergraduate chair, Dr. Natalia Firenze, convene a task force to plan the curriculum revisions in response to the evaluation. Dr. Firenze then asked one faculty member from each semester of the curriculum to work with her on the revisions.

Dr. Firenze and the task force worked for 2 months to design a revised curriculum. In that time, they consulted widely with other faculty members within the School of Nursing. Their proposal entailed some significant changes, including course sequencing and educational approaches.

Specifically, the proposal included a resequencing of some nursing theory courses and the corequisite professional practice courses. Courses related to family health would move from the third to the second semester of the curriculum, and courses related to acute care nursing would move from the second to the third semester. The related non-nursing courses would be similarly resequenced.

Other changes included a stronger emphasis on social justice and advocacy within all nursing courses to respond to the community's socioeconomic situation.

If accepted, this will require some revisions within existing courses in class content and opportunities for students to demonstrate learning.

In relation to educational approaches, the curriculum task force recommended a shift from predominately teacher-centered approaches, such as lecturing, to more active teaching-learning strategies that require students to "work with" concepts and content during class. The task force particularly highlighted the value of ideas pertinent to brain-based learning.

Finally, in relation to logistics, Dr. Firenze and the task force recommended that curriculum changes be introduced in 12 months time. Satisfied with their proposal, the group is asking for approval of the revised curriculum plan.

Questions and Activities for Critical Analysis of the Sunset Meadows School of Nursing Case

1. What might be Dr. La Forêt's rationale for requesting that a task force redesign the curriculum? Provide the rationale for other approaches that might have been employed.

2. Identify questions that the task force can expect from their colleagues when the proposal is presented.

3. Consider the logistical arrangements that would be necessary to implement the curriculum revisions in 12 months time.

4. Propose ideas for discussion with healthcare personnel about the changed professional practice placements. What might be the concerns of healthcare personnel?

5. As changes are implemented, there will be a semester when two classes require the same professional practice placements. How could this be managed?

6. Create a plan to prepare faculty members to implement changed teaching-learning strategies.

7. Plan other necessary activities to promote readiness for, and fidelity of, curriculum implementation.

Questions and Activities for Consideration When Ensuring Readiness for Curriculum Implementation in Readers' Settings

1. Describe the critical planning steps for successful curriculum implementation.

2. How can stakeholders be informed of the developing curriculum and implementation plans?

3. Who will be responsible for exploring learning opportunities in new practice sites? For initiating contract discussions? What assistance can be offered to nursing staff so they will be ready for students' learning experiences?

4. Examine the human, physical, and financial resources necessary to ensure fidelity of curriculum implementation. If all necessary resources are not available, what could be done to procure them or to modify the curriculum to match the resources?

5. Who will be responsible for apprising administrative personnel of the scheduling needs within the redesigned curriculum?

6. Propose strategies that might alleviate student concerns about being "guinea pigs" in a redesigned curriculum or being in a curriculum that is being phased out.

7. What are the plans for phasing out the existing curriculum?

8. Which ongoing faculty development activities could be planned?

9. Identify other matters that require thoughtful consideration to ensure readiness for, and fidelity of, curriculum implementation.

10. Suggest questions that might contribute to ongoing appraisal of readiness for curriculum implementation and fidelity of implementation?

11. Describe feasible scholarship projects related to readiness for curriculum implementation and fidelity of implementation.

REFERENCES

Borrego, M., Cutler, S., Prince, M., Henderson, C., & Froyd, J. E. (2013). Fidelity of implementation of research-based instruction strategies (RBIS) in engineering science courses. *Journal of Engineering Education, 102*, 394–435.

Gaberson, K. B., & Oermann, M. H. (2010). *Clinical teaching strategies in nursing* (3rd ed.). New York: Springer.

Goldenberg, D., & Iwasiw, C. (1988). Criteria used for patient selection for nursing students' hospital clinical experience. *Journal of Nursing Education, 27*, 258–265.

Harn, B., Parisi, D., & Stoolmiller, M. (2013). Balancing fidelity with flexibility and fit: What do we really know about fidelity of implementation in schools? *Exceptional Children, 79*, 181–193.

O'Connor, A. B. (2001). *Clinical instruction and evaluation: A teaching resource.* Sudbury, MA: Jones and Bartlett.

O'Donnell, C. L. (2008). Defining, conceptualizing and measuring fidelity of implementation and its relationship to outcomes in K–12 curriculum intervention research. *Review of Educational Research, 78*(1), 33–84.

Penuel, W. R., Fishman, B. J., Yamaguchi, R., & Gallagher, L. P. (2007). What makes professional development effective? Strategies that foster curriculum implementation. *Educational Research Journal, 44*, 921–958.

Peters, K., Halcomb, E. J., & McInnes, S. (2013). Clinical education in general practice: Relationships between practice nurses and tertiary institutions. *Nurse Education in Practice, 13,* 186–191.

Rodger, S., Webb, G., Devitt, L., Gilbert, J., Wrightson, P., & McMeeken, J. (2008). Clinical education and practice placements in the allied health professions: An international perspective. *Journal of Allied Health, 37,* 53–62.

Scales, F. S. (1985). *Nursing curriculum development, structure, function.* Norwalk, CT: Appleton-Century-Crofts.

Schofield, D., Keane, S., Fletcher, S., Shrestha, R., & Percival, R. (2009). Loss of income and levels of scholarship support for students on rural clinical placements: A survey of medical, nursing and allied health students. *Australian Journal of Rural Health, 17,* 134–140.

Wiles, J. (2005). *Curriculum essentials: A resource for educators* (2nd ed.). Boston: Pearson Education.

Woolley, M. E., Rose, R. A., Mercado, M., & Orthner, D. K. (2013). Teachers teaching differently: A qualitative student of implementation fidelity to professional development. *Journal of Education and Training Studies, 1*(1), 55–68.

CHAPTER 15

Planning Curriculum Evaluation

Chapter Overview

Planning curriculum evaluation is an ongoing process, which begins simultaneously with curriculum design. Nursing faculty and administrators are not only responsible for formative and summative evaluation of the curriculum, but also preparation for program evaluation by external organizations. The definition, overview, and purposes of curriculum evaluation, as well as the benefits for those involved, are described. Evaluation models are overviewed and categorized. Attention is given to assessing fidelity of implementation. Planning evaluation, establishing standards, and determining data-gathering approaches are then addressed. This chapter also includes more specific information about planning evaluation of curriculum components, including goal or outcome statements, design, concepts, courses, strategies to ignite learning, and strategies to evaluate student achievement. Evaluation questions are suggested for each component. In addition, consideration is given to evaluation of learning climate, policies, and human and physical resources; and evaluation of actual curriculum outcomes. Judging curriculum quality, reporting results, and reflecting on the process are also included. The relationship of curriculum evaluation to an evidence-informed, context-relevant, unified curriculum is explained. A brief discussion of faculty development, ongoing appraisal, and scholarship related to curriculum evaluation is followed by the chapter summary and synthesis activities.

Chapter Goals

- Value evaluation planning as a component of curriculum development.
- Understand the purposes of internal and external curriculum evaluation.
- Gain insight into models of curriculum evaluation.
- Review evaluation of individual curriculum components and actual curriculum outcomes.
- Consider the merits of assessing fidelity of implementation.
- Appreciate the relationship of curriculum evaluation to an evidence-informed, context-relevant, unified curriculum.
- Reflect on the core processes of curriculum work related to planning curriculum evaluation.

DEFINITIONS OF CURRICULUM EVALUATION AND PROGRAM EVALUATION

Curriculum evaluation is:

> The assessment and judging of the merit and worth of the broad processes, elements, and resultant outcomes encompassed within an educational curriculum. Curriculum evaluation may include curriculum planning and design processes . . . , curriculum implementation . . . , and assessing the effectiveness of the implemented curriculum in creating desired student change. (Sullivan, 2009)

It is an organized and thoughtful appraisal of elements central to the course of studies undertaken by students, and of graduates' abilities. Curriculum evaluation involves establishment of standards, systematic data gathering, application of the standards, and formulation of judgments about the value, quality, utility, effectiveness, or significance of the curriculum (Fitzpatrick, Sanders, & Worthen, 2004). The aspects to evaluate include the philosophical approaches, goal or outcome statements, design, courses, and educational approaches, and strategies to evaluate students' achievement. Also assessed are actual curriculum outcomes, implementation fidelity, resources to support the curriculum, learning climate, and policies. Additionally, it is important to evaluate not just the "written, taught, and learned curriculum, but also the hidden and experienced curriculum" (Parkay, Hass, & Anctil, 2010, p. 357).

In contrast, program evaluation encompasses a wider scope of elements. In addition to all aspects of curriculum evaluation, program evaluation includes attention to institutional support for the school; administrative structure of the school; faculty members' teaching, research, and professional activities; and the school's relationships with other academic units, student support services, research institutes, and healthcare and community agencies.

Curriculum evaluation is utilization-focused evaluation, that is, "evaluation done for and with specific intended primary users for specific intended uses" (Patton, 2008, p. 37). Therefore, the evaluation questions and processes address matters that are significant to the users, most notably students and faculty. The knowledge generated, and the appraisal or judgment (evaluation) attached to the data, are context specific and applicable for a particular point in time (Alkin & Taut, 2003). Further, curriculum evaluation is dependent on participatory and collaborative approaches. Curriculum developers, implementers, evaluation designers, evaluators, and evaluation users are all faculty members who work together, along with other stakeholders, to achieve the evaluation purposes.

OVERVIEW OF THE CURRICULUM EVALUATION PROCESS

Purpose

The first, and possibly the most important, step in planning curriculum or program evaluation is to decide the purposes of the evaluation. Why is the curriculum being evaluated, and how will the evaluation data and conclusions be used? Answers to these questions will lead to the evaluation design.

Members to Involve in Evaluation Planning

Without question, faculty members have the major responsibility in planning for curriculum evaluation. If the evaluation is considered as the curriculum is being designed, all participants in curriculum development are inherently involved in planning curriculum evaluation. However, if planning for evaluation begins after curriculum implementation, it is prudent to consider who ought to be involved in addition to faculty. Students and other stakeholders have perspectives that faculty members might not consider.

Selection of an Evaluation Model

Agreement about the purposes leads to the selection of a suitable evaluation model. This choice is influenced by the curriculum's philosophical orientation, members' familiarity with various models, match between the evaluation purposes and models, and the timespan in which the evaluation must be completed and subsequent decisions made. Then, evaluation questions based on the purpose and consistent with the model are formulated. From this, the precise elements to be evaluated are determined and standards defined.

Creation of an Evaluation Framework

An overall curriculum evaluation framework is required. Typically, what is evaluated is the fidelity of implementation and the outcomes. For process and outcome components, participants, accountabilities, required data, data sources, data-gathering methods, required resources, and timelines are defined. Also included in the evaluation design are the following: a system to manage data, plans to analyze and interpret data, and procedures to report results. An evaluation of the overall process is the final step (Fitzpatrick et al., 2004; Keating, 2011; Patton, 2013; Posavac, 2011). Through this meta-evaluation, participants can identify the learning they have gained from the process, thereby increasing their own capacities (Patton, 2013).

As part of the framework, decisions are made about the necessity of designing data-gathering tools. These may be surveys, interview and observation guides, curriculum maps, and so forth, depending on the philosophical basis of the framework. The use of data that are already available, such as institutionally mandated course evaluations, or student projects, lessens the need to create data-gathering tools, thus reducing the work associated with curriculum evaluation.

Developing an Overall Curriculum Evaluation Plan

Curriculum evaluation should not be a one-time activity undertaken in preparation for external curriculum review. Rather, it should be a regular process that leads to curriculum improvement. Curriculum monitoring, formative feedback, and summative evaluation form part of an overall curriculum evaluation plan within a school of nursing. Ongoing data gathering, analysis, and interpretation are the bases of formative feedback as the curriculum is being implemented and become part of the summative evaluation. It is necessary to develop a plan for ongoing curriculum review and for the resources that are needed to implement the plan. **Figure 15-1** is an example of a summarized evaluation plan, which incorporates university-mandated teaching and course evaluations and the adopted evaluation framework (Relevance-Congruence-Adequacy-Reasonableness).

Implementing and Monitoring the Evaluation Plan

Once a curriculum evaluation plan has been created, it is then implemented. Data are gathered in accordance with the evaluation framework and analyzed, and conclusions are drawn. As the plan is being implemented, the procedures are monitored to assess their quality and comprehensiveness (see *Ongoing Appraisal* later in this chapter).

Reporting Results and Making Decisions

Evaluation results are reported to curriculum participants and external stakeholders. Following discussion about the results, faculty members make decisions with respect to curriculum maintenance, refinement, modification, reorganization, or discontinuance and replacement, and a new cycle of curriculum development or revision begins.

PURPOSES OF INTERNAL CURRICULUM EVALUATION AND EXTERNAL PROGRAM EVALUATION

Purposes of Internal Curriculum Evaluation

Internal curriculum evaluation is conducted by members of a school of nursing to determine the curriculum strengths, weaknesses, merits, and deficits. Additionally, identification of

Figure 15-1   Summary of curriculum evaluation plan.
Developed by Carroll Iwasiw RN, EdD. © Western-Fanshawe Collaborative BScN Program. Used with permission.

DATA FOR FORMATIVE EVALUATION	DATA FOR SUMMATIVE EVALUATION
Annually • Teaching evaluation data • University course evaluations • Student feedback about practice placements • Agency feedback about student placement experiences	**Annually** • Canadian Nurse Registration Exam results • Institutional graduate survey • Nursing graduate survey • Preceptors' perceptions of graduating students' achievement of curriculum goals **Every 4-5 Years** • Review of pattern of annual formative and summative evaluations • External context: demographics; culture; national and regional health profile; nursing practice and nursing education standards and trends; and socio-political-economics • Students' responses to the curriculum, perceptions of implementation fidelity and reasonableness, and suggestions for change • Faculty members' responses to the curriculum, perceptions of implementation fidelity and reasonableness, and suggestions for change • Practice leaders' perceptions of graduating students' achievement of curriculum goals • Nursing leaders': perceptions of BScN graduates, views about nursing in the future, and projections about the abilities necessary to practice nursing in the future

Undergraduate Curriculum Education Committee (receives all data)
- data interpretation according to the curriculum evaluation model
- development of curriculum recommendations
- reporting to faculty members and stakeholders

possible future directions for the curriculum is typically an outcome of the evaluation process (Oliva, 2009). As a quality-control mechanism, the intent of curriculum evaluation is to assure that the curriculum, its courses, the processes undertaken, and student achievement of expectations are meeting the required standards.

More specifically, the purposes of curriculum evaluation in nursing education are to:

1. Determine the extent to which:
   - The curriculum is meeting defined standards.
   - The curriculum is relevant for its context.
   - Unity, logical progression, and conceptual emphases are evident.
   - Implementation fidelity is maintained (i.e., the intended processes are being followed).
   - Outcomes are congruent with the curricular intent and demands of the external context.
   - Students, faculty, graduates, and employers are satisfied.
   - The curriculum likely fulfills approval and/or accreditation requirements.
2. Obtain data that will influence decisions about:
   - Curriculum maintenance, refinement, modification, reorganization, or discontinuance and replacement
   - Resource allocations and requests
   - Faculty development needs

Achievement of these purposes contributes to the ultimate purpose of curriculum evaluation, that is, to improve the quality of the curriculum and thus to improve the quality of the education that students experience.

Formative evaluation is carried out at regular intervals during curriculum implementation. The purpose is to provide evidence about the feasibility and effectiveness of a portion of the curriculum so that ongoing refinements and improvements can be made. Formative evaluation results provide a basis to form the curriculum (Posavac, 2011). Also referred to as *informative assessment* (Tomlison, 2010), formative evaluation is more than mere feedback; it is feedback in relation to a standard.

Formative evaluation involves purposeful data gathering, comparison of the data to a standard, and rendering of a judgment about a gap (if any exists) between the data and the standard. Therefore, standards must be in place so that a judgment can be made about feasibility and effectiveness. The principal data sources are faculty members and students. The audiences for the evaluation results are those who are affected by any subsequent conclusions or decisions (Gaberson & Vioral, 2014). Therefore, faculty, students, administrators, and possibly personnel in professional practice settings are the main audience for formative curriculum evaluation.

Summative evaluation is carried out at the completion of a portion of the curriculum, or the total curriculum. The purpose of this comprehensive evaluation is to judge the effectiveness of the curriculum, and this becomes the basis of recommendations about maintenance, revision, or discontinuance. Evidence is obtained from faculty members, students, graduates, administrators, employers, and other stakeholders. Audiences for summative evaluation results are those who provide evidence, as well as regulatory bodies, funders, consumers (Gaberson & Vioral, 2014), and committees within the educational institution that monitor curriculum quality.

Whether data are gathered for formative or summative purposes, there is an implicit expectation by those providing data that curriculum alterations will be forthcoming. Therefore, in all internal curriculum evaluations, often unstated and possibly unrecognized purposes include assuring all who provided evaluation data that:

- Faculty are committed to ensuring curriculum quality.
- The curriculum is responsive to influences within and beyond the school of nursing.
- Students will graduate from a dynamic and context-relevant curriculum.

Purposes of External Program Evaluation

External curriculum evaluation is undertaken as part of a more extensive program evaluation conducted for approval or accreditation by an outside agency. State or provincial approval and regional or national accreditation are processes by which an external organization evaluates and recognizes an institution or program of study as meeting certain predetermined criteria.

Approval

Nursing program approval is a compulsory evaluation or review process concerned primarily with the protection of public safety. This protection is accomplished by ensuring that a program has met prescribed minimum standards set by a body designated in state or provincial legislation, or according to regulations authorized by that legislation. Every nursing program leading to registration or licensure examinations must meet the standards of the body authorized to regulate nursing. Approval indicates that a nursing program is of a quality sufficient for graduates to be allowed to write the registration or licensing examination. Schools of Nursing cannot operate without approval because graduates would not be eligible to write the examination.

Accreditation

Accreditation is an endorsement of a nursing program by a nongovernmental agency concerned with nursing education; accreditation is understood to connote excellence. The accreditation process is generally voluntary, although in some jurisdictions it is required. It is a rigorous appraisal of a program to determine the extent to which it meets standards set by the profession. Nursing programs undergo accreditation to demonstrate their quality to the consumers of their products, that is, students, alumni, employers (Heydman & Sargent, 2011). Accreditation can be important in attracting students and faculty, and it can influence a school's eligibility for outside funding, graduates' admission to subsequent programs, and students' ability to obtain grants or loans.

BENEFITS OF PARTICIPATION IN PLANNING AND CONDUCTING CURRICULUM EVALUATION

Faculty

Participation in planning for curriculum evaluation and in the evaluation process may lead faculty members, individually and collectively, to increase their awareness and appreciation of curriculum evaluation and its value. They may expand their capacity to design and implement curriculum evaluation processes, and this will have relevance throughout their careers. Importantly, through involvement in evaluation planning and curriculum evaluation itself, faculty members may modify or develop deeper conceptual understandings of certain aspects of the curriculum (Alkin & Taut, 2003), and this could inherently improve their teaching. Additionally, the curriculum evaluation process may extend faculty members' capability to develop practical curriculum recommendations based on systematically gathered data, and this could strengthen their commitment to evidence-informed nursing education and augment their sense of empowerment. These benefits are independent of the evaluation findings (Robinson & Cousins, 2004).

Because it is the faculty who plan and undertake curriculum evaluation, determine recommendations from the evaluation data, and agree on subsequent actions, the value of curriculum evaluation extends beyond improvements to the curriculum itself. The process has rewards. For example, faculty members may experience benefits such as pride in being part of a progressive, dynamic program, or the social rewards and empowerment that accrue from engaging in important activities with colleagues and stakeholders. Moreover, curriculum improvements may yield increased student satisfaction, resulting in an enhanced teaching and learning environment.

Students and Other Stakeholders

All who are involved in planning for curriculum evaluation can experience the same benefits as those described for faculty members. Importantly, students and other stakeholders have the potential of ensuring that matters important to their constituencies are included in the evaluation.

For example, a group of undergraduate nursing students, supervised in a research practicum by two authors (Iwasiw and Andrusyszyn) of the second edition of this text, surveyed all undergraduate nursing students at Western University to determine matters they considered to be important to include in a curriculum evaluation. Students identified items about which they may not be routinely asked, such as the importance of choice in professional practice placements, consistency of professional practice instructors' expectations, course workload, clarity of course assignments, role of graduate teaching assistants, and expenditures additional to tuition (Fisher et al., 2003). Inclusion of matters important to students will yield a broader picture of curriculum implementation, provide information about the hidden and experienced curriculum, and implicitly reinforce the value of student perspectives in curriculum evaluation.

Stakeholders such as professional practice leaders also have ideas about what is important to evaluate in a curriculum, such as the nature of nursing staff–student relationships or the integration of skills learning in the curriculum. Although stakeholders may not be able to participate in the details of curriculum evaluation planning, their ideas can be obtained and integrated into curriculum evaluation processes and materials. In this way, their context-specific perspectives are honored and partnerships are strengthened.

CURRICULUM EVALUATION MODELS

A curriculum evaluation model is a framework that guides the evaluation of a curriculum. Variations in models arise from differing philosophies, and conceptions and definitions of evaluation. Accordingly, models differ in the emphasis placed on the curricular aspects to be examined, the approaches to data gathering, and the basis for judging the quality of the curriculum. The models provide a path for planning and conducting evaluation, not a detailed roadmap.

Evaluation models and approaches range from checklists and suggestions to comprehensive appraisals. Although models and approaches differ, they are all intended to shed light on the processes, outcomes, and value of a curriculum or program (Posavac, 2011). In nursing education, evaluation of the total curriculum is comprehensive, because a holistic evaluation is most appropriate for a unified curriculum. It is typically based on standards of quality and incorporates quantitative and qualitative approaches.

The presence of defined structural components and predetermined criteria generally lead to the use of quantitative approaches, although not exclusively. Examples are Scriven's Goal-Free Model, Provus's Discrepancy Evaluation Model, and program logic models. Questionnaires are typically used to obtain some data.

In contrast, qualitative models are more open. For example, the constructivist (fourth-generation) evaluation model addresses the concerns, claims, and issues of stakeholders, and the methods to examine these are negotiated with stakeholders (Guba & Lincoln, 2001). If the appreciative inquiry model (a fourth-generation model) is used, the focus is to discover what is working well, dream about what could be, design what should be, and then live the destiny that was created. With tenets of positive psychology as the foundation, the goal is to build on the positive through dialogue (Cooperrider, Whitney, & Stavros, 2008). This model has been used successfully in higher education (Cockell & McArthur-Blair, 2012; Harrison & Hasan, 2013). In qualitative approaches, data are obtained through direct observations and interviews, and guidelines for these are required.

Typologies of Evaluation Models

Evaluation models have been categorized into many typologies. Each classification system presents a different perspective on educational and service program evaluation, even though many of the same models are included. For instance, Stufflebeam and Shinkfield (2007) labeled models as:

- *Pseudoevaluations.* These are designed to achieve a hidden or corrupt purpose, or falsely label other activities such as training, as evaluation.
- *Questions- and methods-oriented evaluation approaches (quasi-evaluation studies).* Questions-oriented approaches may employ a range of methods to answer specific questions, while methods-oriented evaluation approaches use only one method.
- *Improvement- and accountability-oriented evaluation approaches.* These comprehensive approaches consider a full range of questions and criteria, including stakeholders' needs, and examine all relevant outcomes, not merely those tied to objectives.
- *Social agenda– and advocacy-oriented evaluation approaches.* These approaches aim to increase social justice through evaluation. Perspectives of stakeholders and experts are included in the investigation and judgment of programs. Qualitative methods and a constructivist orientation are fundamental to these approaches.

See **Table 15-1** for a list of the evaluation models according to this classification. Improvement- and accountability-oriented evaluation approaches are most frequently used in nursing education.

Guba and Lincoln's (1989) typology is a classification of evaluation models as to first, second, third, and fourth generations, according to the evaluation focus. See **Table 15-2** for a summary of the four generations of evaluation models.

Many curriculum and program evaluation models used in nursing education and service are third-generation models. Several are summarized in chronological order in **Table 15-3**.

Table 15-1	Stufflebeam and Shinkfield's Classification of Evaluation Approaches	
Classification	**Examples of Model or Approach**	**Description**
Pseudoevaluations	1. Public relations–inspired studies	The intent is to convince constituents of the value of a program.
	2. Politically controlled studies	Only data that support a covert agenda are released.
Questions- and Methods-Oriented Evaluation Approaches	1. Objectives-based studies	The purpose is to determine if the program's outcomes match the objectives.
	2. Success case method	The intent is to discover, analyze, and document successful aspects of a program so they can be extended to other parts of the program.
	3. Objective testing programs	Individual student scores are compared to local, state, or national norms or model performance.
	4. Performance testing	
	5. Criticism and connoisseurship	Experts in a given field are presumed to be able to provide analysis and evaluation not possible in other ways.
	6. Mixed-methods studies	The purpose is to provide direction for improving programs and to assess their effectiveness. Many evaluation questions are pursued through the use of quantitative and qualitative methods.
Improvement- and Accountability-Oriented Evaluation Approaches	1. Decision- and accountability-oriented studies (e.g., CIPP [Context, Input, Process, Product] Model)	The purpose is to provide information in a systematic way for proactive evaluation and decision making. It is also used for retroactive evaluation to address accountability.
	2. Accreditation and certification	The purposes are to determine if the institution or program meets the required standards and to provide recommendations for improvement.
Social Agenda and Advocacy Approaches	1. Constructivist evaluation (4th generation evaluation)	Evaluators and stakeholders attend to the claims, concerns, and issues, and jointly collect, analyze, and evaluate constructions of reality within and about a program, possibly creating new constructions.
	2. Deliberative, democratic evaluation	Through equitable involvement of stakeholders, dialogue to examine their ideas, and participatory deliberation, a defensible assessment of the program's merit and worth is achieved.

Source: Some data from Guba, E. G., & Lincoln, Y. S. (2001). *Guidelines and checklist for constructivist (a.k.a. Fourth Generation) evaluation*. Newbury Park, CA: Sage; and Stufflebeam, D. L., & Shinkfield, A. J. (2007). *Evaluation theory, models, and applications*. San Francisco, CA: Jossey-Bass.

Table 15-2 Summary of First-, Second-, Third-, and Fourth-Generation Evaluation Models	
First Generation (technical)	*Measurement (prior to WWI):* Students were targeted for evaluation. Tests were developed to measure variables of interest. Student scores were used to determine curriculum success.
Second Generation (description and technical)	*Description (post-WWI):* Curriculum was targeted for evaluation in an objectives-oriented (Tylerian) description approach (patterns, strengths, and weaknesses related to specific objectives). Congruence between student performance and described objectives was assessed. The program, materials, teaching strategies, organizational patterns, and "treatments" were evaluated. Measurement was redefined as one of several tools to use.
Third Generation (judgment-based, description, and technical)	*Judgment (post-1967):* Program goals and performance were targeted for evaluation. Judgments about merit and worth were based on standards. Information gathered depended on the evaluation model, such as decisions (decision-oriented models), experienced "effects" (goal-free models), or internalized guideposts (connoisseurship models).
Fourth Generation (holistic and inclusive)	*Responsive, constructivist, naturalistic (post–late 1970s):* Took into account the claims (values), concerns, and issues of those involved in the evaluation (students, faculty, clients, administrators). It is responsive (determines parameters and boundaries through an interactive, negotiated process that involves stakeholders), constructivist (interpretive, hermeneutic, relates to the methodology employed), and naturalistic (sociopolitical, diagnostic, change-oriented, education process) and rejects the controlling, manipulative, experimental approach. It results in a constructed understanding of needed improvements and changes, based on consensus of all stakeholders.

Source: Some data from Guba, E., & Lincoln, Y. (1989). *Fourth generation evaluation.* Newbury Park, CA: Sage.

Increasingly, however, elements of third- and fourth-generation models are combined to yield richer evaluations. For example, use of program logic models in evaluation is built on concepts underlying Provus's Discrepancy Evaluation Model (Fitzpatrick et al., 2004). This is primarily a third-generation model, because the focus of the evaluation and the indicators are known in advance. However, attention to stakeholders' concerns, claims, and interests may also be negotiated, more like fourth-generation evaluation.

Table 15-3   Summary of Several Third-Generation Evaluation Models and Their Value in Nursing Curriculum Evaluation

Models in Chronological Order	Description	Value in Nursing Curriculum Evaluation
Scriven's (1967, 1972) goal-free	Measures all outcomes/effects of program, regardless of program goals or objectives. There are no pre-specified objectives. May be applied to total or sections of the curriculum.	Access to unintended curriculum outcomes is possible, and, thus, insight into the hidden curriculum.
Donabedian's (1969) quality assurance	Measures efficiency and effectiveness of courses or units of study. Component parts include trial, structure, purpose, and output.	It can be useful for assessing segments of the curriculum.
Stufflebeam's (1971) CIPP	Involves decisions about planning (Context), structuring (Input), implementing (Process), and recycling (Product). Investigates what needs to be done, how it should be done, if it is being done, and if it succeeded. Assesses and reports on merit, worth, probability, significance.	Examination of relationships of curriculum elements is reflective of the integrated nature of nursing curricula.
Provus's (1971) discrepancy evaluation	Compares performance with standards to determine if a discrepancy exists between the two. Includes five stages: definition of program, installation of program, process, product or outcomes, and cost-benefit analysis. Involves intended vs. actual outcomes, and effects.	The process leads to identification of gaps between the enacted and planned curriculum.
Stake's (1972) (countenance) congruence-contingency	Involves congruence (agreement between desired and actual outcomes) and contingency (relationship among variables). Takes into account *antecedents* (characteristics of students, teachers, curriculum, facilities, materials, organization, community), *transactions* (all educational experiences), and *outcomes* (abilities, achievements, and attitudes resulting from educational experience).	Examination of all curriculum components is possible, as is drawing conclusions about curriculum processes and outcomes.

(continues)

Table 15-3   Summary of Several Third-Generation Evaluation Models and Their Value in Nursing Curriculum Evaluation (*continued*)

Models in Chronological Order	Description	Value in Nursing Curriculum Evaluation
Renzulli's (1972) key features	Considers major concerns of groups who have a direct or indirect interest in the program. Key features are prime interest groups and time.	The focus on concerns of particular groups (e.g., faculty or students) gives importance to their perspectives.
Parlett & Hamilton's (1972) illuminative evaluation	Proposes that understanding of the curriculum is possible only in its wider contexts and in the biography of each course. The approach is not predetermined but develops as issues or problems are identified. It is an ethnographic approach with two core concepts: instructional systems (courses) and learning milieu.	The focus on individual courses could lead to improvements within courses.
Stenhouse (1975)	Discloses meaning of curriculum, purposes of courses, problems amenable to solutions, influence of context on curriculum, and whether the evaluation contributes to theory development. Includes five criteria: meaning, potential, interest, conditionality, and elucidation.	A full understanding of curriculum problems is possible.
Eisner's (1977, 1985) connoisseur/critic	Premise is that experts (connoisseurs) can understand and appreciate subtle qualities of the classroom or program, and merits of the teacher and curriculum.	An outside expert can provide insights not evident to curriculum participants.
Starpoli and Waltz (1978)	Includes specific questions of concern to varied audiences, depending on what is being evaluated. Specifies decision makers for each question (i.e., who should be responsible for evaluation activities, and how evaluation will proceed). There are four distinct, interrelated levels of evaluation: school, program, subprogram, course level; and three frames: input, operations, output.	The comprehensiveness of the model allows for full curriculum assessment.

Table 15-3   Summary of Several Third-Generation Evaluation Models and Their Value in Nursing Curriculum Evaluation (*continued*)

Models in Chronological Order	Description	Value in Nursing Curriculum Evaluation
Stufflebeam's (1983) educational decision model (an extension of the original CIPP model)	Educational decision-making model that addresses four concerns: 1) *context*: setting, mission, community, philosophy, internal/external focus; 2) *input*: resources, support systems, learners, program plan; 3) *process*: implementation, teaching/learning strategies and transactions, learning materials, efficiency and effectiveness; 4) *product*: learner outcomes and satisfaction; all to facilitate decision making.	Holistic examination of the curriculum from the perspectives of faculty, students, and stakeholders is possible. Consideration of the processes gives direction for improvement.
Wholey's (1983) program logic model (based on Provus's model)	Compares program progress against predetermined indictors. Assesses logical linkages (as described by the program model) among parts of the program, such as resources and activities, program processes, outcomes, outputs, and impact. Takes context into account.	Indicators of acceptable performance are specified in advance of curriculum implementation, thus self-assessment and improvement could be ongoing.
Stake's (1991) education evaluation model	Is organized around issues and concerns of stakeholders (students, faculty, administrators, parents, employers); goal is to discover merits and weakness of the program. Uses methods to generate data responsive to identified issues and concerns.	Merits and weaknesses of the curriculum can be identified in response to identified concerns.

Source: Some data from Frye, A. W., & Hemmer, P. A. (2012). Program evaluation models and related theories: AMEE Guide No. 67. *Medical Teacher, 34*, e288–e299; Herbener, D. J., & Watson, J. E. (1992). Evaluating nursing education programs. *Nursing Outlook, 40*, 27–32; McLaughlin, J. A., & Jordon, G. B. (2010). Using logic models. In J. S. Wholey, H. P. Hatry, & K. E. Newcomer (Eds.), *Handbook of practical program evaluation* (3rd ed., pp. 55–80). San Francisco: Jossey-Bass; Stufflebeam, D. L. (2007). *CIPP evaluation model checklist*. Retrieved from http://www.wmich.edu/evalctr/archive_checklists/cippchecklist_mar07.pdf; Stufflebeam, D. L., & Shinkfield, A. J. (2007). *Evaluation theory, models, and applications*. San Francisco: Jossey-Bass; Wholey, J. S. (1983). *Evaluation and effective public management*. Boston: Little, Brown.

Rationale for Choice of an Evaluation Model

Each evaluation approach has particular strengths that illuminate different aspects of the curriculum. Therefore, selection of a curriculum evaluation model, or evaluation approach, should be contingent upon the curriculum's philosophical approaches, purpose of the evaluation, questions to be addressed, issues to be taken into account, available resources, and faculty preference for one model over another.

Whichever model(s) can provide the best evidence to answer the evaluation questions deemed important within the resource constraints would be a good choice. If no one model seems sufficient, a combination of relevant concepts from different models can be used (Glatthorn, Boschee, & Whitehead, 2009). This eclectic approach, while not an evaluation model as such, might offer more scope than one model, and also mature, diverse, and sophisticated evaluation strategies (Fitzpatrick et al., 2004). Within a dynamic evaluation approach, elements from different models are selected (eclecticism), with the additional feature that ongoing attention is given to assessment and refinement of processes, even as the evaluation is being conducted (Grammatikopoulos, Koustelics, Tsigillis, & Theodorakis, 2004).

As an alternate to choosing one model or using elements from several models, faculty members can design their own models and derive the subsequent evaluation framework so that local purposes are fully incorporated. For example, the Relevance-Congruence-Adequacy-Reasonableness (RCAR) Framework (Iwasiw, 2008, 2014) was designed specifically to address curriculum evaluation priorities of the Western–Fanshawe Collaborative BScN Program. The model is presented in **Figure 15-2**. **Table 15-4** depicts a portion of the evaluation framework derived from the model.

It is also possible to use published standards and criteria as an evaluation framework. For example, the standards and criteria of the National League for Nursing Accrediting Commission (now the Accreditation Commission for Education in Nursing) have been used as a basis for curriculum evaluation by one school of nursing (Schug, 2012), as have the Institute of Medicine core competencies (Morris & Hancock, 2013).

In accordance with the premises of utilization-focused evaluation, the model or methods selected and the evaluation design created should achieve the purposes determined by the prime users of the evaluation results. The approaches used should be practical, cost effective, and ethical (Patton, 2008). Other factors to consider when selecting an evaluation model are:

- Burden on participants
- Suitability for all levels of the curriculum
- Ability to assess significant aspects of the curriculum, including the hidden curriculum and unintended effects

Figure 15-2   Relevance-Congruence-Adequacy-Reasonableness (RCAR) Curriculum
Evaluation Model (revised).
© C. L. Iwasiw 2008, 2014 (used with permission).

This evaluation model is premised on a philosophy of pragmatism and a belief in the ability of
experienced nurse educators to make sound, evidence-informed judgments about curriculum quality.
From the model, a framework of evaluation questions, indicators, data sources, and data collection
methods has been derived. Four dimensions are encompassed in the model, and these provide the
criteria and framework for curriculum evaluation:

1. *Relevance* of the:
    • Curriculum for the context in which it is offered and in which graduates will practice nursing
    • Outcomes for the context
2. *Congruence* of the:
    • Curriculum design with the curriculum foundations (educational and philosophical approaches,
      core concepts, and key professional abilities)
    • Implementation with the curriculum foundations and design (implementation fidelity)
    • Actual outcomes with the curricular intent
3. *Adequacy* of resources to deliver the planned curriculum
4. *Reasonableness* of the curricular demands on students and faculty

Notes:
      Relevance = applicability to, or suitability for current and anticipated contextual circumstances
      Congruence = logical consistency, agreement
        Adequacy = sufficiency
Reasonableness = the state of being possible or sensible

- Probability of providing information for decision making
- Consideration of the curriculum context (Glatthorn et al., 2009)

FRAMEWORKS TO ASSESS FIDELITY OF IMPLEMENTATION

Frameworks for assessing fidelity of implementation have been developed (e.g., Carroll
et al., 2007; Century, Rudnick, & Freeman, 2010), and these combine third- and fourth-
generation methods. Their purpose is to determine how well an enacted intervention (e.g.,
a curriculum) matches the original planned intervention, so that conclusions can be drawn
about whether outcomes can be attributed to the intervention. These frameworks arise
from studies of medical interventions in which it is essential to assess the integrity of the
treatment to determine its efficacy.

The frameworks provide guidelines for assessing the components of fidelity of implementation: *adherence, duration or dosage, quality of delivery*, and *participant involvement*. In addition to being components of fidelity, these factors, singly or in combination,

Table 15-4 Relevancy Dimension of the Relevance-Congruence-Adequacy-Reasonableness (RCAR) Curriculum Evaluation Framework

Dimension	Main Questions	Indicators	Data Sources	Data-Gathering Methods	Accountability For Activity
Relevancy	1. To what extent do the philosophical approaches reflect a clear connection with the: • Mission and philosophy of the educational institution?	Correspondence between the mission and philosophy of the educational institution and the curriculum philosophical approaches	Institutional documents	Document review	Faculty task group 1
	• Present and anticipated context of nursing practice?	Correspondence between philosophical approaches and context	External contextual data and trends	Web searches Interviews with nursing leaders Documents related to nursing practice standards Literature about nursing practice trends	Faculty task group 2
	2. To what extent do the curriculum outcomes or goals reflect a clear connection with the: • Philosophical approaches	Philosophical approaches explicitly evident in outcomes or goals	Curriculum documents	Document review	Faculty task group 1
	• Present and anticipated context of nursing practice?	Outcomes or goals are relevant to trends emanating from contextual data	External contextual data and trends	Web searches Interviews with nursing leaders Documents related to nursing practice standards Literature about nursing practice trends	Faculty task group 2

Source: © C. L. Iwasiw 2008, 2014. Used with permission of the author.

The contribution of the Western–Fanshawe Collaborative Program Evaluation Committee is appreciated in the refinement of the complete document.

also influence the outcomes (Carroll et al., 2007). It is worthwhile to note that in nursing curricula, the educational interventions are complex and highly influenced by the dynamic nature of learning contexts and interactions. Therefore, outcomes cannot likely be linked to any one intervention, but rather to a constellation of interventions.

A framework that might be adaptable for nursing education is one used to evaluate fidelity of implementation in a science curriculum (Lee & Chue, 2013). In this study, the authors examined the key activities of the science curriculum (including process skills, such as questioning, researching, and report writing; and contextual provisions, such as content knowledge, field trips, and presentations) and then determined:

- Dosage: measurement of the amount of student exposure to the process skills
- Adherence: measurement of actual teaching of the key components against the planned objectives
- Quality of delivery: comparison of actual teaching against quality teaching factors
- Participant responsiveness: determination of student interest and engagement through student interviews

With this approach, the authors proposed that conclusions could be drawn about areas to improve in the curriculum.

An assessment of the fidelity of all areas of a nursing education curriculum would be unwieldy because the educational interventions are multifaceted and dynamic. Furthermore, a detailed analysis is likely unnecessary if students are achieving the desired curriculum outcomes or goals. However, a careful examination would be useful if particular key expectations are not being met. In this case, quantitative and qualitative methods could be used in combination. If fidelity of implementation is being examined, curriculum evaluators need to ask, "What is an acceptable level of fidelity?" (Harn, Parisi, & Stoolmiller, 2013).

PLANNING CURRICULUM EVALUATION

Planning curriculum evaluation is a dimension of curriculum development that should occur simultaneously with curriculum and course design, although in some schools of nursing, attention is not given to evaluation until curriculum implementation is well underway. Because curriculum evaluation is a participatory process with faculty and other stakeholders involved in the planning and implementation, consensus and shared understanding about the purposes and procedures of the evaluation might lead to more willing acceptance of recommendations that result from the evaluation (De Valenzuela, Copeland, & Blalock, 2005; Patton, 2008).

Curriculum evaluation is only one aspect of a school's activities. Therefore, this undertaking should be confined to only that which is necessary to achieve the purposes of the evaluation. Decisions are made about:

- Purposes and audiences of the curriculum evaluation
- Desired similarity between the internal curriculum evaluation and the requirements for external approval or accreditation
- Individual or committee responsibility for coordinating the curriculum evaluation process
- Evaluation model to be used
- Evaluation questions to be addressed
- Components to be evaluated
- Standards and criteria to be employed
- Data essential to answer the evaluation questions
- Methods and timing of data gathering
- Persons responsible for obtaining or providing data
- Repository for the data
- Individuals who will interpret and judge the evidence, and formulate recommendations
- Process to report evaluation results to relevant audiences
- Deadline for completion

Resolution of these matters in advance of curriculum implementation will allow for organized formative and summative evaluation. The ongoing accumulation of data and subsequent curriculum refinements reflect commitment to continuous curriculum improvement. Moreover, if data gathering for curriculum evaluation is viewed as a regular, expected, and normal part of curriculum implementation, then the stress associated with intermittent internal and external evaluations is markedly lessened.

Curriculum evaluation decisions are not made in isolation from one another. Rather, they are made in a more unified fashion and are based on iterative discussions that arise from the following questions:

- What are faculty's beliefs and values about curriculum evaluation?
- Why is curriculum evaluation being undertaken?
- What learning is anticipated about the curriculum? What are the evaluation questions to be answered?
- Which evaluation model(s) is (are) consistent with the curriculum's philosophical approaches?
- What will constitute quality?
- Which aspects of the curriculum should be evaluated?

- How often and when should the curriculum be evaluated?
- What data are required? How can the data be obtained?
- How will evaluation results be used?
- Who will be responsible for managing the evaluation process?

Generally, curriculum evaluation activities are shared among many faculty members. Yet, the overall responsibility must rest with an individual or group, such as the curriculum leader, a curriculum committee, or curriculum evaluation committee, so that efforts are coordinated and complete. Documenting the evaluation efforts and results and subsequent curriculum modifications will provide information important for later internal and external curriculum and program evaluations. Inevitably, evidence of systematic and ongoing evaluation and the results of these appraisals are required for approval and accreditation.

ESTABLISHING STANDARDS, CRITERIA, OR INDICATORS

Decisions about curriculum effectiveness and quality depend on a clear understanding of the standards against which the curriculum is being judged and the criteria used to determine if the standards are being attained. Standards are "something used as a measure, norm, or model in comparative evaluations" (Stevenson, 2010). It is an authoritative statement or example of correctness, perfection, or quality. Criteria are distinguishing characteristics used to judge whether a standard has been achieved. Standards and criteria should be delineated as much as possible.

Specification of precise standards and criteria for all curriculum components may not be possible, necessary, or realistic. Therefore, it may be more appropriate to define indicators, that is, observations or calculations that show the presence or state of a condition. For example, the nature of classroom activities is an indicator of the congruence between the enacted and the intended educational approaches.

Faculty members rely, in part, upon guidelines, standards, and/or criteria for program approval and accreditation when establishing curriculum standards. They might also write standards particular to the school of nursing. Consideration should be given to standards for various curriculum components. For some, such as strategies to ignite learning, the literature is replete with criteria for effective teaching. These can be invaluable in reaching an agreement about school-specific standards. For some components, faculty may have to develop their own standards. As examples, they might view inclusion of evidence about nursing practices in classes as a criterion on context relevance, or the alignment of students' projects with the philosophical approaches as an indicator of unity. These examples would be relevant for assessing the curriculum and individual courses.

The specification of standards, criteria, and/or indicators allows faculty to answer the questions: *Is this a quality curriculum? On what basis can we say so?* It is vital that the standards, criteria, and indicators be specific enough to be understandable and provide direction for gathering data and making evaluative judgments, while not being too extensive or overly time-consuming to create. These can be refined in the future, if necessary. Additionally, experienced and knowledgeable nursing faculty are generally able to recognize the merits and deficits of a curriculum; they are experts, thus their expert opinions have value (Posavac, 2011). As they consider standards, criteria, and indicators, faculty might ask themselves questions such as:

- Are the standards, criteria, and/or indicators consistent with the curriculum intent and with those used by external evaluating agencies?
- Do the number and nature of the standards, criteria, and/or indicators seem reasonable and appropriate?
- Will we be able to exercise economy of data-gathering efforts in assembling the curriculum evidence necessary to apply the criteria and standards?

PLANNING DATA GATHERING FOR CURRICULUM EVALUATION

The standards, criteria, and indicators that have been formulated give direction about which data are necessary for curriculum evaluation and the data sources. Although a wealth of data might be pertinent, only the most significant should be assembled. The same data could provide evidence of the effectiveness of several aspects of the curriculum. For example, students' reflective journals can indicate the extent to which intended course competencies or goals are being achieved and provide evidence of the appropriateness of the methods by which students demonstrate their achievements. In planning data gathering, faculty should consider what is reasonable and feasible.

Data-Gathering Methods

Data-gathering methods are linked to the evaluation purposes, model selected, evaluation questions, and predetermined standards. Typically, qualitative and quantitative methods are employed. The methods and tools should allow for a comprehensive evaluation, be understandable and easy to use, cost- and time-efficient, valid, reliable, and credible.

Quantitative and qualitative data-gathering methods and procedures with which most faculty are already familiar can be employed for curriculum evaluation. Surveys can be used to assess faculty members' and students' satisfaction with the curriculum, their views about strategies used to ignite learning, infusion of the philosophical approaches into the enacted curriculum, aspects of implementation fidelity (such as quality of delivery), and so forth. Interviews (individual or focus groups) can uncover qualitative data from students, faculty, or graduates for similar purposes. Interviews and surveys are also effective in obtaining data from graduates, clinicians, and employers.

Unstructured observations, and annotations about them, can be useful early in the curriculum evaluation process. From these, structured observation based on criteria can be planned. For example, observations of students in professional practice settings can lead to criteria related to students' practice abilities, attitudes, and values, and subsequently to guidelines for structured observations and the acquisition of more specific data. Anecdotal notes can be used to record observations related to course goals or competencies, and, when accumulated, provide evidence about student achievement. An examination of a sample of students' written projects provides insight into the quality of student work and, by extension, their achievement of course expectations. Similarly, peer or expert observation can lead to conclusions about classroom and professional practice teaching-learning encounters and implementation fidelity.

Rating scales, checklists, curriculum maps, and self-reports are other means of obtaining data for curriculum evaluation. Rating scales could be used to measure abstract concepts, while checklists identify expected behaviors or competencies and related student performance. Curriculum maps, completed after course implementation, can be compared to the original plan for the course. Attitude scales can measure how students and faculty feel about a particular subject or situation, such as a professional practice placement or a learning activity. Faculty could use self-reports or journals to record their ideas and insights as they implement the curriculum. Similarly, student narratives can provide information about their reflections, thoughts, fears, progress, successes, actual outcomes, and ideas for curriculum improvement.

It will likely be necessary to develop instruments or guides for data gathering. In this case, time needs to be planned to develop and test them. The tools can be pilot-tested to ensure that they are understandable and face validity can be assessed. The important features of useful instruments for curriculum evaluation purposes are that they:

- Address processes central to the curriculum
- Can be used in several contexts, such as with faculty or students at several levels or placement settings
- Are understandable to users
- Are efficient and cost effective
- Will yield important information to answer the evaluation questions

After being used once, the validity can be further assessed, and refinements made. "However, validity does not rest with any instrument or procedure, but in its use in generating inferences and conclusions" (Stufflebeam & Shinkfield, 2007, p. 563).

Data Sources

Data sources can include faculty, students, graduates, administrators, clinicians, employers, and nursing leaders, as well as curriculum and course documents. Test scores, essays, journals, and other assignments lead to valuable insights about students' knowledge, attitudes, and experiences. Records, such as student grades, attrition rates, or success rates on licensure examinations and other external tests, are useful for curriculum evaluation. Additionally, data can be used from formal evaluation processes already in place, such as institution-wide teaching or course evaluations. Multiple sources produce a fair and balanced system, with the combination making up for the shortcomings of each (Appling, Naumann, & Berk, 2001).

Data-Gathering Schedule

The timing of data gathering is important. It begins with the introduction of the first courses so that formative evaluation is undertaken concurrently with curriculum implementation. In this way, early decisions arising from formative evaluation can stabilize the curriculum and prevent problems that might occur in courses yet to be implemented.

Some scheduling seems self-evident. Student evaluation of courses typically occurs at the completion of each course. However, formal course evaluation mandated by educational institutions is unlikely to address all the questions to which curriculum evaluators seek answers. Additional data gathering is best scheduled when students are likely to provide opinions about courses without fear of penalty for unfavorable comments, or relinquishing time they feel would be better spent on course work. Similarly, it is evident that data gathering about graduates' abilities cannot occur until there are graduates, but timing and frequency require attention.

A reasonable schedule for gathering pertinent data is necessary. It might be decided that some data do not need to be obtained annually. For example, a survey of graduates might be undertaken every 2 years. The intent is to ensure that data are obtained as frequently as necessary to provide an adequate basis for meaningful evaluation, yet not so often that the task becomes unduly burdensome.

Data Management and Interpretation

Early decisions must be made regarding which individuals will be responsible for gathering, managing, and interpreting data. All activities may not be completed by the same individuals. There ought to be consensus about the group that will receive the data analysis and interpretations, formulate judgments about the alignment with standards, and make curriculum recommendations. The volume of data to be collected is usually an important factor in deciding how many and which people are involved in the management and interpretation of data.

A component of decisions about data management is agreement about a system for logical organization and storage of evaluation data and analysis, curriculum recommendations, and subsequent actions. Information about curriculum recommendations and modifications may be required as part of approval and accreditation procedures. Identification of an individual or group responsible for detailing and recording evaluation decisions and curriculum alterations (if any) ensures accountability.

Use of Evaluation Data and Results

The ways in which evaluation data and results might be used, in addition to making curriculum recommendations, is worthy of discussion and agreement in advance of data gathering. An important decision relates to reporting evaluation results. When and to whom should evaluation data and curriculum recommendations be reported?

There is variation among schools of nursing in their reporting procedures and the extent of information provided to interested groups. Some might report a summary of all data and the subsequent curriculum decisions to all groups that provided data. Others might emphasize data from a particular stakeholder group to that group. Understandably, stakeholders want to know how their data contributed to decisions and actions about the curriculum.

A decision must be made about whether data will be used for purposes beyond the curriculum. If so, who will have access to the data? If teaching or course evaluations beyond standardized institution-wide questionnaires are undertaken, discussion is necessary about how the results will be reported and used. If faculty journals or portfolios are requested, who will read them, and how will they be assessed in relation to the curriculum? Who will receive the results? Could school-specific teaching or course evaluations be used for promotion and tenure purposes? Agreement about these and similar questions is necessary before curriculum evaluation activities begin.

Deliberations About Data-Gathering Plans

Planning the data gathering requires attention to the methods to be employed, the scope of data required, and logistics of the undertaking. When developing a plan for data gathering, faculty might anticipate such questions as:

- Who will be responsible for leading the development of an evaluation plan and its implementation? Will it be the same person who is leading curriculum development? Will it be a committee?
- What data are required to ascertain if standards are being attained?

- How can data be obtained expeditiously?
- When, how, and from whom will data be gathered?
- Which established data-gathering tools could be used? Are they appropriate?
- Who will be responsible for developing, pilot-testing, and approving school-specific data-gathering tools?
- Who will be responsible for obtaining the data?
- How often will data be gathered, reviewed, and interpreted, so that conclusions can be drawn and recommendations formulated? Who will participate in this process?
- How and to whom will evaluation results be reported?
- How will evaluation activities, results, and curriculum alterations be documented so that these records can contribute meaningfully to internal summative evaluation and external evaluations?
- Will evaluation data be used for faculty evaluation or faculty development purposes?
- What resources are required to conduct these activities?

PLANNING EVALUATION OF CURRICULUM COMPONENTS

Philosophical Approaches

The philosophical approaches are fundamental to the implementation of the curriculum and to students' beliefs about nursing and clients. For the purposes of curriculum evaluation, it is important to know if the philosophical approaches are being enacted in all learning environments. Essentially, evaluators want to learn the extent to which:

- The written description of the philosophical approaches is understandable to faculty members.
- Students can articulate the philosophical approaches and explain how they act in accordance with these approaches in classroom, professional practice, and peer interactions.
- The philosophical approaches are being enacted in teaching-learning encounters.
- Processes used to assess student learning are congruent with the philosophical approaches.

Curriculum Goal or Outcome Statements

The goal or outcome statements broadly identify the abilities of graduates and incorporate the philosophical approaches and major concepts of the curriculum. The complexity of the abilities should be appropriate for the educational level of the program and be consistent with (or exceed) criteria for approval and/or accreditation.

When planning the evaluation of curriculum goal or outcome statements, faculty want to determine if the outcomes are appropriate and reasonable; in other words, are these the most suitable goals or outcomes? More specifically, faculty are interested in the extent to which the curriculum expectations:

- Reflect the practice and standards of the educational institution, higher education, the nursing profession, state or provincial licensing bodies, and approval or accrediting organizations
- Are relevant to the healthcare context
- Are appropriate to the program level
- Reflect the curriculum foundations

Curriculum Design

When planning evaluation of the curriculum design, the scope of this component becomes evident. The design encompasses the curriculum outcome or goal statements and the configuration of the program of studies, that is, courses, their sequence, interrelationships, and mode of delivery. In addition, it includes faculty and student activities, and policies governing the curriculum. When planning evaluation of the curriculum design, faculty are interested in the extent to which:

- There is internal consistency (i.e., how well the curriculum elements fit together).
- The design reflects the philosophical approaches and is relevant to the context in which the curriculum is offered.
- The configuration of courses supports student achievement of curriculum outcomes or goals.
- There is consistency, congruence, and organization among and within courses.
- Non-nursing courses facilitate achievement of curriculum outcomes or goals and contribute to a well-rounded liberal education.
- Necessary prerequisites are included so students can be successful.
- Students and faculty believe that courses are appropriate and logically sequenced.
- Concepts and substantive context are complete and relevant.
- Course titles present an image of a conceptually unified curriculum.
- The curriculum presents as a unified whole.

Curriculum Concepts

Evaluation of the curriculum concepts involves two dimensions: the appropriateness of the concepts themselves and the extent to which they form a successful foundation for courses and substantive content. Evaluation of the former rests on qualitative data from students and faculty about the meaningfulness of the concepts for learning about nursing and their utility in professional practice. Faculty will have ideas about whether the concepts might require modification, such as synthesis of several concepts or greater analysis of a concept into its constituent subconcepts. They might also have thoughts about missing concepts. Students will have information about their understanding of the concepts and how they used the concepts in professional practice and course work.

The extent to which the concepts formed a successful foundation for courses and substantive content is an area to be evaluated. Faculty will have information about how well they were able to plan classes that were based on the concepts, and how well the concepts and substantive content merged to form significant learning opportunities for students.

In assessing the concepts, curriculum evaluators are interested in whether the curriculum concepts are:

- At an appropriate level for students
- Sufficient in scope to address the important ideas needed in nursing practice
- A useful basis for class planning and implementation
- Meaningful to students
- Perceived by students to have value in their professional practice

Courses

Evaluation of courses is, in some measure, a microcosm of the total curriculum evaluation. All aspects of course design and implementation are considered. Faculty might determine the extent to which:

- Course competencies or goals are appropriate and linked to curriculum outcome or goal statements.
- Expectations of students are reasonable.
- Learning activities are consistent with the philosophical approaches, educational approaches, and intended course competencies or goals.
- Course activities contribute to students' progress.
- Course activities suit the delivery mode.
- Strategies to ignite learning and technologies used are effective in facilitating learning.
- Content is current, evidence-based, related to other fields of study, and logically organized.
- Core curriculum concepts and key professional abilities are evident in written course materials and classes.

- Methods to evaluate student learning are appropriate in nature and number, varied, and clearly linked to course competencies or goals.
- Students have achieved course expectations.
- Each course can be justified within the curriculum.
- Each course has been implemented as originally conceived (i.e., has implementation fidelity).
- There are redundancies or deficiencies among courses.

Educational Approaches and Strategies to Ignite Learning

When planning evaluation of educational approaches and strategies to ignite learning, faculty can be guided by literature that describes effective teaching according to the chosen approach, dimensions of teaching competence, relationships with students, personal characteristics, and evaluation practices. These ideas about effective teaching and effective faculty can be adopted, adapted, or extended to match the educational and philosophical approaches of the curriculum.

In general, faculty seek to answer the following questions:

- What is the nature of student-faculty interactions?
- How do students respond to the strategies to ignite learning?
- In what ways have faculty affected students' growth as individuals and future practitioners?

Faculty will also want to know the extent to which the strategies to ignite learning:

- Are congruent with the philosophical and educational approaches
- Assist students in their progress toward course and curriculum expectations
- Respect student diversity

Finally, an assessment of satisfaction may be appropriate. Are students and faculty satisfied with the educational approaches and learning activities?

Opportunities for Students to Demonstrate Learning and Evaluation of Student Achievement

Appraisal of strategies to evaluate student achievement is another important dimension of curriculum evaluation. The methods by which students are asked to provide evidence of their learning, and how that evidence is assessed, have great significance to them and color their reaction to the curriculum. Considered could be the extent to which students' opportunities to demonstrate learning are:

- Reflective of the curriculum's philosophical and educational approaches
- Logically linked to course goals or competencies

- Perceived to be fair and flexible
- Varied within a course, semester, and year to accommodate students':
  - Diverse ways of knowing
  - Academic workloads
  - Need for formative and summative feedback
  - Desire to have input into evaluation methods
- Suitable for faculty members' academic workloads
- Consistent with faculty members' expertise and preferences

A review of students' submitted work might be undertaken. Part of this review could be an appraisal of the nature of faculty feedback and its alignment with curriculum tenets.

PLANNING EVALUATION OF OTHER ASPECTS OF THE CURRICULUM

In addition to the curriculum components, there are other matters that require attention, because they reflect and affect the enactment of the curriculum. The learning climate, curriculum policies, and resources devoted to curriculum enactment all influence its success.

Learning Climate

The learning climate consists of the social, emotional, and intellectual atmosphere that exists within the school, and within courses offered through distance delivery methods. It is a strong indication of one aspect of fidelity of implementation, specifically, the adherence to the espoused philosophical approaches. The philosophical approaches in action contribute significantly to the learning climate and this strongly influences the satisfaction, psychological comfort, and empowerment of students, faculty, and staff. In planning evaluation of the curriculum's learning climate, faculty determine the extent to which members of the school are satisfied with:

- Available learning opportunities
- Settings in which learning occurs
- Flexibility in the curriculum
- Variety of perspectives in course content, discussion, and readings
- Diversity of backgrounds of authors of required texts and readings
- Fostering of responsibility and accountability
- Relationships with one another
- Perceived freedom to take intellectual risks and make mistakes without repercussions
- Support available when undertaking new challenges
- Sense of belonging and feeling of community

Policies

Curriculum policies are developed to support students' achievement of curriculum outcomes while ensuring that academic standards are maintained. Therefore, in reviewing and evaluating curriculum policies, faculty consider whether the policies are appropriate, reasonable, understood by faculty and students, and applied consistently. Evaluators might also ascertain if there have been situations that might indicate a need for new policies.

Human and Physical Resources

An important dimension of curriculum evaluation is ascertaining if suitable and sufficient human and physical resources are present. When planning curriculum evaluation, faculty are interested in assessing the extent to which:

- Academic and professional practice faculty are sufficient in numbers and academic preparation to maintain implementation fidelity.
- Faculty teaching assignments are aligned with their expertise.
- Staff numbers, roles, and functions are reasonable to support the curriculum.
- Offices and meeting rooms are available and suitable.
- Classrooms are satisfactory in size, structure, comfort, and appearance.
- Classrooms and labs are equipped with appropriate and functional technologies.
- Professional practice placements and experiences match requirements in quality and quantity.
- Library holdings are sufficient in number, scope, and quality.
- Material resources are adequate.

PLANNING EVALUATION OF ACTUAL CURRICULUM OUTCOMES

The purpose of all nursing curricula is to prepare graduates who will practice nursing competently in a changing healthcare environment, thereby contributing to the health and quality of life of those they serve. It is essential to determine if current students are progressing toward this outcome, and if graduates are successful as they begin practice. Evaluation of actual student outcomes is viewed by some as the most important aspect of curriculum evaluation. The overriding question is whether students are being adequately prepared for professional practice.

Success rates on licensure or registration examinations, possibly in comparison to state, provincial, or national results, should be examined, although it is prudent to remember that these examinations test only for the minimum level of safety that is acceptable. Determination of new graduates' successes and sources of difficulty, and employers' satisfaction with graduates' nursing practice is important in evaluating actual curriculum outcomes.

In addition to obtaining data from and about graduates, an examination of students' progress allows for conclusions about actual outcomes within the curriculum. Therefore, curriculum evaluators are interested in the extent to which students:

- Are achieving intended course and curriculum expectations.
- Can articulate philosophical approaches, intended curriculum outcomes or goals, major curriculum concepts, and key professional abilities.
- Can explain how they use curriculum concepts and philosophical approaches in professional practice experiences.
- Perceive themselves to be ready to begin practice at graduation.

JUDGING CURRICULUM QUALITY AND MAKING RECOMMENDATIONS

Each data set is analyzed and compared to the standards, criteria, and/or indicators previously defined. The extent of correspondence or divergence between the findings and the standards is determined. During this process, the strengths and weaknesses of the curriculum become apparent. This work needs to be conducted by individuals with experience in data analysis and interpretation, so that all faculty, students, and stakeholders will have confidence in the analysis.

Then, the analysis findings are synthesized to determine their meaning for answering the evaluation questions and for judging the quality of the curriculum. It is important to remember that with multifaceted, complex interventions, such as a curriculum, it is not possible to assume a linear relationship (cause and effect) between any one curriculum element and outcomes (Frye & Hemmer, 2012). Rather, a more holistic perspective is necessary. From the conclusions drawn, recommendations are formulated about actions required to maintain or improve curriculum quality. Alternately, there could be a recommendation to discontinue the curriculum and begin afresh with curriculum development.

Reviewing and interpreting evaluation data, reaching a judgment, and making recommendations are typically the responsibilities of a committee. Then, the recommendations are generally considered by the total faculty group, and, if accepted, the specified actions are implemented.

REPORTING EVALUATION RESULTS AND RECOMMENDATIONS

Many people are involved in providing data for internal curriculum evaluation, most notably students, faculty, and external stakeholders. They are interested in knowing about the data they and other groups have provided, and what will happen as a result of the evaluation process. Will there be changes to the curriculum? If so, what will they be, and when will they happen? Thus, the evaluation team generally:

- Prepares a comprehensive written report for internal use
- Plans meetings for verbal presentations of the report (Posavac, 2011)

Each school will decide how widely the written report is distributed, and whether it includes firm plans for curriculum alterations.

The total faculty group, students, and external stakeholders appreciate a comprehensive view of the data and the rationale for curriculum recommendations. As broad a view of data as possible will allow individuals to see where their data fit into the big picture, and possibly to understand how their suggestions are integrated into the recommendations, or why their ideas are absent. There needs to be an opportunity to discuss and possibly modify the recommendations before endorsement can be expected.

Although students are involved in the curriculum evaluation process and have a strong interest in its outcomes, they are sometimes forgotten when evaluation results, recommendations, and subsequent actions are reported. Hosting student forums and/or posting information on student websites could be effective ways of disseminating information about evaluation outcomes and endorsed recommendations. Students want to know if and how their ideas will influence the curriculum.

Results of internal curriculum evaluation and actions taken as a result of the evaluation should also be reported to appropriate administrators and incorporated into external evaluation reports. If curriculum revision is to be undertaken as a consequence of the evaluation, the evaluation results will be part of the contextual data for curriculum redevelopment and provide rationale for a request for resources for further curriculum work.

Care is necessary in the reporting process so that unfavorable conclusions are not interpreted as criticism of individuals. Rather, it may be possible to frame the problem area as one that received insufficient support in its development or implementation. In this way, the evaluators, who are faculty members themselves, can minimize the personal hurt, maintain positive relationships with those affected, and indicate that all members have a responsibility for supporting every aspect of the curriculum.

REFLECTING BACK AND LOOKING FORWARD

Although not always undertaken, a meta-evaluation of the curriculum evaluation process can be useful to identify which processes worked and should be retained for future curriculum evaluations, and which were not successful and should be modified or eliminated. This review can also be useful to identify what might be added to future curriculum evaluations, and what may have been unnecessary or redundant and could be eliminated.

Another aspect of reflecting on the process is to identify the individual and collective learning that resulted from participating in curriculum evaluation. For example, some might have a clearer sense of how course components should be linked; others may have more knowledge of curriculum evaluation processes. There could be a collective revisioning of the school as an organization that is progressively working to achieve excellence. Provision of an opportunity for faculty and other stakeholders to reflect on the curriculum evaluation processes, and share their learning, can increase the capacity and empowerment of all groups.

RELATIONSHIP OF CURRICULUM EVALUATION TO AN EVIDENCE-INFORMED, CONTEXT-RELEVANT, UNIFIED CURRICULUM

The curriculum evaluation data and analysis provide evidence for decisions to alter or discontinue the curriculum. If, during the evaluation, the curriculum goals or outcomes, processes, concepts, and content are appraised for their relevance to the context, and the unity within the curriculum is assessed, then these features of the curriculum can be maintained or strengthened as necessary. Further curriculum work can emanate from the evaluation data; thus the curriculum will continue to be evidence-informed, context-relevant, and unified.

CORE PROCESSES OF CURRICULUM WORK

Faculty Development

Faculty development can initially focus on the purposes and processes of curriculum evaluation. Following this, information about evaluation models, approaches, standards, criteria, and indicators can be presented. Through discussion, faculty can formulate evaluation questions to be answered about each curriculum component, and determine data-gathering approaches. Published accreditation or approval guidelines can serve as exemplars during these activities. Through their involvement in curriculum development, novices will understand the curriculum components, but they may need assistance with defining standards and criteria, and limiting the extent of data gathering. Provision of curriculum data will allow faculty to practice interpreting and judging data, and then deriving recommendations. After the curriculum evaluation is completed, methods to help members identify the learning that was gained could include reflective processes such as storytelling, descriptions of changes and progression in members' work, and group development of the meaning that could be derived from the curriculum evaluation process and results (Verdonschot, 2006).

Ongoing Appraisal

As curriculum evaluation is being planned and conducted, many questions can arise that could lead to an improvement of the processes. These questions include the following:

- Are we clear about the purpose(s) to be achieved?
- Have the best processes been selected to obtain the necessary data? Might there be more expedient means to obtain the information?
- How well will processes reflect respect for participants' time?
- Will any important information be missed? What is it?
- Will the available resources be sufficient to develop instruments and guidelines, define standards, and obtain and analyze data? If the resources are not available, what can be modified?
- Are there published materials that would be helpful?
- Have we been diligent in including stakeholders in our processes? How thorough are our plans for reporting evaluation results and recommendations?
- How thorough is our plan for ongoing evaluation?
- What has been missed?
- Are we satisfied with our decisions?

Scholarship

As with other aspects of curriculum work, manuscripts describing the processes undertaken to plan and conduct an internal curriculum evaluation can be instructive to faculty at other schools. Also important could be a description of the preparations for external evaluation, with attention to the timeframe, activities, and participants. Methods of outcome evaluation, particularly successful ways to obtain data from graduates, would be a valuable contribution to the literature. Furthermore, it would be beneficial to prepare manuscripts that illuminate the deliberations involved in analyzing and synthesizing evaluation data, and the decisions that lead to curriculum recommendations.

Evaluation studies of the outcomes of particular curriculum strategies, such as simulation or paired student-staff nurse professional practice work, add to the evidence base for nursing education. Needed, however, are larger scale reports of the outcomes of curricula of a similar nature, such as concept-based curricula or curricula based on a particular philosophy or educational approach, so that results can be compared and conclusions drawn. Importantly, studies of graduates from schools with varying approaches, the ways they practice nursing, and the effects on clients will be the ultimate evaluation of curricula. Although such studies will be complex, it should be possible to arrive at conclusions about which approaches are contributing most effectively to the desired practice behaviors (Iwasiw, Goldenberg, & Andrusyszyn, 2005).

CHAPTER SUMMARY

In this chapter, the definition, overview, purposes of internal and external evaluation, and models of curriculum evaluation are presented, along with benefits to participants. Evaluation typologies are overviewed and attention is given to assessing fidelity of implementation. Planning the overall curriculum evaluation is considered, including establishing standards, criteria, and/or indicators, and planning data gathering. Then, evaluation of individual curriculum components is addressed, with emphasis on evaluation questions that might be considered for each. Evaluation of actual curriculum outcomes is considered. Ideas are offered about judging the quality of the curriculum, reporting evaluation results, and reflecting on the total process. Possible topics for faculty development activities, questions for ongoing appraisal, and ideas for scholarship projects are proposed.

SYNTHESIS ACTIVITIES

The Solomon University School of Nursing case describes a school of nursing that is about to begin planning for curriculum evaluation. The case is followed by questions and activities to facilitate analysis. Then, questions and activities are provided for consideration when curriculum evaluation is planned in individual settings.

Solomon University School of Nursing

Solomon University is a newly established university that came into existence with the "promotion" of a long-existing community college to university status. The former Department of Nursing is now a School of Nursing in the College of Health and Social Services. The nursing faculty members in the former associate degree (AD) program have been retained.

In preparation for offering a bachelor of science in nursing (BSN) program, the following activities were undertaken in the 3 years leading up to the change from college to university status:

- Three master's-prepared faculty began PhD studies.
- The curriculum committee was given the task of "upping" the AD program to BSN level. They have done so, consulting with faculty members about their decisions. The basic tenets of the AD curriculum have been retained.

- A retired faculty member from another university, Dr. Nur Aydin, was hired to advise periodically on curriculum revisions and development.
- The school leader, Dr. Elizabeta Bartello, negotiated for the non-nursing courses with the College of Science and the College of Arts, Humanities, and Social Sciences.
- Frequent faculty meetings were led by the curriculum committee to explain and discuss the BSN curriculum.

The BSN curriculum is to be implemented 4 months from now. Provision has been made for AD students to transfer into the BSN program or complete the program they started.

The curriculum consultant has worked hard to help the curriculum committee understand the differences between college- and university-level education, and has referred them to many documents, including accreditation standards for baccalaureate degree programs. She is concerned about comments from some curriculum committee members and other faculty, such as:

- *We're already doing that.*
- *There really is no difference in the AD and BSN nursing courses.*
- *Students will still be writing the same licensure exam, so we're okay with what we're doing.*
- *The only difference is that we have to do research.*

Dr. Aydin is not convinced that there is a full understanding of baccalaureate nursing education. She believes that some faculty members will rely on what they have done in the past and what they remember of their own undergraduate education. She meets with Dr. Bartello, and together they agree that:

- Faculty development is needed prior to implementation of the curriculum.
- Ongoing formative evaluation will be important so that any required improvements can be made as the curriculum is implemented.

Dr. Bartello asks Dr. Aydin if she will continue as a curriculum consultant and take on the responsibility of planning curriculum evaluation.

Questions and Activities for Critical Analysis of the Solomon University School of Nursing Case

1. Consider how Dr. Aydin might respond to Dr. Bartello's request. Describe the issues and processes she will likely discuss with Dr. Bartello.

2. Assess the situation at the Solomon University School of Nursing with respect to readiness to implement and evaluate the BSN curriculum.

3. With whom should Dr. Bartello begin planning curriculum evaluation? When? How might she gain support for this endeavor as curriculum implementation is beginning? How could she undertake the task of planning curriculum evaluation?

4. Describe suitable faculty development related to baccalaureate education and evaluation of a BSN curriculum.

5. Develop a feasible plan for formative and summative evaluation at the Solomon University School of Nursing. When should each be undertaken?

6. Propose a suitable framework for evaluation of the curriculum. Explain the rationale for choosing an established framework or a locally developed framework.

7. How might faculty members' comments predict the nature of standards and criteria they will articulate for the curriculum?

8. Explain the advantages and disadvantages of having the curriculum evaluated by (an) external reviewer(s) prior to formal approval or accreditation. What might be the critical aspects of the curriculum to assess?

9. What could be the consequences of unfavorable formative and/or summative curriculum evaluation for individual faculty members and the school? The consequences of favorable evaluation?

Questions and Activities for Consideration When Planning Curriculum Evaluation in Readers' Settings

1. For what purposes should curriculum evaluation be undertaken?

2. Decide who should be involved in planning for curriculum evaluation.

3. Which individual or group will be responsible for coordinating the curriculum evaluation?

4. Identify any special features of the curriculum or the School of Nursing that might influence curriculum evaluation. How could these be taken into account?

5. Examine evaluation models and approaches for fit with the philosophical approaches of the curriculum. Choose suitable ones, or suitable aspects of the models, and explain the rationale for the choice(s).

6. Which components of the curriculum will be evaluated?

7. How can standards, criteria, and/or indicators be established?

8. Develop an overall plan for curriculum evaluation.

9. Propose a detailed plan for data gathering, including data to be obtained, data sources, persons to gather data, and frequency of data gathering.

10. Identify tools or guidelines needed for data gathering. Who will develop them? When will they be pilot-tested?

11. How and where will data be recorded?

12. Create a plan for interpreting and judging the data, and making recommendations.

13. How will a record of the evaluation efforts and subsequent curriculum alterations be maintained?

14. When, how, and to whom will data, evaluation results, and recommendations be reported?

15. Develop a plan for review of the evaluation process.

16. Describe any faculty development needed to support curriculum evaluation. What is the basis of this assessment?

17. Are there questions related to ongoing appraisal of the curriculum evaluation, in addition to those suggested in the chapter, that should be asked? If so, what are they?

18. Propose scholarship activities about curriculum evaluation that could be undertaken.

REFERENCES

Alkin, M. C., & Taut, S. M. (2003). Unbundling evaluation use. *Studies in Educational Evaluation, 29*, 1–12.

Appling, S. E., Naumann, P. L., & Berk, R. A. (2001). Using a faculty evaluation triad to achieve evidence-based teaching. *Nursing and Health Care Perspectives, 22*(5), 247–251.

Carroll, C., Patterson, M., Wood, S., Booth, A., Rick, J., & Balain, S. (2007). A conceptual framework for implementation fidelity. *Implementation Science 2007, 2*, 40. doi:10.1186/1748-5908-2-40

Century, J., Rudnick, M., & Freeman, C. (2010). A framework for measuring fidelity of implementation: A foundation for shared language and accumulation of knowledge. *American Journal of Evaluation, 3*, 199–218.

Cockell, J., & McArthur-Blair, J. (2012). *Appreciative inquiry in higher education: A transformative force*. San Francisco: Jossey-Bass.

Cooperrider, D. L., Whitney, D., & Stavros, J. M. (2008). *Appreciative inquiry handbook: For leaders of change* (2nd ed.). San Francisco: Berrett-Koehler.

De Valenzuela, J. S., Copeland, J. R., & Blalock, G. A. (2005). Unfulfilled expectations: Faculty participation and voice in a university program evaluation. *Teachers College Record, 107*, 2227–2247.

Fisher, S., Kowtecki, P., Mandl, T., Roelofsen, J., Singh, J., Whalley, M., & Willoughby, L. (2003). *Undergraduate survey for curriculum evaluation*. Unpublished paper. London, ON: Western University.

Fitzpatrick, J. L., Sanders, J. R., & Worthen, B. R. (2004). *Program evaluation: Alternative approaches and practical guidelines* (4th ed.). Boston: Pearson Education.

Frye, A. W., & Hemmer, P. A. (2012). Program evaluation models and related theories: AMEE Guide No. 67. *Medical Teacher, 34*, e288–e299.

Gaberson, K. B., & Vioral, A. N. (2014). Program assessment. In M. H. Oermann & K. B. Gaberson (Eds.), *Evaluation and testing in nursing education* (4th ed., pp. 365–387). New York: Springer.

Glatthorn, A. A., Boschee, F., & Whitehead, B. M. (2009). *Curriculum leadership: Strategies for development and implementation* (2nd ed.). Thousand Oaks, CA: Sage.

Grammatikopoulos, V., Koustelics, A., Tsigillis, N., & Theodorakis, Y. (2004). Applying dynamic evaluation approach in education. *Studies in Educational Evaluation, 30*(4), 255–263.

Guba, E. G., & Lincoln, Y. S. (1989). *Fourth generation evaluation.* Newbury Park, CA: Sage.

Guba, E. G., & Lincoln, Y. S. (2001). Guidelines and checklist for constructivist (a.k.a. Fourth Generation) evaluation. Retrieved from http://www.wmich.edu/evalctr/archive_checklists/constructivisteval.pdf

Harn, B., Parisi, D., & Stoolmiller, M. (2013). Balancing fidelity with flexibility and fit: What do we really know about fidelity of implementation in schools? *Exceptional Children, 79*, 181–193.

Harrison, L. M., & Hasan, S. (2013). Appreciative inquiry in teaching and learning. *New Directions for Student Services, 143*, 65–77.

Herbener, D. J., & Watson, J. E. (1992). Evaluating nursing education programs. *Nursing Outlook, 40*, 27–32.

Heydman, A. M., & Sargent, A. (2011). Planning for accreditation: Evaluating the curriculum. In S. B. Keating (Ed.), *Curriculum development and evaluation in nursing* (2nd ed., pp. 311–332). New York: Springer.

Iwasiw, C. L. (2008, 2014). *Relevance-congruence-adequacy-reasonableness model of curriculum evaluation.* Unpublished manuscript. London, ON: Western University.

Iwasiw, C. L., Goldenberg, D., & Andrusyszyn, M.-A. (2005). Extending the evidence base for nursing education. *International Journal of Nursing Education Scholarship, 2*(1), Editorial.

Keating, S. B. (2011). Program evaluation. In S. B. Keating (Ed.), *Curriculum development and evaluation in nursing* (2nd ed., pp. 297–310). New York: Springer.

Lee, Y. J., & Chue, S. (2013). The value of fidelity of implementation criteria to evaluate school-based science curriculum innovations. *International Journal of Science Education, 35*, 2508–2537.

McLaughlin, J. A., & Jordon, G. B. (2010). Using logic models. In J. S. Wholey, H. P. Hatry, & K. E. Newcomer (Eds.), *Handbook of practical program evaluation* (3rd ed., pp. 55–80). San Francisco: Jossey-Bass.

Morris, T. L., & Hancock, D. R. (2013). Institute of Medicine core competencies as a foundation for nursing program evaluation. *Nursing Education Perspectives, 34*, 29–33.

Oliva, P. F. (2009). *Developing the curriculum* (7th ed.). Boston: Pearson Education.

Parkay, F. W., Hass, G., & Anctil, E. J. (Eds). (2010). Curriculum evaluation and assessment of learning. In F. W. Parkay, G. Hass, & E. J. Anctil (Eds.), *Curriculum leadership: Reading for developing quality educational programs* (9th ed., pp. 357–368). Boston: Allyn & Bacon.

Patton, M. Q. (2008). *Utilization-focused evaluation* (4th ed.). Thousand Oaks, CA: Sage.

Patton, M. Q. (2013). *Utilization-focused evaluation (U-FE Checklist).* Retrieved from http://www.wmich .edu/evalctr/wp-content/uploads/2010/05/UFE.pdf

Posavac, E. J. (2011). *Program evaluation: Methods and case studies* (8th ed.). Boston: Prentice Hall.

Robinson, T. T., & Cousins, J. B. (2004). Internal participatory evaluation as an organizational learning system: A longitudinal case study. *Studies in Educational Evaluation, 30*(1), 1–22.

Schug, V. (2012). Curriculum evaluation: Using National League for Nursing Accrediting Commission standards and criteria. *Nursing Education Perspectives, 33*, 302–305.

Stevenson, A. (Ed.). Standard. (2010). *Oxford dictionary of English* (3rd ed.). Oxford: Oxford University Press.

Stufflebeam, D. L. (2007*). CIPP evaluation model checklist.* Retrieved from http://www.wmich.edu/evalctr/archive_checklists/cippchecklist_mar07.pdf

Stufflebeam, D. L., & Shinkfield, A. J. (2007). *Evaluation theory, models, and applications.* San Francisco: Jossey-Bass.

Sullivan, L. E. (2009). Curriculum evaluation. The SAGE glossary of the social and behavioral sciences. Retrieved from http://knowledge.sagepub.com/view/behavioralsciences/SAGE.xml

Tomlison, C. A. (2010). Learning to love assessment. In F. W. Parkay, G. Hass, & E. J. Anctil (Eds.), *Curriculum leadership: Reading for developing quality educational programs* (9th ed., pp. 378–382). Boston: Allyn & Bacon.

Verdonschot, S. G. M. (2006). Methods to enhance reflective behaviour in innovations processes. *Journal of European Industrial Training, 30*, 670–686.

Wholey, J. S. (1983). *Evaluation and effective public management.* Boston: Little, Brown.

PART VI

Nursing Education by Distance Delivery

Curriculum Considerations in Nursing Education by Distance Delivery

Chapter Overview

In this chapter, *distance education* and *nursing education by distance delivery* are defined; then the institutional requirements for distance education are described. Ethical considerations, values, and beliefs in distance education are proposed. The sources of decisions to offer nursing education by distance delivery and the consequent nursing curriculum implications are outlined. Curriculum design is briefly overviewed, whereas the section on course design offers considerations particular to nursing education by distance delivery. The integration of pedagogy and technology is emphasized. Addressed are technology, course concepts and content, strategies to ignite learning, features of individual online "classes," opportunities for students to demonstrate learning, faculty evaluation of student achievement, and deciding on course design. Implementation and evaluation of distance courses are addressed. The relationship of nursing education by distance delivery to a context-relevant, evidence-informed, unified curriculum is explained. The core processes of faculty, ongoing appraisal, and scholarship activities related to distance education are presented. The chapter concludes with a summary and synthesis activities.

Chapter Goals

- Understand the definitions of *distance education* and *nursing education by distance delivery*, and the requirements for institutions to offer distance education.
- Gain insight into the values, beliefs, and ethical considerations in distance education.
- Consider the influence of distance delivery on course design, implementation, and evaluation.
- Review teaching responsibilities in distance education to promote learning; strengthen interaction, community, and inclusion; and enhance students' sense of control and confidence in their ability to be successful.
- Appreciate the relationship of distance education to an evidence-informed, context-relevant, unified curriculum.
- Reflect on the core processes of curriculum work related to distance education.

DISTANCE EDUCATION

Distance education is "institution-based, formal education where the learning group is separated, and where interactive telecommunications systems are used to connect learners, resources, and instructors" (Schlosser & Simonson, 2009, as cited in Simonson, Schlosser, & Orellana, 2011). The teaching and learning can be synchronous or asynchronous, or a combination of these. In all cases there are students, an instructor, geographic distance between them, a telecommunication system, and learning resources, all within the context of a formal educational offering.

Although the term *distance education* may be used synonymously with *online learning* and *e-learning*, it is more encompassing. All can include broadcast systems, electronic or telecommunications systems, and the Internet, but distance education is more than the dispersal of educational materials and provision of links to resources. It requires interaction between and among participants. Thus, correspondence courses are not considered within the definition and discussion of distance education in this chapter.

Distance education is built in part on the concept of *flexibility*. This concept suggests suppleness, elasticity, and nimbleness, adjectives that capture the idea of nonlinearity, consistent with teaching-learning processes. The term *flexible delivery* is used to contrast it with traditional face-to-face delivery, which is time and place dependent. Flexible delivery, therefore, implies single or combined use of delivery methods that are adaptable to a wide variety of students and expected learning outcomes. There is flexibility in the delivery methods employed, in addition to when and how they are used.

The delivery technologies used in distance education are generally web-based, multifaceted learning management systems (LMSs) with provision for private and two-way communication between and among teachers and students. The LMSs used by educational institutions allow for learning resources to be embedded and for external connections to podcasts, vodcasts, learning objects, experts in distant locations, and so forth. Through these means, the learning experience can be extended beyond an online course site. Moreover, the increased sophistication and reliability of technologies, such as videoconferencing systems or desktop videoconferencing, provide even greater opportunities for flexibility in the delivery of all or part of distance courses. However, in all instances, the "delivery" of the teaching and subsequent learning occur when teachers and students are not physically together.

Web technologies are increasingly becoming a part of distance education, although not typically as the sole medium. Web-based utilities and technology tools (e.g., blogs, wikis, social networking sites, instant messaging, cloud computing sites, podcasts, and vodcasts) allow students and faculty to communicate, collaborate, create content, generate knowledge, and share information online (Chu & Kennedy, 2011). Use of these technologies is consistent with a constructivist theory of learning (Greener, 2012; Paily, 2013).

Distance delivery, with or without the inclusion of web technologies, can be employed for complete courses, as convenient and effective adjuncts to on-campus, face-to-face courses, or as part of courses with hybrid delivery. Typically, back-channel digital communication (e.g., email, text messages, Twitter) is used to support connections between students and faculty.

The integration of digital computers and a worldwide telecommunications network to connect them has led to computer-based distance education becoming feasible in much of the world (Amirault, 2012). Therefore, geographic distance, by itself, is no longer an obstacle to education. Nonetheless, there are individuals for whom computer or mobile device ownership is not possible, Internet access is absent or slow, and efficacy with technology is lacking. Accordingly, technology-based distance education cannot yet be a sure solution for advancing the education of nurses worldwide.

NURSING EDUCATION BY DISTANCE DELIVERY

Nursing education by distance delivery is the provision of a complete nursing curriculum or part of a curriculum by distance methods. Within a degree curriculum, it is formal education based in an educational institution. Certificate-level nursing education by distance delivery can be based in educational institutions or other certificate-granting bodies. Continuing nursing education by distance education is provided by educational institutions, professional bodies, clinical specialty groups, and so forth. In all cases, the learning group and faculty are separated, and interactive telecommunications systems are used to connect students, resources, and faculty.

The educational offering can be synchronous, asynchronous, or a blend of the two. The nature and range of delivery technologies can vary, as can the type of interaction between and among learners and faculty. However, education via communication technology is a common feature of degree, certificate, and continuing nursing education.

INSTITUTIONAL REQUIREMENTS FOR DISTANCE EDUCATION

Distance education for an entire curriculum, individual courses, or hybrid courses can be considered only if suitable supports are in place. Without them, the desire of nursing faculty to extend the curriculum beyond the classroom will be unfulfilled. Therefore, the nature, quality, and extent of the supports become parameters for curriculum and course design.

Infrastructure

The structural features, processes, and procedures of an institution's LMS should be robust enough to accommodate a wide variety of learning and course management functions and contain the necessary security and backup features so that information is protected. The availability of authoring and graphics software is also important. An institutional technology plan and centralized maintenance of the technology system are necessary (Cheawjindakarn, Suwannatthachote, & Theearoungchaisri, 2012).

From the perspectives of students and faculty, the LMS needs to:

- Have intuitive navigation and a built-in help feature
- Accommodate the desired teaching, learning, assessment, and testing activities
- Allow for interaction between and among faculty and students, collectively and privately, synchronously and asynchronously
- Be comprehensive enough to preclude the need for use of systems external to the LMS
- Accept podcasts, vodcasts, and embedded links to external websites
- Include a recordkeeping system for marks associated with course activities and assessments

Reliable access to library databases, journal articles, and ebooks is necessary for faculty and students. Additionally, the institution is responsible for obtaining and maintaining the necessary licenses for the use of copyrighted material within course sites.

Resources to Support Distance Education Design and Teaching

Although the prevalence of distance education is growing, the acceptance rate of online education among faculty declined from 34% in 2007 to 31% in 2009 (Allen & Seaman, as cited in Liu, 2012). In a meta-analysis of research about barriers to distance education, increased time commitment, difficulty keeping up with technological changes, and lack of support staff to help with course development were identified by faculty (Berge & Muilenburg, as cited in Simonson et al., 2011). The decline in faculty acceptance of distance education, and the reported barriers point to a need for improved and sustained support for faculty who offer curricula or courses by distance technologies.

Faculty Development

Faculty development related to every aspect of distance education is essential once a decision has been made to offer all or some of a course, or an entire curriculum, by distance delivery. Specific ideas about faculty development are presented in a later section of this chapter.

Instructional Design Assistance

Essential to the successful development of distance courses is assistance from instructional designers and possibly media specialists. In order for students to achieve the goals or outcomes of a nursing course or curriculum, the interactions and engagement normally expected of on-campus students should be incorporated into the courses, using the most suitable technology. The creation of a smooth, productive, and comprehensive learning experience for students may require the expertise of instructional designers and media specialists until faculty members acquire experience and skill in distance education.

Assistance with Technology

Concomitant with assistance from instructional designers or media specialists is orientation to, and assistance with, the technology. Faculty members need to learn to use the technology, have access to expert help as they learn, and importantly, have immediate assistance when problems arise during course implementation.

Faculty, like students, may be present in computer-based distance courses at almost any time; therefore, a telephone help line is essential. Ideally, the help line would be available 24 hours a day, but it should be operational late into the evening at least. It is imperative that the help line is staffed during times that online examinations are being conducted. Help-line personnel ought to have the authority to enter the course site on the LMS to perform the necessary technological functions to resolve problems quickly.

Resources to Support Distance Learning

Paul and Cochran (2013) have proposed a model of interactions for distance programs (or courses), based on research about online learning. The components of the model include various interactions associated with distance education. Two of these are:

- *Student–technology interaction.* Necessary are student-centered and intuitive systems, along with orientation to the system and access to help with technology.
- *Student–institution interaction.* This includes the provision of online support services comparable to those available to on-campus students.

These components of the model are shared responsibilities of the institution and the school of nursing. The following ideas respond to those responsibilities.

Orientation to Distance Education

Students require assistance to learn to use the technology and processes that will form their learning environment. Orientations to technology can be accomplished through on-site sessions, provision of written material or instructional websites before courses begin, peer-tutoring systems, and so on. Of importance is the inclusion of information about the technological requirements (activation of an account, computer requirements, software, Internet speed, etc.). Additionally, the orientation could address attention to best practices for social media use (Schmitt, Sims-Giddens, & Booth, 2012).

Orientation to distance learning can address more than technology. It can include attention to:

- The nature of online learning
- Time commitment required for success
- Expected interactions and participation
- Assessment of readiness for distance education
- Self-directed learning skills
- Time management skills (Blackman & Major, 2012; Brown, Hughes, Keppell, Hard, & Smith, 2013; Cho, 2012)

Further, students should be informed of the resources for help available to them, and that use of these resources is both common and expected.

Technological and Academic Support

Prompt assistance from personnel at 24-hour technical and library help desks, and from faculty members about course matters, will reduce stress and build confidence. Access to telephone help desks is essential when students experience technological problems, and this becomes even more important during exam periods. Support for academic success, such as online tutoring and timely responses to student questions about courses or academic requirements ought to be readily available. Student frustration and discouragement, negative instructor ratings, and ultimately, attrition, can be consequences of lack of timely assistance when students experience academic and technological problems (Lee & Choi, 2011; Tallent-Runnels et al., 2006).

Access to learning materials is vital to support course-related work for faculty and students unable to visit or be physically present in the on-campus library. Therefore, reliable access to library materials, reference services, and resources (Zhu, McKnight, & Edwards, 2006) and assistance with navigating and troubleshooting online library systems are essential.

Students require access to all services available on campus, such as assistance with course registration and study skills, financial aid, and career and personal counseling. Similarly, academic counseling is important, and this will likely be provided by the school of nursing rather than by the educational institution. Student support could be available online, via email or desktop videoconferencing, or by telephone. The support will likely be available through a combination of these methods.

Policies

Suitable institutional polices are needed to support distance education. These require frequent review as the distance education landscape is constantly developing, presenting new opportunities and challenges for institutions.

Workload adjustments and monetary incentives to compensate for the time required to build online courses and to teach them could be a provision of faculty contracts. Additionally, guidelines related to class size and examination processes to ensure safety, security, and rigor should be in place (Vaughn, 2007). Another consideration is the intellectual property rights and ownership of courses authored for distance education, and this may be addressed in faculty contracts.

Policies addressing ethical behavior in distance education warrant attention (Simonson, 2012). Institutional policies related to plagiarism, cheating, and deceptive actions might require modification for distance courses. For example, there might be a specific policy about online test taking.

Policies related to the use of web technologies are also important. To illustrate, the use of social networking sites necessitates that students and faculty join the site and provide personal information. Is it appropriate for institutions to require this as a condition of teaching or course enrollment? Another example is the use of a cloud-computing site for collaborative student assignments. Questions arise about who owns the work: the students or the organization hosting the cloud site? Within schools of nursing, issues of privacy and confidentiality become important when there are references to client or agency situations in private and public sites. Although web technologies are ubiquitous, familiar to many students and faculty, and possibly acceptable to them for use in courses, policies or guidelines about their use would clarify acceptable practices.

ETHICAL CONSIDERATIONS IN DISTANCE EDUCATION

As distance education and the incorporation of web technology into distance and on-campus courses continue to grow, so do the ethical considerations that institutions, faculty members, and students must take into account. In the sections that follow are some interrelated ideas that require discussion and clarification, and possibly policy development. The ideas are listed in alphabetical order, but no hierarchy of importance is intended.

Academic Integrity

Educational institutions have policies related to academic integrity and consequences for breach of the policy. Policy modifications or procedures may be necessary for distance courses to prevent "e-cheating," particularly procedures for online testing. When students are located in their homes, completing unproctored examinations, it is possible for them to use textbooks when exams are not meant to be "open book," consult with one another via telephone or text messaging, or have someone else complete the examination. Should the possibility of cheating exclude the use of online examinations? How can deceitful actions be minimized? How can students be helped to understand that cheating is unacceptable and antithetical to professional nursing values? Should institutions require students to be physically present for testing, or to use software, such as "Secure Software Remote Proctor, which uses biometric verification as well as visual identification to log on to the testing site" (Bedford, Greg, & Clinton, 2011)?

Archiving of Online Courses

Are all course participants aware of the archiving practices of the institution? For what length of time are courses archived and why? Who has access to the archives, and in what circumstances? Consideration of these and similar matters is warranted.

Confidentiality and Privacy

Confidentiality and privacy are important in nursing courses where client information might form the content of some aspects of a course. They are also significant issues in relation to personal information or information about healthcare agencies that students might disclose. Confidentiality and privacy are heightened concerns when technology external to the LMS is incorporated into a course. Should educational dialogue occur only on institution-based sites? Course participants need to be fully informed about their responsibility in relation to confidentiality and privacy of course discussion, client information, and so forth. They ought to be made aware of professional requirements in relation to privacy and confidentiality and be familiar with professional guidelines about the use of web technology. It is necessary to promote professional dialogue and to ensure that only secure sites are used for course purposes.

Full Disclosure

Several questions about full disclosure can be kept in mind. Is there a moral obligation for institutions to disclose to faculty members and students that course sites may be archived? Are students aware that an LMS can track their participation and visits to the course site? Do faculty and students know who has access to the site and why?

Information Posted on the Internet

An important consideration in relation to the content of posted information is accuracy, particularly if material created is, or will be, publicly available. If, for example, the creation of a wiki entry or blog is a course requirement, and there are inaccuracies in it, who bears or shares the moral responsibility for providing incorrect information to the public? How can procedures be built into courses to prevent such occurrences? What if social media sites (used within or external to a course) become a location for comments about the course, the faculty member, or classmates? With whom do responsibility and accountability rest?

Ownership of Archived Courses

With interactive courses, the content has been created by students and faculty. Furthermore, student projects submitted within an LMS have been created by students. This gives rise to the following questions:

- Who owns the archived course, the institution or all those who participated in the course?
- Do students and faculty have any rights of ownership over the completed courses? If so, what are those rights?
- Should the contributions of students who withdraw from a course be expunged or remain as part of the course archive?
- Who has the authority to give consent for use of the archived material for research or reporting purposes?

Use of Communication Tools, Internet Sites, or Media External to the Educational Institution

Many questions can be posed about the use of communication tools, media, and Internet sites external to the course site. Some of these might be:

- Can the use of communication tools or media external to the educational institution be a course requirement if course participants are required to provide personal information in order to use the site or media?
- If these sites are used, who owns the posted information: the account holder or the site provider?
- Should external sites be used for course work that relates to clients or healthcare agencies? Can postings be removed?
- Can the purchase of mobile devices and applications be required, in addition to personal computers? Should only free, web-based applications be used, if the use of external sites is acceptable?
- Does the use of communication tools, Internet sites, and media external to the LMS subtly convey the idea that all material on the Internet is of equal academic rigor and value?
- Are there external agencies that might have authority to view the material posted on private sites? If so, is it acceptable to use those sites?

It is evident that many questions remain unanswered with regard to the implications of using technology in the delivery of education. These questions are worthy of full discussion by educational institutions.

VALUES AND BELIEFS INHERENT IN A COMMITMENT TO NURSING EDUCATION BY DISTANCE DELIVERY

A commitment to nursing education via distance technology reflects nursing faculty members' values and beliefs about themselves, nursing education, and the nursing curriculum. These include acceptance and openness to advances in educational methods and technology, readiness to learn new pedagogical and technological skills, willingness to engage students in technological learning environments, and belief in the importance of accessible education for nurses. Additional values and beliefs inherent in the provision of distance education in nursing are:

- Belief that quality nursing education is possible through the use of technology
- View of active participation and interaction as essential characteristics of learning (i.e., support of constructivism and brain-based learning)
- Appreciation of students' need for ongoing guidance and support
- Dedication to the development of learning communities and supportive class cultures
- Trust in students' autonomy and desire to learn
- Confidence in students' ability to achieve course competencies or goals without the faculty member's physical presence
- Respect for diverse learning styles
- Commitment to maximizing student learning through own ongoing virtual presence

SOURCES OF DECISIONS TO OFFER DISTANCE EDUCATION AND CONSEQUENT NURSING CURRICULUM IMPLICATIONS

A decision to offer distance courses in a nursing curriculum can arise from three different circumstances. Each has implications for subsequent nursing curriculum and course development.

First, during curriculum development, the analysis of contextual data can lead to the logical decision that educational approaches should include distance delivery for all or part of a nursing curriculum. In this situation, the total faculty group endorses the idea, and this decision will be a significant parameter in subsequent curriculum and course development.

Secondly, apart from a formal curriculum development process, nursing faculty members may decide to initiate or expand the use of distance technologies within existing programs in response to student characteristics, desire to increase enrollment or access, conviction that quality learning outcomes can be achieved, and so forth. This choice will result in modifications in course design and implementation, within the existing curriculum design. The number of courses involved will determine the extent of necessary development activities. Thirdly, there can be a strategic decision by the educational institution to increase access to educational programs through distance delivery. As a consequence, the school of nursing is obligated to support the institution's strategic plans. This situation can result in the development of a completely reconceptualized nursing curriculum, or modifications within the existing curriculum.

NURSING CURRICULUM DESIGN INCORPORATING DISTANCE DELIVERY

Curriculum design, explicated as the configuration of a program of studies, includes the courses selected, their sequencing and delivery, relationships between and among them, and associated curriculum policies. The curriculum design process entails all activities and decisions that result in the creation of the actual program of studies, that is, the completed curriculum. The design process for curricula employing distance delivery parallels that for traditional, campus-based, face-to-face delivery.

The starting point for nursing curriculum development is the context in which the curriculum will be offered and in which graduates will practice nursing. The aim is to develop a curriculum that is evidence-informed, context-relevant, and unified; provides opportunities for students to achieve intended outcomes or goals; is congruent with curriculum foundations; and has internal consistency, logical flow, and unity. There should be planning to maximize implementation fidelity and to prepare for formative and summative evaluation of students' achievement and the curriculum components. These fundamental considerations are necessary in all curriculum development, regardless of the delivery method.

Designing Nursing Courses for Distance Delivery

Designing nursing courses for distance delivery includes planning all components of traditional courses: title, purpose, description, competencies or goals, strategies to ignite learning, content, classes, opportunities for students to demonstrate learning and faculty evaluation of student achievement, and the relationships between and among these components. Only the details of course design that require particular consideration for distance delivery are presented in this chapter.

A defining characteristic of course design for distance delivery is the confluence of pedagogy and technology. The skillful integration of these gives vitality to courses, and achievement of a satisfactory convergence might require assistance from instructional design and media experts.

Design Parameters

Course designers are mindful of parameters that influence all course design, such as characteristics of students, educational and philosophical approaches, curriculum outcomes or goals, major curriculum concepts, placement of courses in the curriculum, and so forth. For courses offered by distance delivery methods, the institution's LMS, the availability of web technologies, and policies about distance education are major parameters of course design.

Course designers also consider factors within distance courses that influence student success: student–faculty interaction, student–technology interactions, student–institution interaction (Paul & Cochran, 2013), student–content interaction, student autonomy and control, and student social presence (sense of connectedness; Shearer, 2013). Although these are considerations in traditional courses, they are highlighted in distance courses because of the physical separation of participants and the greater likelihood of some students feeling isolated.

Another possible parameter is temporality. An *a priori* decision may be made about whether course delivery will be synchronous or asynchronous, or include elements of both. This decision will influence the design. Alternately, this decision may emerge during the design process.

Design Process

Designing distance courses is not a matter of trying to recreate a face-to-face class online (Dennen, 2013). Rather, it requires beginning with the course goals or competencies, and creating a course that takes into account the factors that influence student success, the curriculum foundations, the available technologies, and the temporal nature of student participation. Course design is facilitated by collaboration with instructional designers, media specialists, consultation with experts, and access to materials that capture best practices in distance education.

Once the course purpose, description, and competencies or goals have been prepared, the next logical next step is to consider the other components of nursing courses, as described in the following section. Iterative thinking, discussion, and ongoing appraisal are necessary about the course components and their relationship to the available technology.

It is important to emphasize that nursing education courses offered by distance delivery are not designed in isolation from other courses in the curriculum. Each course is part of a larger whole whose aim is to facilitate students' development as professional nurses. Thus, it is essential that course designers consider the placement of each course within the curriculum and ensure that there is logical and conceptual unity within and among courses.

Selection of Technology

The technological aspects of course design are most pronounced when considering strategies to ignite learning and opportunities for students to demonstrate learning. The LMS and web technologies that are used should serve and support learning and teaching in as seamless a fashion as possible and never overwhelm students or distract them from the course purpose.

An institution's LMS provides a consistent organizational template for course materials and teaching-learning processes, while allowing choice in the features that are used, and in the teaching, learning, and assessment processes. Incorporation of learning activities requiring web technologies is possible, if there are no policy prohibitions about this. The template provides a standardized look across courses and this facilitates students' familiarity with, and timely access to, commonly used course elements such as syllabi, discussion groups, timetables, and web links (Halstead, 2005). Additionally, the standardized look contributes to the curriculum's visual unity.

Course Concepts and Content

As in traditional courses, the course concepts and content are determined by the curriculum mapping that is part of curriculum development. Skillful facilitation may be necessary to ensure that concepts are addressed in the desired depth in online discussion, and that discussion focuses in a balanced fashion on concepts and substantive content. Additionally, in courses that employ web technology, faculty ought to plan carefully to ensure that learning to use the technology, and the technology itself, do not overshadow student attention to concepts and content.

Strategies to Ignite Learning

Strategies selected to ignite learning are intended to move students toward achievement of course competencies or goals in a way that is assisted, not hampered, by the technology in use. An LMS allows for strategies normally used in classrooms and additional strategies associated with electronic communication and links. All, or nearly all, can be available simultaneously so students can access course information, resources, and strategies pertinent to them at any time. Because distance education is premised on a belief in the value of active learning and constructed knowledge, the strategies to ignite learning typically require students to engage in divergent thinking, discussion, and collaborative work.

The strategies to ignite learning ought to encompass the three types of interaction previously described: student–faculty, student–student, and student–content (Moore, as cited in Bernard et al., 2009). A fourth type of interaction also requires attention: student–self interaction. This is two-way interaction between the inner/personal self and the academic/professional self through reflection. Revisiting and analyzing insights through individual and shared reflection can lead to deeper learning (Andrusyszyn & Davie, 1997). Therefore, strategies to ignite and sustain reflection are often incorporated into nursing courses offered by distance delivery.

Embedded opportunities within courseware for social interaction, synchronous and asynchronous discussion, and collaboration on practice issues or case studies perceived as authentic by students will promote disciplinary discourse and allow student engagement with the content and the process of knowledge construction (Dunlap, Sobel, & Sands, 2007; Larreamendy-Joerns & Leinhardt, 2006; Martens, Bastiaens, & Kirschner, 2007). Within large classes, small groups can be formed and their discussion segmented from other groups' discourse. Access to each group discussion could be open to all class participants, or only to designated group members.

With courses delivered through an LMS, didactic material and links to other learning resources can be posted electronically. These presentations can be designed with technological enhancements to overcome limitations of written text and static presentations. The learning resources could consist of videos, journal articles, material posted on other websites, supplementary notes, and so on.

Other strategies might involve an online live discussion or a real-time virtual classroom with lectures and demonstrations, if these features are part of the LMS. Such strategies are convenient for guest lecturers and practice experts, and add immediacy and authenticity to the learning. Student presentations are also possible in this way, or through didactic postings. Full use of LMS components allows for a wide range of strategies to ignite learning and responses to a variety of learning styles.

The range of activities can be extended through the use of web technologies. **Table 16-1** includes some of these technologies and ideas about their use in nursing education. Of note is that use of blogs or sites such as Google Drive allows for tracking of contributions, possibly enhancing participation in collaborative work and reducing the "missing in action" phenomenon (Bento and Schuster, as cited in Booth, Andrusyszyn, & Iwasiw, 2011) in online courses.

Countless combinations and permutations of strategies and technologies are possible, and are limited only by faculty members' imagination, creativity, time, and expertise, and the institution's technology infrastructure and support. In an expanding technological world, it is most critical to select strategies to maximize achievement of curriculum outcomes or goals, and to respect student diversity and multiple ways of knowing.

Individual "Classes"

Guidelines for student learning activities can be prepared for sessions in distance education courses, as they are for traditional courses. These provide direction to learning, assisting students to focus on the ideas and processes that lead to achievement of course goals

Table 16-1   Examples of Web Technologies and Possible Uses in Nursing Education

Examples of Web 2.0 Technologies	Possible Uses in Nursing Education
Blogging web software (e.g., Blogger, WordPress)	Creation of collaborative blogs with contributions identified by students' names, and visible to all course participants (Agosto, Copeland, & Zach, 2013), for example, construction of a health information or advocacy site relevant to course topics
Cloud computing (e.g., Google Drive)	Creation of collaborative projects
Desktop conferencing (e.g., Skype audio only or audio and video)	Discussion by course groups
	Consultation or advisement by faculty member with individuals or small groups
	Live class sessions in courses with small enrollment
Online mind-mapping software (e.g., Mindmeister, Mindomo)	Creating individual concept maps, group brainstorming
Podcast and vodcast preparation (e.g., Audacity)	Delivery of mandatory or supplementary course content, including simulations
	Avenue for students to create and share knowledge
Reference management software (e.g., Mendeley, which also provides academic social networking)	Shared reference management
	Collaboration on academic topics
Social networking services (e.g., Facebook)	Tutorial sessions
	Discussion and/or question and answers as examination preparation
Social networking/microblogging services (e.g., Twitter)	Communication among and between students and faculty
	Organizer for class discussions (Bristol, as cited by Schmitt et al., 2012)
Video posting applications (e.g., Youtube)	Posting of course-related videos by faculty or students
	Source of course-related videos
Virtual reality simulators (immersive worlds)	Replacement or adjunct for some professional practice experiences
Web conferencing	Tutorial sessions
	Group discussions and problem-solving
	Consultations with experts
Wikis	Student development of collaborative projects or wikis related to health topics

or competencies. In addition, the guidelines for learning activities, prepared in a consistent format throughout the curriculum, give unity to the course and link the course visually to the rest of the curriculum.

When planning for individual classes, it is necessary to decide exactly what constitutes the temporal span of a "class" in a course that employs ongoing discussion. For example, will the class start on Monday at 9:00 a.m. and continue to Friday at 4:00 p.m.? Will it continue for 7 days a week? When will the summary and transition to the next topic occur? Will discussions be closed at a specified time, or will they remain open for the duration of the course?

Another aspect of temporality is the differences in students' time of participation in asynchronously delivered courses. Design considerations might include whether:

- It is acceptable for some students to contribute their ideas at the end of the discussion period, perhaps on weekends after most students might consider the discussion to be finished.
- Students' obligation to contribute to classmates' learning through timely and regular participation can justify a requirement about the timing and frequency of participation, thereby overriding the premise that distance education is time-independent.

Class design decisions also include matters such as which discussions require small-group work and which would involve the whole class. If small groups are completing learning tasks, is it necessary for them to report back to the total group? If so, the timing of the reporting back would dictate the timing of the small-group work.

Consideration may be given to whether or not students will share responsibility for facilitating discussion in small groups and in the total group. Typically, students manage their own discussion in small groups, with limited involvement of the faculty member, as in traditional classes. Sharing facilitation with the faculty member for the large-group discussion may be desirable if the activity aligns with course expectations and if the logistics can be organized so that all students have an opportunity to do so.

The need for faculty presence in online environments is important for student guidance and learning. Therefore, a suitable balance between faculty presence and student autonomy is considered when courses are designed.

Opportunities for Students to Demonstrate Learning and Faculty Evaluation of Student Achievement

In all courses, students will be expected to demonstrate, and faculty to evaluate, achievement of course competencies or goals. The choice of methods for students to demonstrate learning is related to consistency with philosophical and educational approaches, course competencies or goals, and the like. As always, a variety of methods is preferred. The appropriateness of giving grades for participation remains controversial.

When deliberating about methods for students to demonstrate achievement, faculty members examine factors such as:

- Compatibility of ideas with curriculum foundations and the available technology
- Student access to the necessary resources and supports to demonstrate learning
- Balance between individual and group demonstration of learning
- Potential for timely feedback
- Scheduling of examination sessions (synchronous or asynchronous)
- Security and ease of testing and assignment-submission system
- Opportunities afforded by technology

The opportunities available for students to demonstrate their learning can occur within the bounds of the LMS, or extend beyond this. In all cases, the effort required by students to create the work, and by faculty members to evaluate it, should be commensurate with the extent to which the completed work will demonstrate an integrated achievement of course goals or competencies.

Demonstration of Cognitive, Affective, and Psychomotor Learning

Cognitive learning can be demonstrated through test responses, concept mapping, e-portfolios, peer critique, discussion, and creation of individual or collaborative term papers, projects, presentations, or case analyses, and so forth. Affective learning can be made evident through discussion, creation of video role plays, responses to ethical dilemmas, online debating, and so forth (Oermann & Gaberson, 2014).

Demonstration of psychomotor learning may be less straightforward, because faculty are unable to observe the psychomotor performance in person. However, students can engage in virtual simulations and submit videos of psychomotor skill performance. Attention needs to be given to the possibility of technical problems with video quality, or uploading to an LMS (Strand, Fox-Young, Long, & Bogossian, 2013).

When students are asked to create health-related or issue-related videos, blogs, or wiki entries, they are usually eager for these to become public. Thought should be given to how faculty can assess these learning products quickly and give feedback so students can make necessary revisions within the timeframe of the course. An additional consideration in the work that students submit is the limit on the file size allowed by the LMS. It may not be possible for them to upload large files, such as videos (Kirkwood, 2011). Therefore, the video would have to be located on an external Internet site, such as YouTube. If this is the case, it is wise to consider what could appropriately be made available on a public site.

Academic Integrity

With computer-based testing, security can be strengthened with the use of tightly timed examinations, online proctoring systems, randomized distribution of several forms of the exam, and randomization of test items and response options (Bedford et al., 2011; Caudle, Bigness, Daniels, Gillmor-Kahn, & Knestrick, 2011). Alternately, consideration can be given to the use of examination centers that all students must attend.

Whether or not online testing is used, the creation and support of an environment of academic integrity is an important element of all courses. Clear explanations of what constitutes academic honesty and dishonesty, why it is important to cite sources (including those from the Internet), what plagiarism is, and when collaboration is (and is not) appropriate, are part of developing a context of honesty (Conway, Klaassen, & Kiel and Hart & Morgan, as cited in Oermann & Gaberson, 2014). Significantly, these ideas form part of the course syllabus. Explanations and discussion about how academic honesty relates to professional values and ethics can add importance to ideas of academic integrity for students. Further, the matter of academic integrity can be raised as submission dates for student work approach.

DECIDING ON COURSE DESIGN

Decisions about course design are similar for traditional courses and those offered through distance delivery, with the added feature that an instructional designer and media specialist may be part of the process. Recursive and integrated discussion occurs about course competencies or goals, content, strategies to ignite learning, choice of technology, and possibilities within the technology. Some matters that faculty members and course designers consider are:

- The "look and feel" of the course. Consistency among courses eliminates the need for students to learn new navigation with each course, and contributes to the visual unity of the curriculum.
- The convergence among the course competencies or goals, content, and technology. In what ways is it possible for students to achieve the expectations through the technological environment? Which features of the available technologies would best advance achievement of which course expectations? Is there economy of technology so that learning to use web tools does not supersede students' substantive learning?
- Strategies to ignite learning. Which are possible via technology? How much variation is reasonable? Which can be incorporated while maintaining ease and transparency of navigation within the technologies?
- Moderating discussion. Will faculty and teaching assistants do this entirely, or will students also be expected to be discussion moderators?
- Methods for students to demonstrate learning. Which match the course expectations and are possible and reasonable within the technologies?
- Release of course components. Will all components be available at the beginning of the course, or will some be accessible later as the course progresses? Why?

- Provision of guidelines, rubrics, and self-assessment tools to help students develop confidence in their learning progress (Dunlap, 2005).
- Faculty preferences and efficacy with the LMS and other technologies.
- Anticipated student comfort with the technologies.
- Course etiquette. How, when, and by whom should expectations be determined?
- Teacher availability to respond to messages and requests for assistance.
- Participation patterns for students. Daily? Thrice weekly? As students deem suitable, as negotiated, or as specified by the faculty member?
- Participation pattern for faculty and teaching assistants.
- Time commitment for students, faculty, and teaching assistants.
- Ethical issues inherent in distance education.

Discussion points for hybrid courses incorporating distance technology could be:

- Choice of delivery mode(s) in addition to face-to-face delivery
- Selection of learning activities to be conducted in the face-to-face setting, online, and/ or with web technologies
- Provision of lectures, and preparatory and/or supplementary materials via a website, podcasts, streaming media, and so on (Which material? Which media?)
- Use of web tools for learning activities and completion of opportunities to demonstrate learning

A finalized course design will result when nursing faculty members, instructional designers, and media specialists are satisfied that they have achieved a reasonable convergence of pedagogy and technology. The result should be a course that

- Engages students
- Moves them toward achievement of curriculum expectations
- Is based in technology whose navigation is smooth and transparent
- Incorporates evidence-informed design and teaching
- Is philosophically, educationally, and conceptually consistent with the curriculum foundations
- Contributes to the overall rigor and unity of the curriculum

Summary of Curriculum and Course Design Process for Nursing Distance Education by Distance Delivery

The curriculum and course design process for nursing education by distance delivery is the same as designing for traditional delivery. The difference lies in the influence of the delivery technology on course design. Involvement of an instructional design expert, and, if possible, a media specialist, is often necessary until faculty develop expertise in creating distance education courses. Nonetheless, all decisions and deliberations are based on the curriculum foundations, that is, the philosophical and educational approaches, the major curriculum concepts, and the key professional abilities, along with curriculum goals or outcomes. Important to remember is that the process of design is iterative, with the intent of achieving an internally consistent course with a harmonious blending of pedagogy and technology.

IMPLEMENTING AND EVALUATING NURSING EDUCATION BY DISTANCE DELIVERY

Exemplary Teaching in Online Nursing Courses

Faculty–student interaction is essential to student achievement in distance education courses. As students are engaging in the learning activities, faculty are responsible for attending to the teaching actions that validate students' participation and learning efforts, offer guidance in learning, support motivation, and provide feedback about achievement (Paul & Cochran, 2013). For students to feel they are part of a community of learners, their social, cognitive, and affective presence requires validation. Faculty can plan for this validation through course design and teaching presence (Stavredes & Herder, 2013).

A critical element of the interaction is the faculty member's clarity of communication. Unambiguous written communication is paramount because verbal clarification may not be possible. Misunderstandings can lead to student frustration and take several subsequent messages to correct.

Exemplary teaching via distance delivery can be viewed as consisting of three inter-related and mutually supportive categories of teaching actions. These categories encompass actions that promote learning; strengthen interaction, community, and inclusion; and enhance students' sense of control and confidence in their ability to be successful. All require a faculty member's continuing presence: "being visible to, engaged with, and caring for the students through every step of the way through the learning journey on which they embark together" (Ekmekci, 2013, p. 34).

Promote Learning

Teaching actions that promote learning include:

- Preparing a well-designed course that includes attention to curriculum concepts and substantive content, grounded in the world of nursing
- Stating clear expectations that lead students to perform beyond their initial perspectives of what they would achieve (Edwards, Perry, & Jansen, 2011)

- Using intentional processes within the course so that student learning can be expanded and expressed
- Intervening in a timely fashion, for example, by questioning or refocusing discussion to guide or scaffold learning
- Including course concepts in dialogue with students (Siemens, 2010) and in feedback about student submissions, making important ideas omnipresent
- Asking heuristic questions to help students make connections among concepts, to previous learning, and to nursing practice
- Offering comments that invite reflection, higher order thinking, metacognition, and meaning making (e.g., *I wonder about . . .* ; *Help me to understand how X relates to Y; Tell me how these ideas fit together; Please share your understanding of . . .*)
- Limiting the variety of technologies used, so that learning about technology does not overshadow content and process learning
- Using authentic assessment techniques that reflect a balance of individual and group activities
- Providing prompt feedback (to individuals and groups) that serves as a learning scaffold
- Including activities that intentionally promote reflection, higher order thinking, metacognition, and meaning making

Strengthen Interaction, Community, and Inclusion

Strengthening interaction, community, and inclusion can be advanced by the following teaching actions:

- Informing students about the nature, quality, and quantity of interaction expected
- Providing or negotiating guidelines for communication, participation, and collaboration (Booth et al., 2011) and explaining or inviting comments about why such guidelines are relevant for nursing practice
- Providing guidance as students develop skill in the necessary interaction styles
- Sensitizing students to professional and ethical aspects of social technology use (Schmitt et al., 2012).
- Planning student–student, student–content, and student–self interaction through small- or large-group discussion, group projects, and so forth
- Responding promptly to personal communication
- Creating a vodcast as the welcoming message to the course
- Sending personal messages to individuals or groups, particularly when personal or learning support is needed (Ivanoka & Stick, as cited in Lee & Choi, 2011)

- Acknowledging stressful times (e.g., as the examination period approaches) and offering encouragement through email, vodcast, or podcast
- Posting frequent acknowledgments of the ideas presented and including the names of contributors
- Ensuring that online messages are understandable, clear, unambiguous, inclusive, and free of expressions that might be offensive to some

Enhance Students' Sense of Control and Confidence

Many of the teaching actions previously listed contribute to students' sense of control and confidence in their ability to be successful in the course and in nursing, such as specifying expectations and providing prompt feedback. Additionally, teaching actions in this category can include:

- Organizing and managing the course effectively
- Testing the online course site to ensure that navigation is smooth, course material is visible, and embedded links are working
- Testing external sites (e.g., social networking or document preparation sites) to ensure that students will be able to engage in the planned activities
- Ensuring that textbooks to be purchased and online resources are available
- Referring students to sites for orientation to distance learning and/or technology as necessary
- Responding rapidly to requests for help
- Creating guidelines about how to be successful in the course
- Explicating the purpose of course activities, for example, explaining that discussion is meant to promote meaning making, not reiterate textbook content (Dennen, 2013)
- Providing guidelines and rubrics for projects, and self-assessment tools to help students determine their achievement (Dunlap, 2005)
- Attending consistently to the relationships between course learning and students' participation in the practice of nursing
- Marking and returning course work with meaningful feedback promptly
- Creating incremental opportunities for students to demonstrate learning
- Including opportunities for students to explore the networked world beyond the course site
- Incorporating student choice about projects and/or course activities
- Providing opportunities for peer teaching via online student presentations, student leadership in discussions, creation and posting of videos, and so forth
- Being open to renegotiation of due dates for course work in response to individuals' life events

In summary, exemplary teaching in online nursing courses encompasses the elements of effective teaching in classroom and professional practice environments. In all nursing education contexts, it is necessary to:

- Design a sound learning experience that incorporates interactivity and well-structured content that is relevant to students (Lee & Choi, 2011)
- Incorporate authentic activities that allow for student creativity, enhance motivation, and support success
- Provide "persistent presence" (Siemens, 2010, p. 5), that is, be active, involved, and responsive

Exemplary Teaching in Distance Nursing Courses via Web-based Conferencing

Courses taught via web-based conferencing have many characteristics of traditional classes:

- Faculty and students are present at one time.
- The class is time-limited.
- Slide presentations, live presentations and demonstrations, and dynamic interactions are possible.

The teaching challenge is to attend to all participants, while not being the sole focus of attention. Of importance are the teaching activities of promoting learning; strengthening interaction, community, and inclusion; and enhancing students' sense of control and confidence in ability to be successful. Class size will determine the precise ways these are accomplished, although, in general, the teaching actions cited for online courses are relevant. All aspects of personal communication with individuals and groups remain highly important.

Systems such as WebEx allow for simultaneous visual and audio presentations, and text chat by participants. The faculty member has a multitasking role: leading the session, interacting with the presenter and students, answering questions, and dealing with comments in the text chat (Seddon, Postlethwaite, James, & Mulryne, 2012). Alternately, the faculty member might be the presenter and respond to student questions and comments either during or after the presentation. Because of the time required to type messages, the faculty member needs to attend carefully to succinct, accurate communication.

Blackboard Collaborate offers a feature that allows for live audio chat by participants. Faculty members have the role of moderating the discussion, responding to requests to speak. To be effective leaders of learning, they ought to do more than enable the audio transmission by individuals, but to intervene as appropriate, posing questions and adding thought-provoking comments.

Useful for graduate seminars or small undergraduate classes are desktop videoconferencing services such as Skype, which allow all participants to share the screen for formal presentations and to see and hear one another in real time. In this case, faculty members' activities are most like those in traditional classrooms. Seeing students' nonverbal behavior assists a faculty member to identify when a teaching intervention is required in the discussion.

Web videoconferencing can also be used to link groups of students when each group is physically together. Examples of international linkages of graduate students include joint videoconference seminars by Canadian and Norwegian students (Iwasiw et al., 2000) and American and British students (Daley, Spalla, Arndt, & Warnes, 2008) to discuss topics related to care management. In these examples, exemplary teaching included arranging for technology connections, planning of course and/or seminar purposes and processes by international partners, supporting student facilitation of discussion, surfacing issues of local and international significance, and planning for evaluation.

In summary, there are many web-conferencing systems available, with varying features. The range of teaching activities will be affected, in part, by the system(s) supported by the educational institution. In all cases, however, courses are designed and teaching is undertaken to build connections among students, advance their learning, and contribute to students' achievement of course and curriculum outcomes or goals.

Evaluating Nursing Education Offered by Distance Delivery

Faculty members continually engage in appraisal of curriculum and course design. The design of the course evaluation should be completed before the course is implemented and be consistent with the evaluation plan, model, and procedures in use in the full curriculum.

There may be a need to clarify the purpose of course evaluation specific to distance delivery, if the entire curriculum is not offered in this way. Criteria or standards for courses offered by distance delivery could be necessary, if not already part of the overall curriculum standards. Once the evaluation is completed, reporting of evaluation results may extend to instructional designers, who are now stakeholders in the nursing curriculum.

All aspects of course evaluation ought to be included in the evaluation of courses delivered via technology. Useful information specific to the pedagogy–technology interface include students' feedback about matters such as:

- Sense of connectedness with peers and faculty, feeling of control over technology, perceptions of the contributions of the course design to their learning, and time on task
- Ease of navigation in the LMS and use of system features, such as email and submission of completed work
- Fit between specific learning activities and technologies

- Reasons why they did or did not engage in specified activities (TLT Group, 2011)
- Suitability of technologies for learning about a person-centered, practice discipline
- Authenticity of learning activities and opportunities to demonstrate learning
- General satisfaction with course delivery

The results of organized and regular course evaluations contribute to ideas about subsequent course refinement or revision. When offering courses by distance delivery, or incorporating technology into on-campus courses, it is incumbent on nurse educators to expand ideas of course evaluation to explicitly include features of the technologies used and their intersection with learning about nursing.

If an entire curriculum is being offered by distance delivery, the considerations noted earlier continue to apply. Additionally, all features of planning curriculum evaluation are essential.

RELATIONSHIP OF NURSING EDUCATION BY DISTANCE DELIVERY TO AN EVIDENCE-INFORMED, CONTEXT-RELEVANT, UNIFIED NURSING CURRICULUM

Nursing education courses may be offered by distance delivery in addition to, or instead of traditional nursing courses. In either case, they ought to be visually and conceptually consistent with other courses in the curriculum. In other words, nursing courses offered by distance technology are not separate from the school's curriculum but an integral part of it. Therefore, if the curriculum as a whole has been developed to be evidence-informed, context-relevant, and unified, individual distance education courses will fit into the curriculum framework and form part of a unified whole.

If an entire nursing curriculum is intended to be offered by distance delivery, its development, implementation, and evaluation should follow the processes of the Model of Evidence-Informed, Context-Relevant, Unified Curriculum Development. If this is done, the evidence-informed, context-relevant, and unified nature of the curriculum will be assured.

CORE PROCESSES OF CURRICULUM WORK

Faculty Development

Faculty development and support are necessary in relation to designing and implementing courses offered by distance delivery. Faculty development can be led by technology specialists, instructional designers, and media experts, as well as faculty members experienced in distance education.

Course Design and Technologies

The overall goal of faculty development as it relates to curriculum and course design is to advance members' appreciation, understanding, and knowledge of distance methods and their intersection with pedagogy. Essential is the development of proficiency in use of the institution's LMS. Importantly, it is incumbent upon faculty to learn about current web technologies, social media, and their potential for use in nursing education.

Faculty development can include individual, micro-level assistance with course development, based on faculty members' comfort, knowledge, and expertise with distance delivery. Broader discussions could be undertaken with faculty from nursing and other disciplines about possible opportunities for students to demonstrate learning in distance courses, the right balance of various technologies, academic integrity in courses, or the ethical considerations of distance education.

Learning opportunities with a wider scope might include centrally offered workshops to address strengths and limitations of selected delivery methods, or informal dialogue among faculty about successes and frustrations with specific delivery or communication methods. Sharing circles with novice and experienced faculty could encourage discussion among those who are tentative about the effectiveness of distance education and those who are convinced of its value. Such perspectives and experiences might provide a balance between positive and negative views.

Guided workshops for faculty converting courses to distance delivery could include brainstorming about course reconfiguration to incorporate different technologies. This may have relevance for faculty wanting to incorporate technology into on-campus classes. In addition, novices might be observers in distance courses being offered and could be mentored by experienced peers as they develop their own courses for distance delivery.

Teaching via Distance

A critical aspect of preparing for teaching via distance technologies is an understanding of the faculty role in course implementation. For some faculty, a shift is needed from being the *playwright*, *active director*, and *featured actor* of in-class learning activities, to being a combination of *playwright*, *minor player*, and *prompter*. The playwright in traditional and distance courses creates the course structure, and develops and makes available necessary resources and processes. As a minor player, the nursing faculty member in distance courses contributes to the unfolding dialogue and learning but becomes the central focus rarely and only for brief periods. The prompter's presence is persistent and known to students, who receive support and assistance as needed. This may represent a significant change in teaching style for some faculty; therefore, faculty skilled in classroom teaching may need support in shifting their teaching style (Johnson & Meehan, 2013).

Facilitation of online courses or web-conferencing courses is a skill that involves knowing when to intervene, where to intervene (in the public discussion forum or privately via email), how to phrase ideas so the intent is conveyed clearly, and when to observe without comment. Development or refinement of these skills can be facilitated through review and analysis of examples of online discussion (used with participants' permission). The nature and tone of the facilitation ought to be consistent with the philosophical and educational approaches that form part of the curriculum foundations.

Another faculty development activity might be to consider the evidence-informed teaching practices that faculty members are using in the classroom and consider how they could be transformed into teaching actions in distance education. An introduction to best practices and research about teaching in distance education courses would strengthen this discussion. Sessions focusing on the transition to distance teaching could include faculty members from other disciplines and/or members of the institution's teaching support center.

Shared teaching with experienced distance education faculty can be a way to ease the transition from classroom to distance teaching. Ongoing mentoring can be useful to novices as they encounter teaching challenges in distance education. Regular discussions among faculty about topics such as online teaching, web conferencing, the use of web technologies, social media, and so forth can be of help to experienced and novice faculty in distance, hybrid, and traditional courses. Furthermore, faculty members' self-assessment, course evaluations, and student feedback all contribute to the development of faculty leading nursing education courses delivered by distance technology.

Ongoing Appraisal

The ongoing appraisal processes of curriculum development, implementation, and evaluation for nursing education by distance delivery includes all the appraisal questions posed during curriculum development of traditional courses. Additional areas of appraisal relate to the intersection of learning and technology. Faculty might ask themselves questions such as those that follow:

- Are the plans for student engagement sufficient to stimulate motivation and learning?
- Are the learning activities commensurate with the curriculum foundations, the selected technology, and the timeframe of the course?
- Will the learning activities require active involvement by all students, or is there potential for some students to be "missing in action"?
- Will the need to learn new technologies create undue stress for students?
- Is a suitable variety of technologies used across courses? How many are really necessary?

- Has sufficient attention been given to matters of privacy and confidentiality in course work?
- Is there sufficient academic and technical support available for students and faculty?
- What are the plans to respond to technological problems (of individual students or the LMS) during weekly sessions, project submission, and testing? Are the plans sufficient?
- Have issues of privacy and confidentiality been addressed and resolved?

Scholarship

Nursing education by distance delivery is an area of scholarship requiring development beyond expository literature and reports of the learning outcomes of individual courses. If comparisons are made between face-to-face and distance courses, the variables that influence learning outcomes (student time on task, class size, course processes, course materials, nature and amount of feedback, interactions, student and faculty characteristics, etc.) should be accounted for so that supportable conclusions can be drawn from the results (Liu, 2012; Simonson et al., 2011).

Significantly, attention should be given to the wealth of scholarship about distance education generally, and the following question should be asked: *What is particular about distance education in nursing that requires explication or investigation?* Qualitative studies that examine how, and how well, students learn about a person-oriented profession, develop professional values, and are acculturated to nursing in courses with no face-to-face contact, would deepen an understanding of effective learning strategies and activities in nursing education.

In addition, student engagement and "interaction patterns in courses and how these contribute to the overall learning environment" (Simonson et al., 2011) might be studied, along with the affective learning that accompanies the patterns. The results of investigations such as these would provide insight into effective course design in nursing.

One topic worthy of development is ethics and values in distance courses. For example, an exploration could be undertaken of the perspectives of nursing faculty and students about the ethical issues inherent in the use of external websites and web tools for course work in which client information forms the basis of discussion. Results could be compared to the perspectives of students and academics in other health disciplines to determine if there are shared values and beliefs. This could have implications for interprofessional education by distance. Another example of a scholarship project that could be of value is a survey of student beliefs about academic integrity in a course that relies on student access to and use of Internet resources. It would also be relevant to determine if Internet-based learning results in student perspectives on nursing professional values and academic values that are the same or different from those in traditional courses.

To expand the evidentiary foundation for nursing education by distance delivery, a school of nursing might adopt a single theory or group of theories upon which to base their studies. In this way, a theory-based body of knowledge would be developed.

CHAPTER SUMMARY

Distance education and nursing education *by distance delivery* are defined, and the institutional requirements for offering distance education are explicated. Ethical considerations, values, and beliefs pertinent to distance education are described. The sources of decisions to offer nursing education by distance and implications for nursing curriculum are summarized. Curriculum design is briefly overviewed. Highlighted is the fact that the design process for distance and traditional courses in nursing is the same. However, considerations particular to nursing courses offered by distance technologies are described. Discussed are course components of concepts and content, strategies to ignite learning, features of individual classes, and opportunities for students to demonstrate learning and faculty evaluation of student achievement. Deciding on course design is addressed, as are implementing and evaluating nursing education by distance. The relationship of nursing education by distance delivery to a context-relevant, evidence-informed, unified curriculum is explained. The core processes of curriculum work in relation to distance education in nursing are described.

SYNTHESIS ACTIVITIES

The Cardol College School of Nursing is undergoing an imminent change in the delivery of the registered nurse to considering further integration of distance delivery into the bachelor of science in nursing (BSN) curriculum. Questions are provided for analysis of this case. Then, questions and activities are suggested for readers' deliberation when planning, implementing, and evaluating distance education in nursing.

Cardol College School of Nursing

Cardol College School of Nursing has a 45-year history of offering nursing programs responsive to the community. The 4-year, integrated BSN curriculum is offered by hybrid and traditional delivery. The incorporation of web technology is evident in some courses. Some non-nursing courses are offered by distance delivery.

Several faculty members are fully committed to the incorporation of distance delivery and web technologies into nursing courses. Others believe that such activities create psychological distance between and among faculty and students. Moreover, they contend that if nursing is taught through technology, the message is conveyed that clients are merely learning objects and not individuals who are important as persons.

Faculty members who are enthusiastic about nursing education by distance delivery are proposing that some current hybrid courses be redesigned to be offered fully by distance delivery and that some traditional courses be offered through hybrid delivery. They suggest that, as a minimum, all theory courses incorporate the use of web technologies.

There is resistance to the proposal. Some faculty members believe strongly in the importance of personal contact to fully socialize students into nursing. They cannot conceive how they could role-model interpersonal communication, empathy, and respect in an online environment, or how students could engage in these behaviors without regular face-to-face encounters. Moreover, they see the need for the continuing online presence of faculty as representing a significant change in their pattern of working, specifically as an intrusion on research and personal time. Finally, this group is concerned that those wanting to offer their courses by distance delivery will work mainly from home, making themselves unavailable for the committee activities in the school.

The university's strategic plan includes a commitment to increase ease of access to all programs. The school leader, Dr. Grace Ingersmith, is supportive of this direction and would like to see the use of distance technology integrated more strongly into the school's programs. Furthermore, she believes that students need to learn to use web technologies in a professional manner and that some guidance by faculty members is required.

At a meeting of faculty, Dr. Ingersmith declares that the school must follow the university's strategic plan, and that the proposal is worthy of consideration. She further states that there must be a thoughtful integration of technology and pedagogy, with the ultimate aim that students are given opportunities to achieve the curriculum goals. She suggests, therefore, that the Curriculum Committee take on the task of determining the appropriateness of increasing the use of distance delivery and web technology in the curriculum. She asks the group to consult as necessary and report back in 3 months with specific recommendations, and rationale for the recommendations.

Questions and Activities for Critical Analysis of the Cardol College School of Nursing Case

1. Hypothesize about the factors that might have led some faculty to propose a greater emphasis on technology-based courses.

2. Propose questions that the Curriculum Committee might ask of themselves, the school leader, and faculty members as they undertake their work.

3. Develop a plan for the Curriculum Committee's work that will lead to sound recommendations.

4. What are the advantages and disadvantages for students and faculty of increasing technology-based learning?

5. Consider the possibility of offering some undergraduate nursing theory courses completely through distance delivery. Does this seem reasonable? Explain the rationale for and against this idea.

6. Is it educationally sound to ask that all nursing theory courses incorporate some web-based technology? Why or why not?

7. How realistic are faculty members' concerns about the workload associated with distance courses? How might the workload be managed?

8. Consider the advantages and disadvantages of synchronous and asynchronous delivery of some courses for both students and faculty.

9. Describe the supports that might be necessary to expand the use of web-based technology in the undergraduate curriculum.

10. If the proposal ultimately forms the Curriculum Committee's recommendations, what might be the implications for the curriculum, students, and faculty?

11. Consider the scholarship activities this group might undertake if they accept the proposal.

Questions and Activities for Consideration When Planning, Implementing, and Evaluating Nursing Education by Distance Delivery in Readers' Settings

1. Analyze the factors that are propelling the school of nursing toward offering nursing courses by distance delivery.

2. What resources are available within the educational institution and the school of nursing for offering nursing education by distance?

3. What institutional policies are in place to support distance education initiatives?

4. Are additional policies and resources needed to support distance education? If so, policies about what? What types of resources?

5. How can the distance courses be developed and implemented so they are conceptually and visually consistent with the entire curriculum?

6. Analyze the general comfort level of faculty with the integration of web technology into traditional and distance courses.

7. Consider some web tools that might form part of a course. How could they contribute to student learning?

8. Propose ideas for learning activities that reflect a creative and learning-focused integration of technology and pedagogy.

9. What faculty development activities might be effective to support faculty movement toward offering distance education?

10. In addition to the questions suggested in the chapter, what other ongoing appraisal questions should be asked?

11. Suggest scholarship activities that could be undertaken about the development, implementation, and evaluation of nursing education courses and curricula offered by distance delivery.

REFERENCES

Agosto, D. E., Copeland, A. J., & Zach, L. (2013). Testing the benefits of blended education: Using social technology to foster collaboration and knowledge sharing in face-to-face LIS courses. *Journal of Education for Library and Information Science, 54*, 94–107.

Amirault, R. J. (2012). Distance learning in the 21st century university: Key issues for leaders and faculty. *Quarterly Review of Distance Education, 13*, 253–265.

Andrusyszyn, M. A., & Davie, L. (1997). Facilitating reflection through interactive journal writing in an online graduate course: A qualitative study. *Journal of Distance Education, 12*, 103–126.

Bedford, D. W., Greg, J. R., & Clinton, M. S. (2011). Preventing online cheating with technology: A pilot study of Remote Proctor and an update of its use. *Journal of Higher Education Theory and Practice, 11*(2), 41–58.

Bernard, R. M., Abrami, P. C., Borokhovski, E., Wade, C. A., Tamim, R. M, Surkes, M. A., & Bethel, E. C. (2009). A meta-analysis of three types of interaction treatments in distance education. *Review of Educational Research, 7*, 1243–1289.

Blackman, S. J., & Major, C. (2012). Student experiences in online courses: A qualitative research synthesis. *Quarterly Review of Distance Education, 13*, 77–85.

Booth, R. G., Andrusyszyn, M. A., & Iwasiw, C. L. (2011). Student perceptions of online participation in baccalaureate nursing computer-conferencing courses. *CIN: Computers, Informatics, Nursing, 29*, 191–198.

Brown, M., Hughes, H., Keppell, M., Hard, N., & Smith, L. (2013). Exploring the disconnections: Student interaction with support services upon commencement of distance education. *International Journal of the First Year in Higher Education, 4*(2), 63–74.

Caudle, P., Bigness, J., Daniels, J., Gillmor-Kahn, M., & Knestrick, J. (2011). Implementing computer-based testing in distance education for advanced practice nurses. *Nursing Education Perspectives, 32,* 328–332.

Cheawjindakarn, B., Suwannatthachote, P., & Theearoungchaisri, A. (2012). Critical success factors for online distance learning in higher education: A review of the literature. *Creative Education, 3*(Supplement), 61–66.

Cho, M.-H. (2012). Online student orientation in higher education: A developmental study. *Education Technology Research and Development, 60,* 1051–1069.

Chu, S. K.-W., & Kennedy, D. M. (2011). Using online collaborative tools for groups to co-construct knowledge. *Online Information Review, 35,* 581–597.

Daley, L. K., Spalla, T. L., Arndt, M. J., & Warnes, A. M. (2008). Videoconferencing and web-based conferencing to enhance learning communities. *Journal of Nursing Education, 47,* 78–81.

Dennen, V. P. (2013). Activity design and instruction in online learning. In M. G. Moore (Ed.), *Handbook of distance education* (3rd ed., pp. 282–298). New York: Routledge.

Dunlap, J. C. (2005). Workload reduction in online courses: Getting some shuteye. *Performance Improvement, 44*(5), 18–25.

Dunlap, J. C., Sobel, D., & Sands, D. I. (2007). Supporting students' cognitive processing in online courses: Designing for deep and meaningful student-to-content interactions. *TechTrends, 51*(4), 20–31.

Edwards, M., Perry, B., & Jansen, K. (2011). The making of an exemplary online educator. *Distance Education, 32,* 101–118.

Ekmekci, O. (2013). Being there: Establishing instructor presence in an online learning environment. *Higher Education Studies, 3*(1), 29–38.

Greener, S. (2012, October). *How are Web 2.0 technologies affecting the academic roles in higher education? A view from the literature.* European Conference on e-Learning: 183-X. Kidmore End: Academic Conferences International Limited.

Halstead, J. A. (2005). Promoting critical thinking through online discussion. *Annual Review of Nursing Education, 3,* 143–164.

Iwasiw, C., Andrusyszyn, M. A., Moen, A., Östbye, T., Davie, L., & Buckland-Foster, I. (2000). Graduate education in nursing leadership through distance technologies: The Canada-Norway Nursing Connection. *Journal of Nursing Education, 39,* 81–86.

Johnson, A. E., & Meehan, N. K. (2013). Faculty preparation for teaching online. In K. H. Frith & D. J. Clark (Eds.), *Distance education in nursing* (3rd ed., pp. 33–52). New York: Springer.

Kirkwood, A. (2011).Transformational technologies: Exploring myths and realities. In E. Burge, C. C. Gibson, & T. Gibson (Eds.), *Flexible pedagogy, flexible practice* (pp. 285–297). Edmonton, Canada: AU Press.

Larreamendy-Joerns, J., & Leinhardt, G. (2006). Going the distance with online education. *Review of Educational Research, 76,* 567–605.

Lee, Y., & Choi, J. (2011). A review of online course dropout research: Implications for practice and future research. *Educational Technology, Research and Development, 59,* 593–618.

Liu, O. L. (2012). Student evaluation of instruction: In the new paradigm of distance education. *Research in Higher Education, 53,* 471–486.

Martens, R., Bastiaens, T., & Kirschner, P. A. (2007). New learning design in distance education: The impact on student perception and motivation. *Distance Education, 28*(1), 81–93.

Oermann, M. H., & Gaberson, K. B. (2014). *Evaluation and testing in nursing education* (4th ed.). New York: Springer.

Paily, M. U. (2013). Creating constructivist learning environment: Role of "Web 2.0" technology. *International Forum of Teaching and Studies, 9*(1), 39–50, 52.

Paul, J. A., & Cochran, J. D. (2013). Key interactions for online programs between faculty, students, technologies, and educational institutions: A holistic framework. *Quarterly Review of Distance Education, 14*(1), 49–62.

Schmitt, T. L., Sims-Giddens, S. S., & Booth, R. G. (2012). Social media use in nursing education. *The Online Journal of Issues in Nursing, 17*(3), 2.

Seddon, K., Postlethwaite, K., James, M., & Mulryne, K. (2012). Towards an understanding of the learning processes that occur in synchronous online seminars for the professional development of experienced educators. *Education and Information Technologies, 17*, 431–449.

Shearer, R. L. (2013). Theory to practice in instructional design. In M. G. Moore (Ed.), *Handbook of distance education* (3rd ed., pp. 251–267). New York: Routledge.

Siemens, G. (2010). *Teaching in social and technological networks.* Retrieved from http://www.connectivism .ca/?p=220/September16th2010

Simonson, M. (2012). Ethics and distance education. *Distance Learning, 9*, 64–65.

Simonson, M., Schlosser, C., & Orellana, A. (2011). Distance education research: A review of the literature. *Journal of Computing in Higher Education, 23*, 2–3, 124–142.

Stavredes, T. M., & Herder, T. M. (2013). Student persistence—and teaching strategies to support it. In M. G. Moore (Ed.), *Handbook of distance education* (3rd ed., pp. 155–169). New York: Routledge.

Strand, H., Fox-Young, S., Long, P., & Bogossian, F. (2013). A pilot project in distance education: Nurse practitioner students' experience of personal video capture technology as an assessment method of clinical skills. *Nurse Education Today, 33*, 253–257.

Tallent-Runnels, M. K., Thomas, J. A., Lan, W. Y., Cooper, S., Ahern, T. C., Shaw, S. M., & Liu, X. (2006). Teaching courses online: A review of the research. *Review of Educational Research, 76*(1), 93–135.

TLT Group: Teaching, Learning and Technology. (2011). The Flashlight approach to evaluating educational uses of technology. Retrieved from http://www.tltgroup.org/flashlight/Handbook/flashlight_ approach.pdf

Vaughn, N. (2007). Perspectives on blended learning in higher education. *International Journal on E-Learning, 6*(1), 81–94.

Zhu, E., McKnight, R., & Edwards, N. (2006). Principles of online design. Retrieved from http://www .fgcu.edu/onlinedesign/index.html

INDEX

Note: Page numbers followed by *f* or *t* indicate materials in figures or tables, respectively.